Evidence Synthesis in Healthcare

Thanos Athanasiou • Ara Darzi
(Editors)

Evidence Synthesis in Healthcare

A Practical Handbook for Clinicians

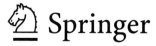 Springer

Editors
Thanos Athanasiou, PhD, MD, FETCS
Department of Surgery and Cancer
Imperial College London
St. Mary's Hospital Campus
London, UK

Prof. Ara Darzi, PC, KBE, FMedSci,
HonFREng
Department of Surgery and Cancer
Imperial College London
St. Mary's Hospital Campus
London, UK

ISBN 978-0-85729-175-2   e-ISBN 978-0-85729-206-3
DOI 10.1007/978-0-85729-206-3
Springer London Dordrecht Heidelberg New York

British Library Cataloguing in Publication Data
A catalogue record for this book is available from the British Library

Library of Congress Control Number: 2011921693

Cover design: eStudioCalamar, Figueres/Berlin

Printed on acid-free paper

Springer is part of Springer Science+Business Media (www.springer.com)

Preface

Modern healthcare is now fundamentally dependent on decisions that are based on the best evidence available. The current era of evidence-based healthcare has led to a revolution in our understanding of diseases and their treatments. It has also transformed modern medical practice and the training of all levels of healthcare workers. As a result the enhancement of clinical skills is unavoidably intertwined with a basic knowledge of research and methodology.

Acquiring the best evidence is not always straightforward as there is a wide heterogeneity between types of evidence and the variability for each distinct disease, environment and patient population. Sometimes, the evidence is totally non-existent for a specific complaint, whilst other times a large discrepancy exists between evidence sources. The increased application of robust statistics to healthcare research led to a tipping point in our realisation of diseases processes and their management.

The introduction of techniques such as meta-analysis and systematic reviews permitted the mathematical amalgamation of several quantitative studies to derive a unified overall result or treatment conclusion from a variety of data sources. The dissemination of these techniques was gradually appraised by the healthcare community and led to an increased appreciation of different study types and methodologies.

Integrating the results from multiple healthcare studies can be challenging and arduous in view of the complexity of data types and research designs. More importantly, however, the application of older techniques such as meta-analysis is largely dependent on the use of comparative studies presenting quantitative data, which is not always possible. This occurs as there is no appropriate data to combine for some particular diseases (for example the lack of randomised treatment studies in emergency cases which are constrained by ethical limitations). The point of disruptive innovation has however been achieved through the overarching medium of evidence synthesis. Here numerous study types (quantitative or qualitative) can be powerfully amalgamated to derive answers to complex healthcare questions. The application of such methods into evidence-based practice has been traditionally limited to a few individuals and centres that until now have had the expertise to carry out these advanced decision-making approaches.

This book has been designed to offer all healthcare workers the opportunity to understand, carry out and realistically perform a broad range of evidence synthesis techniques. It uniquely offers the reader both practical hands-on knowledge coupled with the theoretical comprehension of evidence synthesis techniques to derive answers for healthcare questions. It covers traditional areas that have been enhanced with cutting-edge advances including the performance of meta-analyses with standard access software. Importantly however, it offers experience and familiarity with several newer evidence synthesis procedures including cost-effectiveness analysis and decision analysis coupled with workable real-life examples using available software.

We also aim to equip readers with a full scientific grounding in understanding the process of modern evidence synthesis which in turn provides a comprehensive approach to identifying and deriving the best evidence for evidence-based medicine as also assessment of relevant uncertainty and inconsistency. The style of this book is to describe the concepts of these approaches which are then complemented by a step-by-step 'how to do it' methodology. The reader should therefore gain all the skills necessary to study and research evidence whilst also obtaining quantitative knowledge of these from the myriad of sources available.

The broader context of evidence synthesis is also described, as this book is not only intended for clinicians to provide evidence synthesis for the healthcare community, but rather for providing evidence that will have impact for the whole of society. At the highest level, evidence synthesis can provide expert knowledge for healthcare workers, but also the media and policy-makers. Evidence synthesis can guide national and international governmental decisions which as a result carry a heavy impact on worldwide healthcare. Providing the tools to achieve robust evidence synthesis at these levels can empower modern day health staff to offer powerful improvements to healthcare practice.

We hope that readers will benefit from the techniques described in this text to fulfil the ultimate goal of improved healthcare through the provision of radical innovation and superior quality. These can be exposed through a universal evidence-based approach that this text offers. Equipping individuals and institutions with the techniques described herein provides a direct route to translational medicine where bedside questions can be answered at a local, national and international level.

Adopting these evidence synthesis techniques can encourage enhanced learning and understanding of patients, diseases and the overall healthcare process from primary to quaternary care. A greater understanding of evidence synthesis by a larger proportion of the healthcare community can offer greater communication and an earlier adoption of successful treatments. The universal ability to perform evidence synthesis empowers the whole healthcare community to contribute to global information and expertise in evidence such that patient outcomes can be improved and healthcare practices can be strengthened.

The nature of many of the techniques within this book is not static as there are several synthesis methods to answer each question. The reader will be able to choose the most appropriate test or tests for each scenario such that they will have flexibility in their thoughts and decision making. This aspect affords the reader a freedom of thought allied with autonomy and self-determination such that patients can benefit from global trends in healthcare in addition to the best personalised healthcare possible.

The powerful ability of evidence synthesis to integrate data from variable sources whilst decreasing the uncertainty of the result will allow an increased confidence of decision making for clinicians and policy-makers. This renders evidence synthesis not only a powerful tool, but an obligatory constituent of best medical practice for now and the future. The reality of evidence synthesis is unquestionably prevailing; this book aims to offer the opportunity of its use for all healthcare providers with the ultimate aim of better quality of care for all.

Acknowledgements

The editors would like to specifically forward their appreciation to a number of individuals without whom this book would not have been possible. We thank **Beth Janz** who tirelessly managed the book from its inception, devoting long hours in communication with contributors and editors to bring this book to completion. Special thanks also go to **Hutan Ashrafian** who worked with energy and skill to co-ordinate many of the authors in keeping this project on track. We would also like to recognise **Christopher Rao** for dedicated graphical support on many of the chapter figures.

Biographies

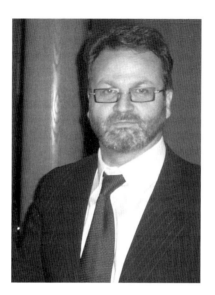

Thanos Athanasiou, M.D., Ph.D. FETCS Reader in Cardiac Surgery and Consultant Cardiac Surgeon

Thanos Athanasiou is a Consultant Cardiothoracic Surgeon at St Mary's Hospital, Imperial College Healthcare NHS Trust and a Reader of Cardiac Surgery in the Department of Surgery and Cancer at Imperial College London. He specialises in complex aortic surgery, coronary artery bypass grafting (CABG), minimally invasive cardiac surgery and robotic-assisted cardiothoracic surgery. His institutional responsibility is to lead academic cardiac surgery and complex aorta surgery. He is currently supervising ten MD/ PhD students and has published more than 275 peer-reviewed publications. He has given several invited lectures in national and international forums in the field of technology in cardiac surgery, healthcare delivery and quality in surgery. His specialty research interest includes bio-inspired robotic systems and their application in cardiothoracic surgery, outcomes research in cardiac surgery, metabolic surgery and regenerative cardiovascular strategies.

His general research interests include quality metrics in healthcare and evidence synthesis including meta-analysis, decision and economic analysis. His statistical interests include longitudinal outcomes from cardiac surgical interventions. He has recently developed and published a novel methodology for analysing longitudinal and psychometric data.

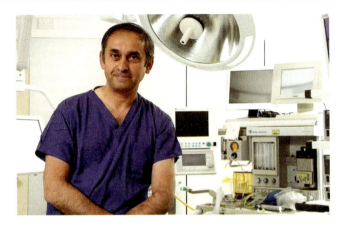

Professor Lord Ara Darzi of Denham PC, KBE, FMedSci, HonFREng

Professor Lord Darzi holds the Paul Hamlyn Chair of Surgery at Imperial College London where he is Head of the Department of Surgery and Cancer. He is an Honorary Consultant Surgeon at Imperial College Hospital NHS Trust and the Royal Marsden Hospital. He also holds the Chair of Surgery at the Institute of Cancer Research.

Professor Lord Darzi and his team are internationally respected for their innovative work in the advancement of minimal invasive surgery, robotics and allied technologies. His research is directed towards achieving best surgical practice through both innovation in surgery and enhancing the safety and quality of healthcare. This includes the evaluation of new technologies, studies of the safety and quality of care, the development of methods for enhancing healthcare delivery and new approaches for education and training. His contribution within these research fields has been outstanding, publishing over 500 peer-reviewed research papers to date. In recognition of his outstanding achievements in research and development of surgical technologies, Professor Lord Darzi was elected as an Honorary Fellow of the Royal Academy of Engineering, and a Fellow of the Academy of Medical Sciences.

Following a Knighthood in 2002 for his service to medicine and surgery, Professor Lord Darzi was introduced to the House of Lords in 2007 and appointed as Parliamentary Under Secretary of State at the Department of Health (2007–2009). At the Prime Minister's request, Professor Lord Darzi led a review of the United Kingdom's National Health Service, with the aim of achieving high-quality care for all national healthcare patients.

He was awarded the Queen's approval of membership in Her Majesty's most honourable Privy Council in 2009. Professor Lord Darzi is currently Chairman of The Institute of Global Health Innovation.

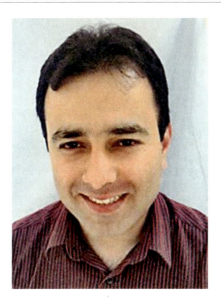

Kamran Ahmed is a Research Fellow and General Surgeon at Imperial College London. His areas of interest include research into tools for continuing medical education and methods for assessment of specialist clinical practice. This entails expert opinion, observation at workplace, evaluation of skills within simulated environment and outcome-based assessment of competence and performance.

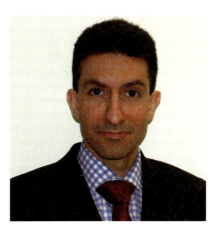

Hutan Ashrafian is a Clinical Lecturer in Surgery and a Wellcome Trust Research Fellow at Imperial College London. His work focuses on the surgical resolution of metabolic syndrome, obesity-related cardiovascular disease, novel techniques in evidence synthesis and the development of precision performance metrics in medical science and academia. His research interests include the development of innovative strategies and bio-inspired regenerative technologies in healthcare.

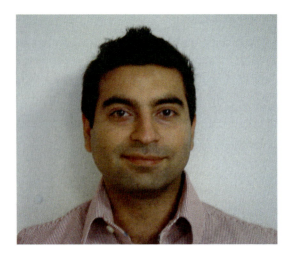

Sejal Jiwan is Technology Manager for the Division of Surgery Imperial College. His interests focus on Business Analysis and Corporate Governance.

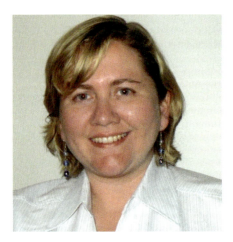

Catherine Jones is a radiologist, having trained in Australia, the United Kingdom and Canada. She is a trained statistician and is experienced in the use of medical statistics. Catherine has been a clinical research fellow with the Department of Surgery at Imperial College since 2006. Her special interest is diagnostic accuracy methodology and its role in expanding the medical literature, particularly in primarily diagnostic specialties such as clinical radiology. Her current areas of research interest include the diagnostic accuracy of cardiac imaging.

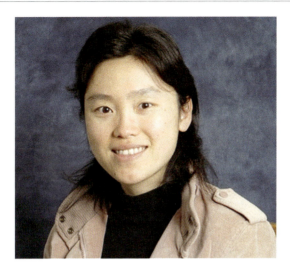

Melody Ni is a Project Manager and Decision Researcher in the Department of Surgery and Cancer at Imperial College London. She studied Decision Sciences at the London School of Economics. At Imperial College, she applied Bayesian networks to investigate the uncertainties embedded in the checking procedures of nasogastric feeding tubes. Her current research focuses broadly on (a) understanding risk perceptions and behaviours in response to dreadful events and (b) using decision analysis to improve the quality of clinical decision making.

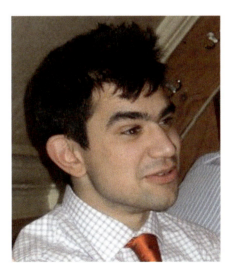

Christopher Rao is a Surgical Trainee and Clinical Research Fellow at Imperial College London. His work has focused on the economic and clinical evaluation of novel surgical technology. He is currently completing a PhD investigating the cardiovascular applications of pluripotent stem cells funded by the Wellcome Trust.

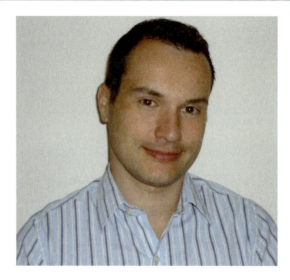

Srdjan Saso is a trainee in Obstetrics and Gynaecology and is currently working as a Clinical Research Fellow at the Institute of Reproductive and Developmental Biology, Imperial College London. His research interests lie in the fields of reproductive medicine and gynaecological oncology, with his most up-to-date work focusing on advancing our knowledge of uterine transplantation.

Contents

Contributors

Kamran Ahmed, MBBS, MRCS
Department of Surgery and Cancer,
Imperial College London,
St Mary's Hospital Campus,
London, UK

Hutan Ashrafian, MBBS, BSc (Hons.), MRCS (Eng.)
Department of Surgery and Cancer,
Imperial College London,
St Mary's Hospital Campus,
London, UK

Thanos Athanasiou, PhD, MD, FETCS
Department of Surgery and Cancer,
Imperial College London,
St Mary's Hospital Campus,
London, UK

Prof. Ara Darzi, PC, KBE, FMedSci, HonFREng
Department of Surgery and Cancer,
Imperial College London,
St Mary's Hospital Campus,
London, UK

George B. Hanna, PhD, MD
Department of Surgery and Cancer,
Imperial College London,
St Mary's Hospital Campus,
London, UK

Catherine M. Jones, MBBS, BSc, FRCR
Department of Surgery and Cancer,
Imperial College London,
St Mary's Hospital Campus,
London, UK

Sejal Jiwan, BA (Hons.)
Department of Surgery and Cancer,
Imperial College London,
St Mary's Hospital Campus,
London, UK

Zhifang Ni, PhD
Department of Surgery and Cancer,
Imperial College London,
St Mary's Hospital Campus,
London, UK

Sukhmeet S. Panesar, MBBS, BSc.(Hons.) AICSM
National Patient Safety Agency,
London, UK

Lawrence D. Phillips, PhD
The Department of Management,
London School of Economics,
London, UK

Christopher Rao, MBBS, BSc (Hons.), MRCS
Department of Surgery and Cancer,
Imperial College London,
St Mary's Hospital Campus,
London, UK

Srdjan Saso, MBBS, BSc (Hons.),
Institute of Reproductive &
Developmental Biology, Imperial College
London, Hammersmith Hospital Campus,
London, UK

Nick Sevdalis, PhD, MSc, BSc
Department of Surgery and Cancer,
Imperial College London,
St Mary's Hospital Campus,
London, UK

Weiming Siow, MBBS, BSc (Hons.),
North Middlesex University, NHS
Hospital, London, UK

**Kathie A. Wong, MBBS, BSc (Hons.),
MRCS**
Department of Surgery and Cancer,
Imperial College London,
St Mary's Hospital Campus,
London, UK

Evidence Synthesis: Evolving Methodologies to Optimise Patient Care and Enhance Policy Decisions

1

Hutan Ashrafian, Ara Darzi, and Thanos Athanasiou

Abstract Evidence synthesis is a term applied to a group of assessment techniques that integrate the data from variable evidence sources. These techniques are used to provide best evidence in healthcare. Evidence synthesis has several advantages when compared to single studies and traditional data integration through meta-analysis. The complexities of combining heterogeneous data sources such as the amalgamation of both qualitative and quantitative data sources can be successfully overcome by applying these techniques. Evidence synthesis can summarise data by classifying each individual source according to its quality whilst it can also quantify the degree of uncertainty in synthesis results. In this chapter, we discuss current evidence synthesis methods and consider their application for medical practitioners, scientists and policymakers. We identify the future trends and increased importance of utilising evidence synthesis for evidence-based medicine. The versatility of evidence synthesis renders it a powerful tool in attaining the ultimate goal of improved health outcomes, innovation and enhanced quality of patient care.

1.1
The Theoretical Aspects of Evidence and Evidence Synthesis

> Knowledge, the knower and the object of knowledge, these are the three incentives to action.
> Bhagavad Gita – Chapter 18, Verse 18

The scientific experimental paradigm is a fundamental principle of modern academic research. This paradigm is designed to provide us with an ability to answer questions. It accounts for a system which is based firstly on experiments of observation and secondly on the theory to acquire true knowledge which is objective, unbiased and just. These experiments generate 'raw data' which require refinement and contextualisation with previous knowledge to provide us with an independent sample of evidence (Fig. 1.1).

H. Ashrafian (✉)
Department of Surgery and Cancer, Imperial College London,
St Mary's Hospital Campus, London, UK
e-mail: h.ashrafian@imperial.ac.uk

T. Athanasiou and A. Darzi (eds.), *Evidence Synthesis in Healthcare*,
DOI: 10.1007/978-0-85729-206-3_1, © Springer-Verlag London Limited 2011

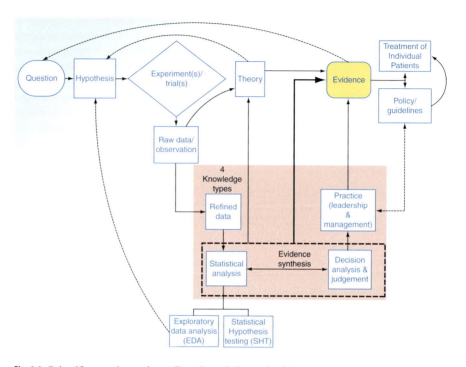

Fig. 1.1 Scientific experimental paradigm, knowledge and evidence

Evidence is defined by the *Oxford English Dictionary* as 'information or signs indicating whether a belief or proposition is true or valid'.[1] It is the language of science where we communicate true facts that are derived from the component elements of true knowledge,[2] namely:

- Knowledge from research (refined data or evidence)
- Knowledge of measurement (statistical methodology)
- Knowledge from experience (judgements and decision)
- Knowledge of practice (leadership and management)

The application of statistical methodology is critically important in refining data to provide the best possible evidence. As a result, two broad techniques have been developed to augment the process of evidence accrual. Firstly, statistical hypothesis testing (also known as confirmatory data analysis) provides a technique to statistically accept or deny a hypothesis. Secondly, exploratory data analysis (EDA) evaluates data to provide research hypothesis for analysis.

As the volume of raw data increases from an increased number of experiments, there is now a concomitant rise in available evidence.[3,4] Some consider that we are inundated with evidence 'overload', whilst others would argue that more evidence can only enhance our understanding of diseases and their treatments. Either way, it is clear that it is necessary to

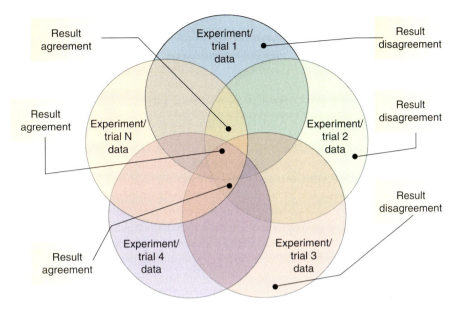

Fig. 1.2 The concept of evidence synthesis – deriving 'best evidence' through the integration of data sets

identify areas of agreement and disagreement between studies (Fig. 1.2) and integrate the results of all the available studies in one field into interpretable results. The word 'synthesis' (derived from ancient Greek) represents such an integration and refers to the combining of two or more entities to form something new.

'Evidence synthesis' is the synthesis (or integration) of variable data to produce information in the form of best evidence. It provides a set of methodologies to identify areas of agreement and disagreement in qualitative and quantitative data sets. By integrating data sets, this methodology may calculate the concordance and magnitude of effects from multiple studies.

The aim of evidence synthesis is to address questions by providing the best evidence derived through the integration of data and knowledge to present information of factual integrity and least uncertainty.

In this chapter, we describe the current approach to evidence synthesis and outline relevant cutting-edge techniques that integrate studies to discern best evidence in healthcare. We also outline the limitations and strengths of other techniques of evidence extrapolation and present the advantages and disadvantages of evidence synthesis. We consider the history, philosophy and ethics of this methodology in order to fully contextualise the application of modern evidence synthetic techniques. This chapter presents the role of evidence synthesis within the scientific experimental paradigm, and discusses its role in patient care, health policy and evidence-based medicine (EBM).

Although one of the key roles of evidence synthesis includes the determination of answers to healthcare questions at an individual or group level, there is also a significant

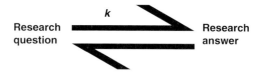

Fig. 1.3 The relationship between research questions, answers and evidence synthesis. k = reaction equilibrium constant = quality and type of evidence synthesis

aspect of evidence synthesis which provides further research questions (Fig. 1.1). A comparable analogy includes the answering of a research question to a chemical reaction, where evidence synthesis acts as the enzyme to catalyse a reaction. Here, equilibrium is achieved between a research question and its answer. As each chemical reaction has an equilibrium constant, each research question has an equilibrium constant of evidence that is determined by the quality and nature of the evidence synthesis (Fig. 1.3).

Evidence synthesis can determine the strength of an association between a disease and its supposed causative agent or associations considering prognosis, diagnosis and treatment. A set of inference criteria used to describe these associations was introduced by Sir Austin Bradford Hill in 1965. These remain in use today and are termed eponymously as the Bradford Hill criteria[5,6] for causation in healthcare:

1. Analogous evidence
2. Consistency
3. Coherence
4. Experiment
5. Strength
6. Specificity
7. Plausibility
8. Temporality
9. Biological gradient

Although addressing association strength is a key consideration of studies, the methodology of achieving the data is also of paramount importance. Different research methods can be ranked according to the validity of their findings according to a pre-defined hierarchy of evidence.

The aim of such a hierarchy is to provide a mean where evidence from a range of methodologically different studies which can be categorised and ranked. These can also provide a logical outline that can be utilised for designing or setting up a research study so as to provide the best available evidence for evidence synthesis. A widely acknowledged hierarchy of evidence is the one developed at the Centre for Evidence-Based Medicine at the University of Oxford (Fig. 1.4).[7] This classification categorises non-experimental information at the lowest levels of an evidence pyramid and randomised control trials at a much higher level. The highest level of evidence represents evidence sources where data from multiple randomised trials are integrated and appraised in the form of meta-analyses and systematic reviews.

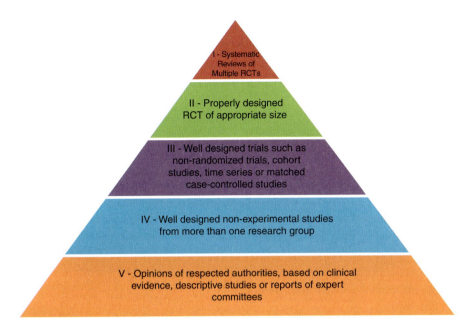

Fig. 1.4 Hierarchy of evidence pyramid based on the levels advocated by the Oxford Centre for Evidence-based Medicine (May 2001)

1.2
Limitations of Single Studies

A single study carries an inherent risk of achieving false conclusions. This is because each individual study is subjected to design and trial completion by an individual group of researchers within the construct of a local healthcare environment and personal predispositions. Single studies may be subject to statistical errors that are usually classified in type I error (also known as α) and type II error (also known as β).

Type I errors occur when the null hypothesis of a study is rejected (by a statistically significant probability p) when it is actually true, and a Type II error occurs when a null hypothesis is false, but fails to be rejected. One analogy to this is the conviction of a criminal by a court of law, where the concept of null hypothesis is equivalent to the innocence of a defendant. Type I error can be likened to a legal error when an innocent person goes to prison, and type II error when a guilty individual is released as a result of 'inadequate evidence'.[8]

Typically type II errors result from inadequately powered studies with low numbers of subjects, a common problem in numerous research studies. One study assessing the extent if type II errors in clinical studies revealed that the probability of missing effects in a true population series for these studies was greater than 10% for 67 of 71 trials.[9] In reality, small differences in treatment effects can be translated to much larger ones at a population level. However to prove these small differences, trials with extremely large numbers of participants[10] are required, which is usually unfeasible by one study group running a single centre trial.

1.3
Advantages of Evidence Synthesis

Evidence synthesis provides a framework of techniques to appraise and integrate study results within the context of a broad number of variables including methodology, size and design. In view of its ability to combine extensive volumes of both qualitative and quantitative data, it can provide evidence with increased accuracy and less uncertainty compared to other studies (Fig. 1.5). Evidence synthesis can evaluate knowledge from[11]:

1. Study design
2. Effect size
3. Quantification of research heterogeneity
4. Time trends
5. Impact of covariates adjustment
6. Quality of studies
7. Research gaps
8. Variability in study populations

The techniques of combing studies in meta-analysis are traditionally based on studies from the highest levels of the evidence hierarchy (primarily randomised controlled trials). If these were not available, then researchers would go down sequentially to the next tear of evidence (Fig. 1.4) ranging from observational studies to anecdotal reports.[12] Researchers adhered to the principle that when using 'weaker' evidence, the study reporting would be

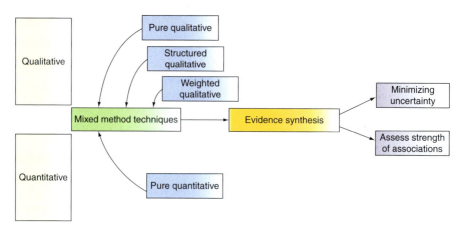

Fig. 1.5 Multiple sources in evidence synthesis

performed with more depth to clarify areas of research agreement and heterogeneity. In evidence synthesis however, all data and data sources can be assessed. Each study requires classification and is quantified by a weighting process to allow accurate comparisons. This enables the synthesis to achieve 'best evidence' by utilising all available knowledge within an appropriate context.

The integration of the described factors is required to fulfil some fundamental outcomes[13] of evidence synthesis (the CONE principle):

Causality – The establishment of causality within the null hypothesis (in healthcare this typically requires the clarification of the association between disease resolution and treatment).
Outcome predictors – The clarification of dependent and independent predictors of outcome
New hypotheses generation
Effect quantification (of treatment)

To achieve these outcomes, evidence synthesis compares favourably to traditional techniques of systematic review and meta-analysis in providing a rigorous modelling technique that provides statistical rigour in answering a healthcare question, but also has the ability to quantify evidence uncertainty (Table 1.1).

1.4
Current Evidence Synthesis Methods

The current techniques of evidence synthesis can be used to derive knowledge from clinical facts, clinical studies and also decision or policy directives. Although traditionally there has been a strong focus on synthesising data from randomised control trials and quantitative studies, in current era there is a wealth of synthesis techniques that can also be used for qualitative studies as well (Fig. 1.5). The choice of evidence synthetic technique has become progressively more complex as medical choices and policy decisions are not always suitably supplied by quantitative evidence or randomised control trials. Increasingly medical decisions are based on qualitative studies and consensus opinions,[14] and therefore techniques of evidence synthesis are required to robustly reflect the information from these data sources.

Although the concept of integrating multiple, variable data sources to synthesise accurate evidence can be an attractive notion, there are nevertheless arguments that consider these as controversial and untenably idealistic. According to *relativists*, research provides several truths, all of which can coexist at the same time. As a result, they consider that applying a method to integrate disparate research to achieve one single answer as invalid. *Realists* however defend evidence synthesis[15] as this provides a pragmatic method of delivering complex answers with evidence gained from numerous and sometimes disparate studies which would not have been possible using the individual studies alone.

As a result, the complexities of overcoming disparities between groups of qualitative and quantitative studies were gradually achieved and recent methodological developments have provided techniques to overcome the analytical differences between qualitative and quantitative studies. As a result of current evidence synthesis techniques, research data no

Table 1.1 Comparison of systematic reviews, meta-analysis and evidence synthesis

	Systematic review	Meta-analysis	Evidence synthesis
Search strategy and sources	Pre-defined databases	Pre-defined databases	Diverse – open to all knowledge media
Study inclusion	Systematic (Empirical and Qualitative)	Empirical only	Comprehensive (all available evidence)
Heterogeneity	Quantified	Quantified and limited (resulted in only a few analyzable studies)	Quantified and applied/accounted in study results and conclusion
Study quality	Quantified	Quantified	Quantified and applied/accounted in study results and conclusion
Bias	Yes as a result of subjectivity	Limited only	Quantified
Analysis	Subjective	Objective	Objective
Logic	Inductive	Deductive	Bayesian
Interpretation	Comparative and relativist (multiple truths)	Aggregative	Combinative integration
Uncertainty	Difficult to quantify	Small but limited to small number of studies	Quantified
Precision	Dependent on input (Garbage-In-Garbage-Out)	Dependent on input (garbage-in-garbage-out)	Input screened and moderated to deliver optimum answers
Result conclusiveness	Rare	Occasional – limited by only a few analyzable studies	Expected
Hypotheses generation	Rare	Rare	Frequent
Ability to directly answer medial and policy questions	Sometimes	Sometimes	Frequently

longer focus on whether the data is qualitative or quantitative, but allow the statistical capability to measure the strength of findings and the degree of uncertainty.

Whilst the underlying concepts of most synthetic techniques provide attractive processes to integrate wide-ranging data sources, the practicality of performing these techniques requires a rigorous adherence to scientifically address each research question whilst maintaining a powerful analytical pragmatism.

As a result, evidence synthesis can provide a *spectrum of results* that can answer questions ranging from those of pure scientific knowledge and clinical trial queries to those of focussing on management and decision making (Fig. 1.6). This spectrum can be termed as the *knowledge–decision* spectrum, which comprises pure knowledge at one pole and decisions at the other pole. The knowledge spectrum between these poles comprises varyingly of knowledge supports and decisions supports which are in turn derived from the research studies included in each synthesis. Varying quantities of these knowledge supports and decision supports provide different knowledge types and evidence.

Knowledge support types are defined as three types[16] according to Hammersley:

- Aggregative (data collection and accrual)
- Comparative or replicative (comparative studies, A versus B)
- Developmental (hypothesis generating, explanation and mechanism identification)

Decision support types however consist of:

- Guidelines and consensus statements
- Expert opinions

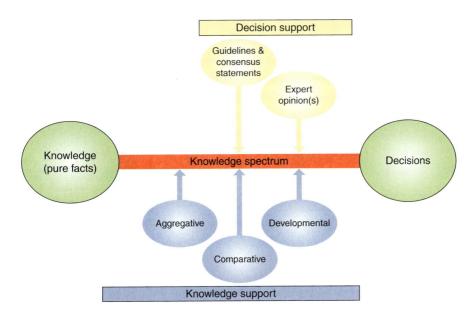

Fig. 1.6 Knowledge–decision spectrum derived from evidence synthesis

Traditionally, there has been a division between knowledge support and decision support such that scientific studies should be based on knowledge support, whereas decision strategies should be derived from decision support. Although this holds true for some examples of research, the knowledge spectrum is in reality a continuum where each individual study will have a balance between knowledge supports and decision supports to answer the questions for each evidence synthesis review.

The knowledge for each individual study used in an evidence synthesis exercise falls somewhere along the knowledge spectrum as does the evidence from each individual synthesis. Evidence types can be broadly defined as quantitative or qualitative, but can be further classified into:

- Pure qualitative or 'narrative' studies
- Structured qualitative studies
- Weighted qualitative studies
- Pure quantitative studies

Evidence synthesis can provide the analytical techniques to provide answers for the whole spectrum of the knowledge–decision spectrum (Fig. 1.7). Combining and integrating the evidence from these different study types requires two broad categories of synthesis:

1. *Integrative synthesis* – Here evidence from individual sources or studies are integrated or combined to formulate a data summary. A traditional example includes study comparison and data pooling to achieve an amalgamated statistic such as those provided by meta-analysis.[17] This type of synthesis has conventionally been considered for quantitative studies. Although this is usually the case, it should not preclude the application of integrative synthesis to qualitative studies (Fig. 1.8), where data integration may reveal

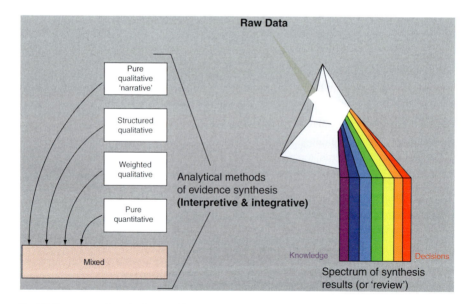

Fig. 1.7 Spectrum of results from evidence synthesis

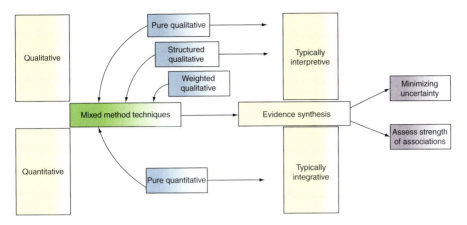

Fig. 1.8 The ability of evidence synthesis to interpret and integrate both qualitative and quantitative studies

useful quantitative values and summaries regarding qualitative data sets.[18] For example, evidence synthesis could correlate the degree of similarity between different national guidelines designed to address the same disease condition.

2. *Interpretative synthesis* – Here evidence from individual sources or studies is assessed and considered according to refined theoretical construct.[17] The descriptive accounts from studies are re-described into a common frame of reference for comparison. This type of evidence synthesis is regarded as synthesising results from several data sources not to define fixed concepts of data aggregation, but rather to present a rigorous theory accurately derived from all data sets.[18]

Clearly, not all syntheses can be divided into these polar extremes of integrative and interpretative, but rather many fall along a spectrum between these concepts. However, in order to describe the wide range of evidence synthetic techniques currently available, we have therefore plotted them on a matrix categorised by qualitative and quantitative and integrative and interpretative (Fig. 1.9).

1.4.1
Narrative Review

Narrative reviews consist of subjective data collection that are then described and interpreted through the personal opinions of the individuals performing the review. This type of evidence is descriptive and narrative. The results of such a review are therefore reflective on the subjective opinions of the authors. Historically such reviews were only undertaken by experts in the field of study, though more recently these can be openly performed by any researcher.

These reviews communicate the knowledge of their specialist field descriptively by the selection and presentation of the most relevant facts for a particular subject. By definition,

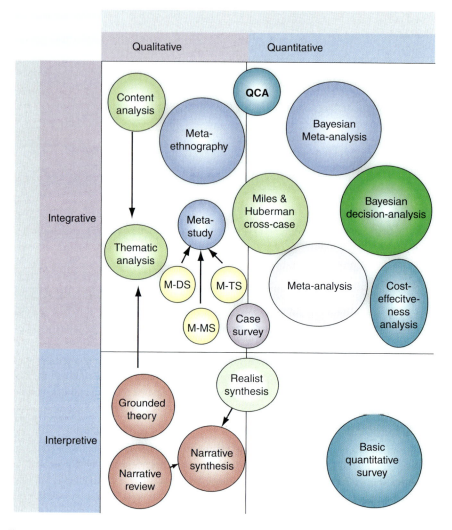

Fig. 1.9 Matrix of evidence synthesis types

therefore, narrative reviews are subjective and are therefore prone to bias and error.[19] Specifically, they can be limited by an individual's academic or personal flaws and may also be influenced by personal conflicts of interest.

In areas of research controversy, narrative reviews can on occasion reflect the biases of an individual reviewer rather than deriving the best evidence from a research area. In many narrative reviews, conclusions are derived from listing and counting studies subjectively.[20] The application of a simple counting process is inherently flawed in view of the exclusion of methodological considerations, sample size and effect size.

As narrative reviews lack a formal structure of data interpretation and communication, the knowledge they provide only represents a superficial analysis of a particular field. Specific areas of deficiency include a lack of rigorous examination of:

- Study design and surgical methodology
- Sample size and power of a study
- Effect size
- Consistency of results

As a result of the subjective selection of data, interpretation and conclusion, narrative reviews are considered to be akin to extended commentaries and consist of the lowest levels of the evidence hierarchy. Their application is increasingly limited as data extraction for narrative reviews is not necessarily systematic. Nevertheless, they can be an important contribution to complex fields where data may be difficult to integrate. Furthermore, on occasion the opinion of an expert performing such a review can reveal highly relevant summaries and insights into a complex field.

1.4.2
Narrative Synthesis and Systematic Reviews

Narrative synthesis is considered to be 'typical systematic review', with clearly defined inclusion criteria and exclusion criteria in selecting and interpreting textual evidence. Increasingly however, this is combined with more complex methods including realist synthesis and meta-techniques.

It requires the following steps[16]:

A. Preliminary synthesis of included studies
B. Identifying research result relationships
C. Evaluating the quality of the synthesis produced

In summary, narrative synthesis identifies the following elements from research studies[16]:

- Organisation
- Description
- Exploration
- Interpretation
- It attempts to identify explanations for the cumulative results of these research findings

The advantages of narrative synthesis include its transparent ability to identify the heterogeneity between studies, although it is not always certain that it can identify areas of commonality in data sources.[21]

1.4.3
Meta-analysis

Meta-analysis integrates the results of a number of research studies that consider related research hypotheses. It uses meta-regression techniques to detect common effect sizes. It allows the calculation of overall averages and can control for study characteristics. Applying this technique, meta-effect sizes can be calculated from directed study averages which subsequently provide evidence that is more precise than the accrued effect sizes

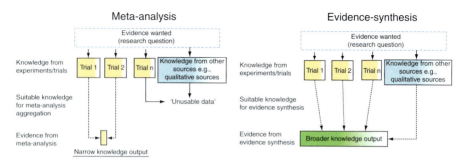

Fig. 1.10 Comparison of meta-analysis and evidence synthesis

from single studies. Until the twenty-first century the term evidence synthesis was used synonymously with the term meta-analysis.[11] The ideal example of a meta-analysis is one that incorporates high-quality, large, randomised controlled trials.

When assessing heterogeneity in meta-analysis, if the studies reveal consistent homogeneity between effects, this implies a sampling variation and a *fixed-effect model* is useful. If there is a large variation of results, then a *random effects model* should be applied. This may lead to statistically weak answers, as null hypotheses are rarely answered[22] (Fig. 1.10).

When combining evidence sources it is almost an inevitability that a researcher will be confronted by a degree of heterogeneity in studies. Contrary to common belief, the presence of heterogeneity does not always imply a weakness of data integration. It is however necessary to consider the source of heterogeneity. *Heterogeneity of the study population, heterogeneity of methods* and *heterogeneity of results* are three distinct areas that need distinctive assessments.

In evidence synthesis, heterogeneity requires careful consideration. Factors such as study design, data measurement and subject demographics all require attention. These are best addressed well before any analysis has taken place and heterogeneity analysis should be included in the original study protocol.

When study results demonstrate consistency in the context of large heterogeneity of study populations, then one can infer a robustness of effect which remains reliable despite the large variation of study subjects. Whereas in meta-analysis the application of heterogeneity may lead to a lack of power in rejecting or accepting null hypotheses, evidence synthesis can provide the means to overcome this statistical power effect, to answer study questions.

1.4.4
Grounded Theory

Grounded theory (GT) is a systematic evidence synthesis technique used for qualitative data applying concepts that work inversely to the 'standard experimental paradigm' typically applied in social research. Here, textual data is collected, comprehensively read and then categorised by coded variables identified from the assessment of the text. Any inter-relationships between categories are also noted.[23-25] A typical use for grounded theory includes the analysis of interview data.

For example, a text fragment studied might include the following statement: Metabolic surgery is an effective treatment for patients with a body mass index above 40, or those with a body mass index above 35 who also suffer from obesity-related co-morbidities such as diabetes and sleep apnoea. In these patients, it is considered that the quality of life and mortality benefits of metabolic surgery outweigh that of medical therapy for at least 15 years post-operatively.

From this statement, the following are implied regarding metabolic surgery:

- Its *application* is based on weight category (body mass index)
- It is *effective* when compared to medical therapy in some circumstances
- There may be a *duration* of effect
- There are other *treatment methods* to manage these patients (medicine)

Although this is a straightforward example, such an analysis can reveal concepts of application, effectiveness, effect duration and an overview of therapies when studying large volumes of documents. These concepts can then be assigned a certain code and can be used to summarise a large corpus of texts. As such, the technique is named grounded theory as it openly analyses text 'ground up' using inherently identified points rather than the traditional technique of above below, where all texts are usually compared to a preset selection of ideas from set hypothesises.

The codes can represent pure data, first level analysis (open coding or substantive coding), second level analysis (selective coding) or even those based on theoretical models (theoretical coding).[23,26]

Once all texts are coded, they are then sorted and re-written and placed in the correct context for defined readers. Accordingly, one of the founders of grounded theory purports that it offers research freedom and time efficiency due to its elements of 'No pre-research literature review, no taping and no talk'.

According to the technique's originators, the results of grounded theory evidence synthesis are neither wrong nor right, but consist of the elements of (1) fit – how closely a model resembles real life, (2) relevance of the study, (3) its workability at a practical level and (4) the modifiability of the underlying theory.[23,26]

The advantages of GT include its ability to offer the systematic analysis of large volumes of text; it can convert quantitative data to qualitative data, comparative data. The disadvantages of GT include its inability to provide inclusion criteria, weighting for studies, although it is systematic, the interpretation of studies remains subjective.

1.4.5
Content Analysis

Content analysis is also a systematic evidence synthesis technique used for qualitative data that relies on accurate data categorisation depending upon an accepted set of categories. Typically, it is used to record interview transcripts.[27]

It considers data validity and objective transparency (so that multiple team members can apply the same codes). Every content analysis requires the answering of the following questions[27]:

- Which data are analysed?
- How are they defined?
- What is the population from which they are drawn?
- What is the context relative to which the data are analysed?
- What are the boundaries of the analysis?
- What is the target of the inferences?

Content analysis has the advantages of being objective and reproducible whilst providing the ability to transform qualitative to quantitative data. Its disadvantages include its effects to oversimplify and generalise complex data whilst the application of frequency-counting may lead to inappropriate weighted results.

1.4.6
Thematic Analysis

Thematic analysis is a systematic evidence synthesis technique used for qualitative data. It shares some characteristics of both narrative reviews and content analysis. Rather than focussing on the categorising data by specific content types, it summarises data through the interpretation of larger themes that can be presented in tabular and graphical form.[18,28] It is typically utilised in interview studies.

This technique can be systematic, transforming qualitative data to quantitative data from broad fields.[29] It is also considered that thematic synthesis has a powerful capability in hypothesis generation when compared to other techniques such as narrative synthesis.[21] Occasionally however, the concept of a theme may be very similar to that of the contents within content analysis and so there can be some confusion between the use of thematic analysis and content analysis.

1.4.7
Realist Synthesis

This is a systematic evidence synthesis technique primarily used to for qualitative data but can also be used for quantitative studies. According to the realist theory approach, it offers analysis from a broad range of data sources including scientific publications, media and policy statements.[18,30] Realist synthesis is typically used for studying the effects of policy changes on outcomes (e.g., what is the impact of increasing the number hospital doctors in the NHS?), and is considered to be an intermediate alternative between meta-analysis and narrative review.[31]

It has the advantages of offering the systematic analysis of both qualitative and quantitative studies from a broad range of data sources, where it can convert qualitative data to quantitative data. However, it cannot easily weight studies according to importance and significance.

1.4.8
Meta-ethnography

Meta-ethnography is an evidence synthesis technique used for assessing qualitative data between similar studies.[16-18] Following the acquisition of data, there are several levels of analysis:

1. First order – extraction of concepts and metaphors by themes and contents (basic analysis)
2. Second order – analysis of the first-order results (aimed for scientists and can be mathematical)
3. Third order – occasionally analysing the second-order results

The techniques used to achieve these analyses include:

- Reciprocal translational analysis (RTA) – identifies common themes, concepts and metaphors between studies
- Refutational synthesis – identifies incongruities between these, concepts and metaphors between studies
- Lines of argument synthesis (LOA) – identifies common arguments and interpretations between studies

Meta-ethnography is typically used to convey the results of scientific studies to policy-makers. For example, how do the UK results on prostate cancer surgery outcomes compare to those in the USA. It offers the systematic and hierarchical analysis of qualitative studies. Nevertheless, it has the disadvantage that result interpretation remains subjective.

1.4.9
Critical Interpretive Synthesis

Critical interpretive synthesis is a systematic evidence synthesis technique that has been designed to provide a rigorous multi-disciplinary and multi-method approach for both qualitative and quantitative studies. It is derived from a combination of meta-ethnography and grounded theory.[25,32] The uses of critical interpretive synthesis can be broad. One example would be to clarify the national benefits of recertification on physician/surgeon practice. This technique is new, but can be used successfully in areas of healthcare where there are few studies of complex patients published in dissimilar and separate sources.

1.4.10
Meta-study

Meta-study is the process of applying statistical analyses to integrate qualitative data from research studies.[18,25,33] It systematically breaks down the techniques of data acquisition, assessment and integration through three techniques. These include the following:

- Meta-data synthesis
- Meta-method synthesis
- Meta-theory synthesis

This is a relatively novel evidence synthesis method and should not be confused with the similar sounding meta-analysis. It is an evidence synthetic technique utilised to integrate data from quantitative studies. According to the meta-study's originator, there are no 'absolute truths'; however, the aim of this technique is to dissect layers of research hierarchy. This is because primary research can be considered as one layer of a research construct, and therefore secondary research is a further layer of research construction rendering it a 'construct of a construct'.[25] A typical example includes the benefits and problems of the changes in postgraduate medical education from the point of view of practising doctors. Meta-study was therefore designed to identify the original nature of differences between studies.

1.4.11
Meta-narrative

Meta-narrative is an evidence synthesis technique specifically designed to provide solutions for complex policy decisions.[25,34] It is based on the concept that knowledge types are derived from assumptions of legitimacy regarding research questions. As a result, multiple studies can be broken down through their concepts of research paradigms or traditions. Each of these consists of[25,34,35]:

- Historical roots
- Scope
- Theoretical basis
- Research questions posed
- Methods and materials
- Main empirical findings
- History and development of knowledge base
- Strengths and weakness of research paradigm

Studying research manuscripts using these traditions could allow each manuscript to be scored into a number of 'meta-narratives'. An example would be to study the benefits of water fluoridation according to medical and public perceptions. These can be used to achieve a result of several research themes which can then be included in an evidence synthesis review.

1.4.12
Miles and Huberman Cross-Case Analysis

Miles and Huberman cross-case analysis[36] can be applied to both qualitative and quantitative studies. This consists of a highly systematic methodology that orders data into clustered data representations including meta-matrices and time-ordered displays.

The use of these displays can facilitate the comparison of data types to identify areas of correlation or disagreement. An example of its use includes studying the local and national benefits of the 4-h rule in accident and emergency departments. It has the advantage of using visual data analysis coupled with a strong systematic approach. Its disadvantages include data selection for studies that are poorly specified and not easily stratified according to quality. Highly systematic application of this technique can be work intensive.

1.4.13
Framework Synthesis

Framework synthesis is a technique derived from Miles–Huberman analysis to provide a condensed summary value to large volumes of qualitative text by applying a systematic framework of numerical codes and graphical representations. An example of its application includes the measurement of patient satisfaction following the introduction of online healthcare assessed through online feedback questionnaires. Although it is a newer technique, it has proved highly valuable in studying research fields with large volumes of textual data in a manageable time frame. As a result, it has powerful applicability for policymakers.[25,37,38]

1.4.14
Case Survey

Case survey is a systematic evidence synthesis technique used to collate data from a large set of qualitative studies to derive quantitative results.[18,39] Data from qualitative studies are extracted from extensive pre-formulated data question sheets. An example of its use includes the local and national assessment of surgeon's preference to a new surgical instrument. The technique can be extended to provide results in the form of a meta-analysis. Its disadvantage however is that it lacks sufficient flexibility to consider the much of the interpretive aspects for qualitative studies.

1.4.15
Qualitative Comparative Analysis

Qualitative comparative analysis (QCA) is one of the most widely used evidence synthesis techniques and provides a method to derive quantitative data from qualitative studies.[2,18,40] This is performed through the use of Boolean logic, where study data is categorised into 'truth tables' and Boolean algebra is the applied to identify quantitative scores for qualitative variables.

Each variable will be given a binary score of 1=present and 0=not present, this will then correspond to an outcome which is also scored with a binary number (Table 1.2). As an example, we can consider an integrative study of surgeons identifying good operative performance. The literature in this field consists of studies that list the following explanatory variables (A–C) associated with good surgical technique (Table 1.2).

Table 1.2 Example Boolean truth table in qualitative comparative analysis (QCA)

Explanatory variables			Dependant variables	
Variable A = anatomical knowledge	Variable B = physiological knowledge	Variable C = technical dexterity	Outcome D = surgical performance	Number of studies
0	0	0	0	12
1	0	0	1	33
0	1	0	1	25
0	0	1	1	37
1	1	0	1	16
1	0	1	1	42
0	1	1	1	12
1	1	1	1	67

In this hypothetical set of manuscripts, the Boolean equation follows that D (the dependant variable) = A + B + C. Thus, it can be seen that good surgical performance can result from any or all of: knowledge of anatomy, knowledge of physiology and technical dexterity.

This technique can be applied to much more complex scenarios, revealing more complex truth tables. However, the Boolean mathematics can derive powerful answers from studies. Recently also, the application of 'fuzzy Boolean logic' has been used to identify trends across qualitative studies using this technique.

The advantages of QCA include the Boolean approach which offers a simple, low-intensive method to derive quantitative data from qualitative score. However, the binary score given to variables can make it difficult to adequately weight each variable and the technique lacks sufficient flexibility to consider many of the interpretive aspects for qualitative studies.

1.4.16
Bayesian Meta-analysis

Bayesian meta-analysis is an evidence synthetic technique that applies Bayesian mathematics to traditional meta-analytical synthesis.[16,18,41-43] The Bayesian concept is based on the premise that for a given question, there is a prior belief which carries a probability close to the mean probability of the answer.

It requires the following components:

• Prior distribution – the probability of a parameter based on previous experience and trial data

- Likelihood – probability of a parameter based on data from the current research study or trial
- Posterior distribution – the updated probability of a parameter based on our observation and treatment of the data

With this methodology, all data can be converted into a quantitative constructs and then applied to a pre-defined probabilistic model. The Bayesian concepts are robust and practical, though their underlying mathematics is powerful though complex. The technique can offer both qualitative and quantitative synthesis and can readily be used in conjunction with other synthesis techniques.

The Bayesian technique offers evidence synthesis for the following:

- Designing a study
- Interpreting a study
- Reporting a study
- Decision making

Bayesian meta-analysis specifically offers particular strengths in decision making and judgement analysis. The probabilistic models can feed into simulations which allow the derivations of optimal decisions and judgements. As such, Bayesian meta-analysis is a particularly powerful evidence synthesis tool for policymakers and politicians. An example of Bayesian meta-analysis includes the comparison of Treatment A versus Treatment B. Although traditional meta-analysis would consider randomised trials comparing A versus B, Bayesian meta-analysis allows the inclusion of non-randomised data (such as prospective and retrospective studies), and has the advantage that it can mathematically score the strength of each of these study types (according to the hierarchy of evidence) and therefore weight them accordingly in the analysis. As a result, Bayesian meta-analysis can integrate the data from a broad range of sources to achieve an answer derived from the quality of the data sources.

Its advantages include a broad application to quantitative and qualitative data by applying Bayesian mathematics. It can importantly consider the weighting of different interpretative elements. The disadvantages of the technique include the generation of complex results that may require extensive training in this technique. Furthermore, complex judgements may need to be assigned relative weighting and this is not always straightforward.

1.4.17
Ecological Triangulation

Ecological Triangulation is an evidence synthetic technique of qualitative studies where research evidence from various vantage points can achieve best data synthesis through the 'triangulation' of knowledge sources.[25,44] A typical example of its use includes the assessment of whether the introduction of Drug A is beneficial to a health authority or country. To answer this question, data from trial meta-analysis and questionnaires from doctors and patients can all be 'triangulated' to identify themes of concordance between these sources.

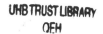

In essence, it aims to reveal the best knowledge, by revealing it from several 'angles'. This occurs through the collective analysis of diverse data sources to expose mutually interdependent relationships between:

- Behaviour
- Individuals
- Environments

1.4.18
Qualitative Meta-summary

Qualitative meta-summary is a recent evidence synthetic technique[25,45] of qualitative studies where results are cumulatively aggregated and measured according to their frequencies. One example of its use includes the identification of perspectives on spirituality at the end of life.[46] In this technique, a higher frequency of a particular finding reflects increased result validity.

1.4.19
Cost-Effectiveness Analysis

Cost-effectiveness analysis (CEA) is an evidence synthesis technique derived from economic analysis that is specifically designed to synthesise cost-benefit effects. As healthcare costs constitute a fundamental element of healthcare management, CEA has an increasingly pivotal role in healthcare policy and decision making.[47,48]

Deriving accurate financial knowledge regarding treatment strategies can be highly complex and typically requires the consideration of several hierarchical interactions. These include models of how costs are accrued and how these are balanced against short-term and long-term monetary gains or losses. The data for many of these models are limited by a lack of direct evidence. In order to overcome these problems of direct costing, Bayesian techniques are now increasingly used to successfully utilise indirect cost data for evidence synthesis models of cost-effective analysis.[47,48]

1.4.20
Meta-interpretation

Meta-interpretation is a recent evidence synthesis technique of qualitative studies that provides strong potential for use in policy and decision making. It provides the following[25,49]:

- Exclusion criteria that are ideographic and not pre-defined.
- There is a clear aim to contextualise synthesis results.
- Assessment of raw data.
- Iterative approach to theoretical sampling.
- A transparent audit trail.

One example of its use includes the analysis and summary of the results from a nationwide questionnaire.[50] This technique offers the generation of objective summaries from complex literature-based data.

1.5
Selection of Evidence Synthesis Approach

Choosing the best method for evidence synthesis is a critical requirement of attaining best evidence in response to a question. Each type of question requires a specific type of synthesis methodology. Ideally, each synthesis technique will be tailor-made to the question that needs answering.

The choice of questions can vary from the need of pure factual knowledge to the attainment of judgement and decision (Fig. 1.11). These two are not polar opposites, but fall at opposite ends of a question spectrum that broadly includes the following:

- Knowledge of facts
- Comparison of treatments
- Time considerations

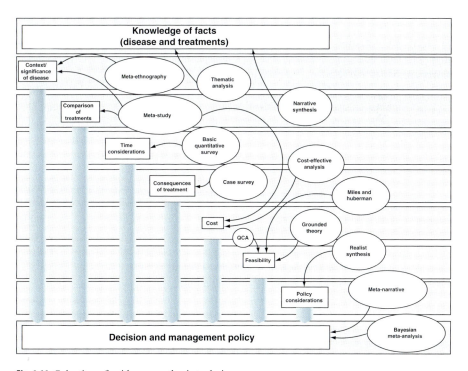

Fig. 1.11 Selection of evidence synthesis technique

- Consequences of treatment
- Cost
- Feasibility
- Policy considerations
- Decision information

In order to adequately provide knowledge for the question types, different techniques of synthesis need to be applied individually to provide the best evidence.[16,18,51,52] Several techniques have a broad application to a variety of different questions; however, when performing a synthesis it is necessary to objectively appraise each technique and to select the ideal synthesis model for the underlying study aim and question. At an epistemological level, two broad types of evidence synthesis are present. (a) Idealist studies are iterative and consider sources with large heterogeneity resulting in an exploration of questions, whereas (b) realist evidence synthesis is linear with little heterogeneity between selected studies and offers answers to questions.[25]

Knowledge of facts, such as whether a particular disease process is important or not, can be suitably answered by narrative review which can bring broad conclusions and is flexible in knowledge accrual. Conversely, decisions and judgements are particularly suited to Bayesian meta-analysis as this can identify hierarchical logic used in the process of medical judgements, whilst meta-narrative can offer policymakers a practical summary of the relevant research literature.

Considerations of a disease course or timing can be done by a standard quantitative survey, whereas consequences of treatment can be identified through case survey of actual patient outcomes, even for rare conditions. Contextualising a disease by comparing different treatments according to specialist can be performed through meta-study, whereas feasibility of both quantitative and qualitative studies can be performed by QCA, grounded theory and Miles and Huberman techniques (Fig. 1.11).

On occasion, no one single technique will offer all the required results, and in these cases a combination approach may identify the best evidence synthesis approach. This may only be realised after a primary evidence synthesis is performed (Fig. 1.1), and that it is realised that another 'evidence synthesis loop' requires completion. Alternatively, however two or more techniques can be used at the same time or in quick succession, or rarely even a new technique introduced to answer a rare synthesis problem.

Recently, there have been a number of techniques introduced to account for uncertainty in cost-effective models, which can also be increasingly applied to other forms of evidence synthesis.[53] Calculating the sensitivity of a decision according to its level of uncertainly has become a central theme. Sensitivity analysis can be measured through 'scenario' analysis performed using extreme values of expert opinions or probabilistic sensitivity analysis (PSA). The application of PSA has found increased favour as a result of easily interpreted analyses using distributions by Monte Carlo simulation.

Therefore, PSA can offer decision solutions based on modelling that would be impossible with scenario modelling. Monte Carlo simulation can be very well suited to Bayesian posterior distributions, and there is now a number of easily accessible software programmes (such as WinBUGS) that cater for the highly applicable Markov Chain Monte Carlo (MCMC) models. These include the following:

- Evidence structures that induce parameter correlation (mixed treatment comparisons, Markov models of disease and correlation uncertainty)
- Methods for multi-parameter synthesis

The use of these simulation models in evidence synthesis has revolutionised the use of synthesis away from the classical non-linear models in cost-effectiveness and random effects in meta-analysis. The additional consideration of uncertainty in these synthesis techniques therefore provides an increased level of flexibility and precision when interpreting the results of evidence synthesis.

1.6
Quality of Sources

Sources for evidence synthesis can be highly variable, including qualitative and quantitative data sets, but also novel knowledge sets including national guidelines, web pages and media articles. Defining a scoring for each source according to its quality can have significant implications with regard to study interpretation, but also as a key measurement of uncertainty for presenting the conclusions.

Traditionally, qualitative reviews have focused on measuring quality of sources based on the concept of construct validity which estimates the validity of evidence from a particular experimental set-up by relating it to a theoretical or similar experiment whose evidence is valid. Furthermore, in the UK, the NHS Centre for Reviews and Dissemination based at the University of York outlines the measurement of quality based on validity, bias, quality assessment instruments and hierarchies.[54]

For quantitative studies, the Centre for Evidence-Based Medicine at the University of Oxford identifies a hierarchy of research studies that can be used as a measure for the quality of sources. There are also internally set criteria for the inclusion of studies that consider quality which are specified in statements such as CONSORT, TREND and PRISMA.[55]

Unfortunately however, not all studies comply with these regulations and statements, and on occasion, a study's quality can be unclear and would require a lower ranking according to the evidence presented.

The future guidelines of quality measures in evidence synthesis need to adhere to the established quality measures identified, however these need to be interpreted though the relevance of sources and impact of sources which can in some cases also allude to levels of quality.

1.7
Quantity of Sources

In an ideal scenario, all possible evidence sources will be reviewed for an evidence synthesis question. In reality however, for broader questions, this may not be practical or feasible. Each evidence synthesis team consists of a finite number of members with a finite time within which to perform the synthesis. In reality therefore, people carrying out evidence synthesis need to be aware of the magnitude of their research. One technique used in qualitative research that has potential for application in a broader range of studies includes the concept of theoretical sampling. Here data acquisition continues until there is a consensus that no new data is being acquired. At this time, a theoretical saturation point is identified and the data acquisition is stopped for analysis. This form of sampling is however considered problematic, as it has the possibility of missing out rare, but vital data for complete evidence synthesis. As a result, in order to address this practical issue of potential data overload in the search strategy, it is possible to narrow the focus of the research question for synthesis. Although this may limit the applicability of the results, the evidence synthesis will nevertheless provide the best evidence for the questions asked.

1.8
Stages of Evidence Synthesis

There are a number of important steps required to provide a useful evidence synthesis solution (Fig. 1.12). The first step of evidence synthesis is to gather a group of individuals to clarify the essentials of the evidence synthesis. Ideally, the group will consist of healthcare experts, clinicians, managers and policymakers where appropriate. At this point, it is critical to define the aim of the review and specify a focussed review question.

The context of the review is critical and the outset, and the methodology and type of review selected should be directly stratified according to the audience that will use the evidence synthesis. Therefore, a synthesis for policymakers should be performed with the aim of answering a policy question. Once the selection of synthesis type and method is chosen, a team of multi-disciplinary individuals has to be selected who will ultimately perform the synthesis. Ideally, this will include an expert who has expertise in the type of synthesis in question. It is also vitally important that the people carrying out the evidence synthesis have a clear idea of the nature of the review and its audience. At least one of the team members should come from the same background as the synthesis audience; therefore, if a policy synthesis is being performed, then at least one policy member should be on the synthesis team.

The reasoning and methodology of the review needs to be clear and transparent at all times. Reasons for adopting particular methods or disregarding others should be identified and communicated with other team members and eventually in the text.

Rules of data inclusion, whether qualitative or quantitative require rigorous adherence. All data needs systematic categorisation and should be filed in such a way, that external reviewers can comprehend and access the knowledge of the synthesis. This carries scientific validity and eases the interpretation of methods undertaken. It also allows external reviews or expert to be introduced to the synthesis with ease and without confusion of techniques.

Once a comprehensive data acquisition has been made, it needs to have clear quality assessment and data extracted adequately. It is vital that these two factors are performed as accurately as possible as both will influence the overall conclusions and their interpretation.

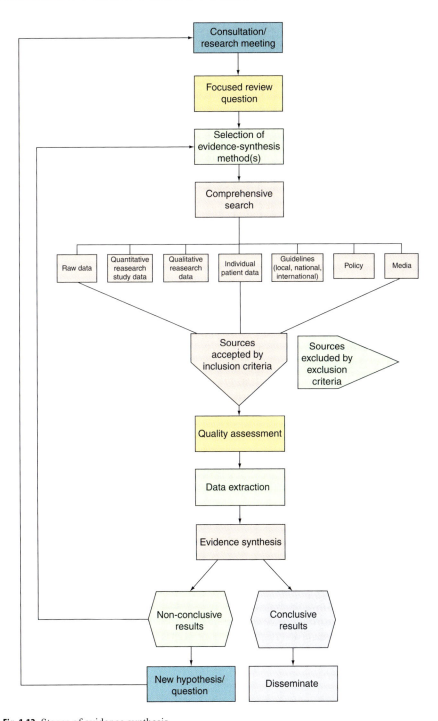

Fig. 1.12 Stages of evidence synthesis

At this point, the actual evidence synthesis takes place. In actuality, if all the previous steps have been performed adequately, and all data sources have been appropriately uploaded, then much of the mathematical aspects of synthesis on computer take only a brief amount of time.

The results of the synthesis need meticulous consideration and factors of data quality and quantification of uncertainly and probability in results needs adequate explanation and analysis. Members of the synthesis team need to assess and discuss the magnitude of synthesis findings and need to place it in the context of the original synthesis question. If the evidence synthesis offers conclusions regarding decisions and judgements, then the mechanisms of these conclusions need clear explanation and identification through summaries of the original data sets. The results should be transparently communicated in the text, both logically and coherently. The final evidence synthesis manuscript should be specifically suited for the target audience, but should nevertheless be accessible by other readers also.

1.9
Policy Considerations

The ultimate aim of evidence synthesis for policy is to provide accurate evidence for a set question and to have clear succinct knowledge to make decisions. The role of policymakers differs significantly from that of scientists and media individuals. Even though researchers ultimately perform much of the evidence synthesis, it is critical to bear in mind, who is asking the question and what type of outcomes are necessary.

For policymakers, the evidence and decisions require the following considerations:

- The questions of evidence synthesis need to apply to realistic policy decisions.
- The evidence synthesis results need to be comprehendible by policymakers.
- The evidence synthesis results require formatting in such a way that allows the knowledge to be communicated accurately to the public.

These policy considerations vary from the evidence needs of media and also those of scientists. Although the media require evidence that is easily communicated to the public, unlike the policymakers, they do not need evidence to necessarily make healthcare decisions.

The requirements of academics can occasionally fall directly in line with those of policymakers; however, their evidence on occasion has the requirements to fulfil the need for pure knowledge independent to transforming this evidence to publicly digestible information. It is therefore necessary to clarify the end points of every synthesis before this is undertaken, as this can have an effect on the results of the synthesis (Fig. 1.13).

1.9.1
Policy Context

The nature of the sources used in evidence synthesis should also be stated when the evidence is referenced, otherwise a disparity can become apparent when used incorrectly.

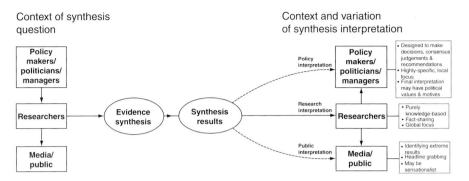

Fig. 1.13 Performance and interpretation of evidence synthesis by various groups

One recent example is that of the UK government's scientist who chaired the Advisory Council on the Misuse of Drugs (ACMD) using evidence from the scientific literature to contextualise the significance of the drug ecstasy (MDMA-3,4-methylenedioxymethamphetamine). He specified that the risks associated with horse riding (1 serious adverse event every ~350 exposures) were higher than those compared to taking ecstasy (1 serious adverse event every ~10,000 exposures). Although numerically, this was correct, the nature of the evidence was not assessed through scientific scrutiny, but rather through public and political fervour. As a result, the implications of the statement were not interpreted through the intended framework, which ultimately resulted in a disparity between scientists and policymakers. This may have been averted, if the origin of the evidence used was inferred for medical analysis, and a specific synthesis had been applied for policy considerations.[56,57]

1.9.2
Behavioural Simulation

The King's Fund, a leading independent healthcare think tank published two reports to identify the broad needs and challenges of healthcare reform for individuals participating in the reform process. These two projects named Windmill 2007 and Windmill 2009 utilised behavioural simulation techniques to guide their evidence synthesis.[58,59]

The project designers (Loop2) applied behavioural simulation as they felt that traditional evidence synthesis extrapolation were not fully applicable to 'real-world' scenarios where decisions are made in the context of complex social and economic environments. They therefore invited individuals who directly contribute to health decisions for their simulations. These individuals included, senior managers, clinicians, policymakers and regulators who attended a series of workshops and were finally able to contribute to fullblown scenarios of healthcare policy changes. These scenarios would inform policymakers of some of the real-life decisions made by individuals at all levels of the health service in the event of health reforms.

Windmill 2007[59] considered the implications of introducing a more market system to the National Health Service. It had two simulation rounds, one for 2008/2009 and another for 2010/2011. It concluded that (1) health partnerships open new opportunities regarding health delivery, (2) resource constraints were significantly limiting factors in the continuation of providing health reform opportunity and (3) the justification of exclusions in commissioning certain services pushed competition within the health market to a new level.

Windmill 2009[58] considered the implications of the NHS response to the national and international financial storm. This also had two simulation rounds, one for 2009/2010.

This simulation identified three factors that would enable a change to address the financial crisis. (1) There is a necessity for collaboration between providers to achieve a solution. (2) Cross-organisational interaction is required for this collaboration. (3) A new performance management regime would allow institutional interests to be overcome so that broader financial needs could be addressed.

The designers describe behavioural simulation through a mirror analogy portrayed in Michael Schrage in his book *Serious Play: How the World's Best Companies Simulate to Innovate*.[60] Here a hypothetical mirror can reflect (and therefore predict) the effects of particular actions. Although novel, these simulations are not universally accepted, and still require further validation before expanding their use to a variety of different healthcare scenarios.

1.10
History of Evidence Synthesis

Combining complex mathematical results and probabilities was first used by astronomers[61] to coalesce some of their complex observations by applying the seminary work (Fig. 1.14) of Blaise Pascal (1623–1662).[62] His mathematical techniques were initiated in 1654 when Pascal corresponded with Pierre de Fermat to collaborate in a theory of probability, largely inspired by gambling. He worked on the philosophical grounds of work on existentialism to mathematically address issues of uncertainly when assessing the likelihood of an event. These were based on the following observations:

• Uncertainty in all
• Uncertainty in man's purpose
• Uncertainty in reason
• Uncertainty in science
• Uncertainty in religion
• Uncertainty in scepticism

The British Astronomer Royal George Biddell Airy published a textbook in 1861[63] that contained chapters written by Johann Carl Friedrich Gauss and Pierre-Simon Laplace. This contained the first practical mathematical techniques described to summarise the results from several studies.

The British statistician Karl Pearson was asked to study the association between typhoid infection, mortality and inoculation in young soldiers. Having studied Airy's textbook, he combined small data sets from army audits into larger data groups to achieve an accrued overall result clarifying the effects of typhoid inoculation by performing the first known meta-analysis in 1904.[64]

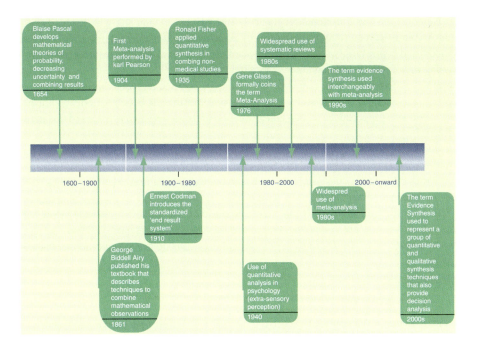

Fig. 1.14 Evidence synthesis timeline

Ronald Fisher had also studied Airy's textbook and performed a meta-analysis of multiple studies concerning the benefits of fertiliser use in agriculture.[65] Fisher's colleague William Cochran formalised this work to introduce a formal random effects model. In his 1977 book *Costs, Risks and Benefits of Surgery*, Cochran used this technique to identify the effects of vagotomy on duodenal ulcers.[66]

By applying the concepts of British physician Sir Thomas Percival (1740–1804), the American surgeon Ernest Codman (1869–1940) developed the first tumour registry in the United States. In 1910, he commenced his standardisation drive through an 'end result system' that was implemented by hospitals throughout the USA. He used this to monitor patient outcomes and identified the most successful aspects of tumour treatment so that all units could study the top centres in order to modify their practice to achieve the best possible results. Codman is considered one of the fathers of evidence-based medicine and healthcare reform. He is noted for introducing outcomes management in patient care through an 'end results system' that tracks patients and their outcomes; essentially creating the first patient healthcare database. He also set up the first mortality and morbidity meetings, and contributed to the founding of the American College of Surgeons and its Hospital Standardization Program.[67]

The first use of data integration for healthcare and biomedicine was used by psychologists in 1940 to identify the effects of extrasensory perception.[68] Further use of these techniques to systematically summarise the data from multiple studies was developed and called quantitative synthesis until 1976, when Gene Glass coined the term 'meta-analysis'.[69]

Amongst the early prominent meta-analytical studies was the study by Peter Elwood and Archie Cochrane (one of the fathers of evidence-based medicine), who performed a randomised control trial to assess the effects of aspirin in reducing the recurrence of myocardial infarctions.[70] Although there was a trend toward the benefits of aspirin, the results were not statistically significant until Elwood and Cochrane included their results into a larger meta-analysis conducted by Richard Peto to confirm the beneficial effects of aspirin.[71] Peto also proposed the testing and estimation of fixed-weighted averages of treatment effects.[72]

Within the social sciences, it was also possible to systematically summarise the data from several similar studies and this was entitled Systematic Review. Since that time, the numerous other techniques used to combine and integrate data from multiple studies have been introduced under the umbrella term evidence synthesis.

As a result, there is currently three terms in common use for summarising the evidence from studies. These are systematic review, meta-analysis and evidence synthesis.

According to Last's *Dictionary of Epidemiology*[73] the following two definitions are given:

Systematic review: The application of strategies that limit bias in the assembly, critical appraisal, and synthesis of all relevant studies on a specific topic. Meta-analysis may be, but is not necessarily, used as part of this process.
Meta-analysis: The statistical synthesis of the data from separate but similar, i.e., comparable studies, leading to a quantitative summary of the pooled results.

Our proposed definition of evidence synthesis includes:

Evidence synthesis is the synthesis (or integration) of variable data to produce information in the form of best evidence. It provides a set of methodologies to identify areas of agreement and disagreement in qualitative and quantitative data sets. By integrating data sets, this methodology may calculate the concordance and magnitude of effects from multiple studies.
    The aim of evidence synthesis is to address questions by providing the best evidence derived through the integration of data and knowledge to present information of factual integrity and least uncertainty.

1.11
Network Analysis and Graphical Synthesis

Traditional medical evidence has focussed on comparing two individual treatments for one disease. This is problematic, as these sources of evidence fail to provide a context for the all the variety of treatments available for a specific disease. These studies are not practical as they can skew the validity, applicability of the interpretation of the evidence. There has recently been a powerful development in network mathematics that has been established information regarding the World Wide Web, industry and even security sectors.[74] Its use in academic medicine is being increasingly recognised; and these techniques can also be powerfully used in evidence synthesis.[2,75,76]

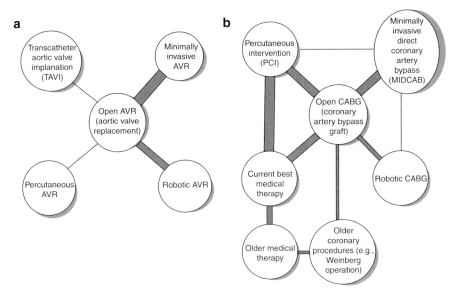

Fig. 1.15 2D Network geometry diagrams of research trials representing (**a**) the surgical treatment of aortic valve disease and (**b**) the management of coronary artery disease. Line thickness represents the number of studies comparing two treatments. These are simplified examples and larger 3D maps can be generated which can subsequently be modelled by network mathematics to generate results for evidence synthesis. Each treatment geometry represents one point in time, and the model structures will change in accordance with changes and updates in treatments and research

The demonstration of these treatments can be in two dimensions (Fig. 1.15) or three dimensions and can be managed by an increasing range of computing hardware and software.[74] Displaying the geometric network of a disease or its treatments can:

- Summarise all the treatments of a disease
- Demonstrate relationship between these treatments
- Contextualise the role of a particular treatment in the overall management of a disease.
- Identify treatments patterns
- Identify novel areas to develop new treatments
- Allow geometric models to be applied for use in establishing new treatments

The increased use of network assessment techniques[77] can help identify the sources of evidence used in systematic strategy. It can reveal underlying associations between evidence sources, research collaborations and the research utility (based on citation and access metrics).

1.12
The Future of Evidence Synthesis in Evidence-Based Medicine

Although the modern concept of evidence-based medicine (EBM) was introduced by the Scottish epidemiologist Archie Cochrane in 1972,[78] its application universally in healthcare has not yet happened at a practical level. Furthermore, although the majority of healthcare providers believe in theory, the application of these principles for all medical decisions does not exist. One healthcare specialist states that 'no one really knows how many people owe their lives to EBM, just as no one really knows how many have died because of it'.[79]

Some researchers continue to argue against the superiority of an evidence-based approach, citing several flaws in the practical issues of adopting EBM but also in the philosophical difficulties in its application. Many of these concepts are based on the limitations of traditional forms of evidence-provision that are primarily focussed on the availability of studies such as randomised controlled trials to fuel decisions. Current and newer evidence synthesis techniques however can generate new echelons of evidence that can address decisions for a larger variety of clinical questions.

1.12.1
Personalised Evidence-Based Medicine

The argument that traditional EBM is disparate from personalised medicine may hold true at some levels, although with modern techniques of synthesis, it is now possible to generate personal evidence-based decisions (Fig. 1.16).

Many aspects of medicine continue as an art form incorporating aspects of morals and emotional intelligence including empathy and compassion. Furthermore, not all surgery is easily definable which on occasion is derived from technical nuances and personal experience. These aspects can be defined as 'personalised medicine'[80] and were traditionally ignored in evidence-based decisions. Evidence synthesis however provides the depth and breadth of mathematical tools to incorporate a personalised aspect to EBM, including its ability to integrate both quantitative and qualitative studies for decision.

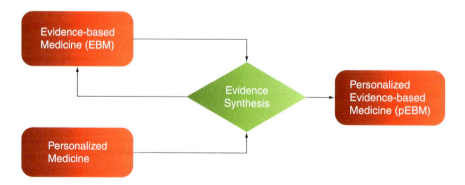

Fig. 1.16 Personalised evidence-based medicine

From a philosophical standpoint, some EMB antagonists question the following:

- What is the evidence for EBM?
- How can we prove that EBM is better than non-EBM?
- If we only have EBM techniques to compare EBM versus non-EBM then are the results for such a comparison meaningless?

Protagonists of EBM however cite the work of Foucault, who defined power as being derived from knowledge, which in turn reproduces and recreates through knowledge, and that those who are against EBM have a paranoia that the knowledge of EBM is too regulatory or powerful.[81,82]

It has been likened to the biblical analogy that if Eve did not know of knowing then why did she eat an apple?

The argument that by abiding to EBM leads to a decrease in one's autonomy[81] of decisions counteracted by positivist and objectivists[83] who state that failing to believe in EBM is an example of Moore's paradox and that it is extremely important for doctors of the future to adopt different types of knowledge. A variety of knowledge-types and styles certainly does not limit ones decision autonomy[84] but allows the adoption of the personalised evidence-based medicine. The integration of all these knowledge types is therefore highly relevant, and is best achieved through evidence synthesis.

The concept of evidence synthesis has been questioned by some in terms of feasibility and acceptability as a result of the variability of methodology in quantitative and qualitative studies. These authors argue that only studies with similar methodologies can be synthesised. As a result, the mixing of methods leads to complexity in objective comparison. These arguments are hardened for synthesising quantitative evidence from qualitative data. This is known as the 'quantitising of qualitative data'. The problems of data quantitising data now been resolved, particularly with the newer techniques of synthesis including Qualitative Comparative analysis (QCA) and Bayesian meta-analysis.

Evidence synthesis is a process that undergoes dynamic evolution and in type will likely incorporate newer knowledge types. It does not represent a static model and carries the strength of offering flexibility in adopting novel and innovative techniques to answer evidence questions. This is constant adoption of newer knowledge types therefore also strengthens the use of evidence synthesis for each generation such that it will continually evolve to provide improved evidence for current and future EBM.

The contribution of evidence synthesis to evidence-based medicine has become increasingly apparent[85,86] and is a direct source of providing powerful health reform.[87] This can be achieved through evidence-based medicine's ability to provide innovation for institutions, physicians and patients through the goal of quality. Evidence-synthesis can therefore identify, disseminate and guide innovation which in turn can reform healthcare institutions to provide the highest level of quality for patients. This has been termed 'Quality at the heart of everything we do'[85] and consists of a strengthening of clinical governance:

1. Bring clarity to quality
2. Measure quality
3. Publish quality performance
4. Recognise and reward quality

5. Raise standards
6. Safeguard quality
7. Stay ahead (new treatments and technology)

1.12.2
Game Theory and Neuroeconomics

Evidence synthesis provides an increasing proportion of the evidence-base used to inform policy debate and support policy making. On occasion, translating the results of evidence synthesis into practical healthcare policy can be challenge. Techniques used to improve qualitative methodologies in the healthcare include both narrative inquiry and discourse analysis. These techniques can offer both organisational priority and direction for the use of evidence synthesis techniques in real-life healthcare settings.[88] Currently clinical practice guidelines poorly integrate evidence on patient preferences and focus mainly on treatment effectiveness.[89] Therefore to offer the best personalised evidence-based medicine, it is incumbent on clinicians and policymakers to ensure a thorough consideration of both treatment efficacy and patient preference.

Potential examples of newer knowledge types derived for evidence synthesis include neuroeconomics and game theory. Neuroeconomics combines elements of experimental neuroscience and economics to better understand individual and group decision making.[90-92] Although it was developed to derive insights into financial decision making, it can be readily adapted to model healthcare decisions also. Better understanding of the mechanisms of decision making may help the presentation and contextualisation of evidence to targeted groups such as physicians and policymakers.

Game theory provides another potential technique for evidence synthesis. It is a theory that studies rational behaviour (game decisions) among interdependent agents (players) and is based on the mathematical study of how these rational interdependent factors interact, strategise and make decisions.[93,94] Although it has also been traditionally applied to economics (receiving eight Nobel Prizes to date) and the social sciences, its ability to model human decisions and interactions offers a powerful tool that can be used in the study of other areas of decision analysis, including healthcare[95-97] and surgical judgements.

The term 'game theory' was coined in 1944 by von Neumann and Morgenstern[94] although there has been sporadic examples of mathematical analysis of decisions well over 2,000 years ago in the Talmud.[98] Each game (or assessment of decisions) consists of the following:

1. Set of players (or participants)
2. Set of actions for each player
3. Set of preferences (picked by each player based on possible outcomes)

The prerequisites of each game include the following:

- Players have a common interest to score as high possible, however.
- Players have competing interests to increase their proportion of scores.
- A player's rational decision requires the consideration of other players' decisions.
- Uncertainty is a fundamental element of these games.

There are a number of set games that have been designed to increase the comprehension of decisions. They typically display their results and findings in game matrix. In the simplest games, there are only two players who each have the same two choices of actions, otherwise known as 2×2 coordination games. The ultimate aim of game theory modelling in healthcare is to identify a dominant solution for a pre-defined game setting. If the dominant solution does not accommodate best evidence, then the set of actions or participants need modification to ultimately provide patients with best-evidence treatments. Evidence synthesis can identify novel actions to alter each game in provide the most suitable treatment strategies.

A participant's best response is the strategy with the highest score, taking into account the strategy choice of other players. A *Nash equilibrium* is said to exist when there is a strategy profile such where every participant's choice is a best response when compared to their other choices. This is essentially when neither participant has anything to gain by changing their choice unilaterally. According to Nash, there is at least one Nash equilibrium within each game that has a definite beginning and ending (finite game).[93,94]

We provide a game theory example for surgery based on the established 'Stag Hunt Game'[99] set by the French philosopher Jean Jacques Rousseau in the eighteenth Century. This game is a coordination game, requiring the interaction of two players and reveals concepts of team working and mutual benefit.

The setting: Two healthcare institutions aim to improve their surgical department. The choices or setting up a robotics programme or replacing current minimally invasive equipment. The only way to set up a robotics programme (the preferred choice) is for the two healthcare institutions to combine resources and work together.

Replacing current equipment is easier and if one of the institutions decides to go for this option, it means that neither will get a robot. If both units simply replace their current equipment, then they each receive half of all new equipment available at that time, whereas if there is a discrepancy between one unit choosing the robot and the other choosing new equipment, then all the new equipment goes to that unit (Table 1.3).

The scoring:

0 – No healthcare benefit to patients
1 – Mild healthcare benefit to patients
2 – Moderate healthcare benefit to patients
3 – Maximal healthcare benefit to patients

In summary, if both units cooperate and acquire the surgical robot, then both score highly, if they both decide to update their equipment, then they both score lowly. However, if there

Table 1.3 Game theory matrix modelling the choices of two hospitals to select a new surgical robot or renewing their current surgical equipment. The scores for Hospital 1 are in bold whereas the scores for Hospital 2 are in standard font

Game theory matrix		Hospital 1	
		Surgical robot	New equipment
Hospital 2	Surgical robot	3, **3**	0, **2**
	New equipment	2, **0**	1, **1**

is a discrepancy between their decisions, then one scores moderately whereas the other does not score at all. The two so-called Nash equilibrium states include both institutions choosing either robot or new equipment.

Although both healthcare institutions would get more benefit from the robot (a 3-3 score), in practice they may opt for the new equipment (a 1-1 score), as it is deemed as 'less risky' although more inefficient. The role of evidence synthesis is to clarify the risk-benefit ratio of the robot, so as to enable decision makers to successfully choose the 'better option' (robot) according to the best evidence available. In the 'real world', not all games have decisions of equal value and when studying individuals or populations decisions are not always binary. In more complex scenarios, probability distributions can be calculated within each matrix (such as using a 'mixed strategy' algorithm) to identify decision outcomes from game theory models.

1.12.3
Decision Making Through Multi-attribute Utility Theory (MAUT)

Multi-attribute utility theory (MAUT) has been recently introduced in the healthcare setting as a technique that can aid healthcare decisions based on evidence synthesis. In this technique, selected objects or tools will receive an overall score of attractiveness (utility) based on the weighted score of each of the object's/tool's benefits.[100] For example, a new surgical instrument can be evaluated through a number of instrument criteria that include safety, ease of use, surgical applicability and patient outcomes.

The overall value for the new instrument can then be compared to an established instrument, where each will receive a relative or weighted score based on the pre-defined instrument criteria using the best evidence available. The scores for each instrument are then totalled in order to identify the value of the new instrument. Of the several decision making tools available, the particular strength of MAUT lies in its ability to robustly calculate certainty and uncertainly in its valuation methodology.

1.13
Interpretation of Evidence Synthesis

Integrating the data from numerous studies increasingly requires the consideration of both heterogeneity and bias. The assessment of heterogeneity in particular can in itself provide a number of evidence insights[101] regarding the nature and effects of a particular surgical technique. Recently, a set of nine suggestions were proposed by Ioannidis as important factors in interpreting a meta-analysis. These points are equally valid for evidence synthesis and encompass the effects of causality and bias for researchers in evidence synthesis researchers[101]:

1. Inferences should not be made based on plain visualisation alone (such as forest or funnel plots).
2. Measures of statistical significance and amount of heterogeneity are important and should be measured. However, it is important to report the uncertainty of these metrics.

3. Strong statements should be avoided with limited evidence.
4. Statistical heterogeneity inferences cannot be translated directly into clinical heterogeneity inferences.
5. The explanation of heterogeneity is an important opportunity to derive new knowledge.
6. There are no single statistical tests that can document or exclude bias with certainty.
7. It is important to consider the prior odds of bias before applying complex statistical tests to detect bias.
8. When any statistical tests are applied, they should be applied using models of that have at a minimum, sound statistical properties.
9. 'In all, perfect evidence is eventually much sought, but hardly ever reached utopia. A meta-analysis is not an effort to generate perfect evidence out of perfect studies. As a systematic effort, it offers actually a prime opportunity to describe limitations and caveats systematically in a body of evidence. Statistical tests may complement and enhance this effort, if used when appropriate and interpreted with due caution'.

1.14
Evidence Consistency and Windows of Evidence

When comparing patient outcomes throughout their whole care pathway for comparison in evidence synthesis (Fig. 1.17a), it is possible to discern that there are a number of steps that lead to patient pathology including genetic background environmental factor and disease process. The subsequent treatment of pathology is also a step that finally results in a measurable outcome.

In a study assessing the complication rates (pathology) of the common sexually transmitted infection (STI) by the bacterium *Chlamydia trachomatis*, van Valkengoed and colleagues[102] demonstrated that comparing Dutch infection data in a cost-effectiveness analysis (CEA) derived from the disease process and pathology (corresponding to data sets 3 and 4 in Fig. 1.17), the estimate for the environmental rate of chlamydial infection (corresponding to data set 2 in Fig. 1.17) was grossly exaggerated when compared to real-life values. This highlighted that there was an inconsistency between the individual data sets and the final result of the evidence synthesis.

Such inconsistency in data sets noted in the study on *Chlamydia* is also a problematic issue in a wider number of studies on evidence synthesis in healthcare.[103] It arises from the piecemeal nature of data collection of synthesis, where each data set is taken from independent registries. As a result, when the data from varying registries are compared, the results do not represent the patient pathway for individual patients throughout their treatment process, or even subgroups of patients with similar backgrounds and treatments. The difficulty in data acquisition has resulted in inconsistent data sets being artificially 'jumbled-together' to achieve evidence synthesis. This leads to the artificial comparison of variable patient subgroups or 'inconsistent data sets' with no accounting of subgroup variability. Inconsistency of data sets can lead to inaccurate results, as for example the environmental factor and disease process (corresponding to data sets 2 and 3 in Fig. 1.1) can vary according to patient age, location and socioeconomic status.

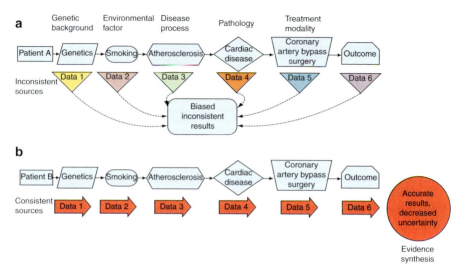

Fig. 1.17 Care pathways of theoretical patients undergoing coronary artery bypass grafts. (**a**) Outcome analysis based on inconsistent sources. (**b**) Analysis based on evidence synthesis

In order to address this problem, it is necessary to utilise consistent data for evidence synthesis, where all data sets correspond to the equivalent subgroups of patients (Fig. 1.17b). This can minimise inaccuracy as it compares groups 'like-for-like' and decreases any 'apples-and-oranges' comparison effects. There are a number of methods to integrate and compare the data sets along the patient care pathway, these include the following:

- Confidence profile method (CPM)[104]
- Bayesian Monte Carlo[105]
- Combination techniques

These techniques have similar methodologies to methods used to combine evidence in industry and the physical sciences, where a variety of estimations are made on calculating processes based on physical constants. The advantage of working with consistent data sources is to provide increased result accuracy and decreased uncertainty. Although standard models of healthcare modelling such as those in Fig. 1.17 are considered to be *deterministic*, meaning that data from each step is determined by the previous data sets. The integrative models mentioned however apply a *probabilistic* technique by utilising probability-weighted scores for each data set which can therefore accurately compare data sets to decrease result uncertainty.

Before combining information however, it is necessary to ensure that the data sources for each parameter are considering the same values before applying the integration technique for any particular model. It is important to consider that 'real-life' data from patients can be very complex and cross-reactive (Fig. 1.18) necessitating the need for clear data accrual and consideration before applying to a model.

Once evidence synthesis has been completed, there is a need to clarify the extent of data consistency when presenting evidence synthesis results. This can be done mathematically by comparing accrued values from data sets to independent data sets from trial and hospital

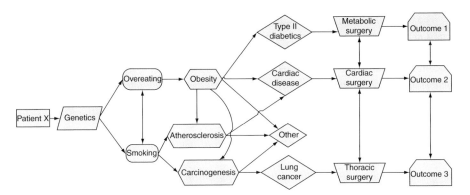

Fig. 1.18   Care pathways of a theoretical patient requiring multiple outcome analysis

registries. High inconsistency in data may result in a biased results and therefore inappropriate evidence. Applying all the available evidence by considering data consistency can provide the best evidence synthesis with the least uncertainty.

1.15
Conclusion

Evidence synthesis has been developed to integrate the knowledge from complex evidence sources to provide best evidence for healthcare practice. The techniques available have increased in number and type where each offers a unique application that corresponds with a specific research question. There is no longer a simple polarity between qualitative and quantitative, but rather a dynamic spectrum that offers these two and many more.

The applications of evidence synthesis are continually broadening and can accommodate academic medical questions, but also those from the media and importantly policymakers. The ultimate role of evidence synthesis therefore is not only to provide evidence for the pure sake of knowledge, but rather to provide evidence that can change practice locally, nationally and internationally. As such, it offers techniques that empower decision-modelling and judgement analysis.

Modern evidence synthesis techniques provide high-precision methods to collate a broad corpus of evidence, and can consider the complexity of healthcare systems in terms of hierarchy and networks. Future analytical methods will increase the ease of data interpretation, but will also account for the organisational design of healthcare systems through techniques of hierarchical modelling and network analysis. Importantly, they will increasingly focus on outcomes that directly consider patients rather than simply hospitals and units. These techniques will therefore provide the ultimate goal of personalised evidence-based medicine that will equip each individual with the best treatment options in addition to an increased ability of knowledge-based treatment choices. Clinicians and policymakers will also benefit from these techniques, as they will be in a position to ask relevant questions and obtain appropriate answers within their respective fields.

The current and future techniques of evidence synthesis will equip physicians, politicians and policymakers with the ability to provide the highest levels of evidence for an increasing number of conditions. This evidence will have an ability to be considered according to individual areas, economic environments, health systems and patients themselves. Evidence synthesis has now become a key element in augmenting future clinical care, providing management guidelines and directing policy at local, national and international levels.

References

1. *Compact Oxford English Dictionary of Current English*. Oxford University Press. Available at: http://www.askoxford.com/concise_oed/evidence?view=uk.
2. Ashrafian H, Athanasiou T. Evidence-based surgery. In: Athanasiou T, Debas H, Darzi A, eds. *Key Topics in Surgical Research and Methodology*. Heidelberg: Springer; 2009.
3. Rebitzer JB, Rege M, Shepard C. Influence, information overload, and information technology in health care. *Adv Health Econ Health Serv Res*. 2008;19:43-69.
4. Revere D, Turner AM, Madhavan A, et al. Understanding the information needs of public health practitioners: a literature review to inform design of an interactive digital knowledge management system. *J Biomed Inform*. 2007;40:410-421.
5. Hill AB. The environment and disease: association or causation? *Proc R Soc Med*. 1965; 58:295-300.
6. van Reekum R, Streiner DL, Conn DK. Applying Bradford Hill's criteria for causation to neuropsychiatry: challenges and opportunities. *J Neuropsychiatry Clin Neurosci*. 2001;13: 318-325.
7. *Levels of Evidence*. Available at: http://www.cebm.net/index.aspx?o=1025.
8. Rogers T. *Amazing Applications of Probability and Statistics: Type I and Type II Errors - Making Mistakes in the Justice System*; 1996. http://www.intuitor.com/statistics/T1T2Errors.html.
9. Freiman JA, Chalmers TC, Smith H Jr, Kuebler RR. The importance of beta, the type II error and sample size in the design and interpretation of the randomized control trial. Survey of 71 "negative" trials. *N Engl J Med*. 1978;299:690-694.
10. Collins R, Keech A, Peto R, et al. Cholesterol and total mortality: need for larger trials. *BMJ*. 1992;304:1689.
11. Mosteller F, Colditz GA. Understanding research synthesis (meta-analysis). *Annu Rev Public Health*. 1996;17:1-23.
12. Slavin RE. Best evidence synthesis: an intelligent alternative to meta-analysis. *J Clin Epidemiol*. 1995;48:9-18.
13. Letzel H. "Best-evidence synthesis: an intelligent alternative to meta-analysis": discussion. A case of "either-or" or "as well". *J Clin Epidemiol*. 1995;48:19-21.
14. Mitton C, Patten S. Evidence-based priority-setting: what do the decision-makers think? *J Health Serv Res Policy*. 2004;9:146-152.
15. Hammersley M. *What's Wrong with Ethnography?* London: Routledge; 1992.
16. Mays N, Pope C, Popay J. Systematically reviewing qualitative and quantitative evidence to inform management and policy-making in the health field. *J Health Serv Res Policy*. 2005;10(Suppl 1):6-20.
17. Noblit G, Hare R. *Meta-Ethnography: Synthesising Qualitative Studies*. Newbury Park: Sage; 1988.
18. Dixon-Woods M, Agarwal S, Jones D, Young B, Sutton A. Synthesising qualitative and quantitative evidence: a review of possible methods. *J Health Serv Res Policy*. 2005;10:45-53.

19. Teagarden JR. Meta-analysis: whither narrative review? *Pharmacotherapy*. 1989;9:274-281. discussion 281–274.
20. Egger M, Smith GD. Meta-analysis. Potentials and promise. *BMJ*. 1997;315:1371-1374.
21. Lucas PJ, Baird J, Arai L, Law C, Roberts HM. Worked examples of alternative methods for the synthesis of qualitative and quantitative research in systematic reviews. *BMC Med Res Methodol*. 2007;7:4.
22. Egger M, Smith GD, Phillips AN. Meta-analysis: principles and procedures. *BMJ*. 1997;315: 1533-1537.
23. Glaser BG, Strauss AL. *The Discovery of Grounded Theory: Strategies for Qualitative Research*. New York: Gruyter; 1967.
24. Strauss A, Corbin J. *Basics of Qualitative Research: Techniques and Procedures for Developing Grounded Theory*. California: Thousand Oaks; 1998.
25. Barnett-Page E, Thomas J. Methods for the synthesis of qualitative research: a critical review. *BMC Med Res Methodol*. 2009;9:59.
26. Glaser BG. *Doing Grounded Theory: Issues and Discussions*. Mill Valley: Sociology Press; 1998.
27. Krippendorff K. *Content Analysis: An Introduction to Its Methodology*. Thousand Oaks: Sage; 2004.
28. Morton RL, Tong A, Howard K, Snelling P, Webster AC. The views of patients and carers in treatment decision making for chronic kidney disease: systematic review and thematic synthesis of qualitative studies. *BMJ*. 2010;340:c112.
29. Baxter S, Killoran A, Kelly MP, Goyder E. Synthesizing diverse evidence: the use of primary qualitative data analysis methods and logic models in public health reviews. *Publ Health*. 2010;124(2):99-106.
30. Pawson R, Greenhalgh T, Harvey G, Walshe K. Realist review – a new method of systematic review designed for complex policy interventions. *J Health Serv Res Policy*. 2005; 10(Suppl 1):21-34.
31. Pawson RD. *Evidence Based Policy: II. The Promise of 'Realist Synthesis'*. ESRC UK Centre for Evidence Based Policy and Practice: Working Paper 4; 2001. http://kcl.ac.uk/content/1/c6/03/45/91/wp4.pdf.
32. Dixon-Woods M, Cavers D, Agarwal S, et al. Conducting a critical interpretive synthesis of the literature on access to healthcare by vulnerable groups. *BMC Med Res Methodol*. 2006;6:35.
33. Paterson BL, Thorne SE, Canam C, Jillings C. *Meta-Study of Qualitative Health Research*. Thousand Oaks: Sage; 2001.
34. Greenhalgh T, Robert G, Macfarlane F, Bate P, Kyriakidou O, Peacock R. Storylines of research in diffusion of innovation: a meta-narrative approach to systematic review. *Soc Sci Med*. 2005;61:417-430.
35. Kuhn TS. *The Structure of Scientific Revolutions*. Chicago: University of Chicago Press; 1962.
36. Miles M, Huberman A. *Qualitative Data Analysis*. London: Sage; 1994.
37. Oliver SR, Rees RW, Clarke-Jones L, et al. A multidimensional conceptual framework for analysing public involvement in health services research. *Health Expect*. 2008;11:72-84.
38. Pope C, Ziebland S, Mays N. Qualitative research in health care. Analysing qualitative data. *BMJ*. 2000;320:114-116.
39. Yin RK, Heald KA. Using the case survey method to analyse policy studies. *Adm Sci Q*. 1975;20:371-381.
40. Ragin CC. *The Comparative Method: Moving Beyond Qualitative and Quantitative Strategies*. Berkeley: University of California Press; 1992.
41. Jansen JP, Crawford B, Bergman G, Stam W. Bayesian meta-analysis of multiple treatment comparisons: an introduction to mixed treatment comparisons. *Value Health*. 2008;11: 956-964.
42. Ojajarvi A, Partanen T, Ahlbom A, et al. Estimating the relative risk of pancreatic cancer associated with exposure agents in job title data in a hierarchical Bayesian meta-analysis. *Scand J Work Environ Health*. 2007;33:325-335.

43. Voils C, Hassselblad V, Crandell J, Chang Y, Lee E, Sandelowski M. A Bayesian method for the synthesis of evidence from qualitative and quantitative reports: the example of antiretroviral medication adherence. *J Health Serv Res Policy*. 2009;14:226-233.

44. Banning JH. *Ecological triangulation: An approach for qualitative meta-synthesis* Colorado: Colorado State University; (not_dated)Post2001. http://mycahs.colostate.edu/James.H.Banning/PDFs/Ecological%20Triangualtion.pdf.

45. Sandelowski M, Barroso J. *Handbook for Synthesizing Qualitative Research*. New York: Springer; 2007.

46. Williams AL. Perspectives on spirituality at the end of life: a meta-summary. *Palliat Support Care*. 2006;4:407-417.

47. Ades AE, Sculpher M, Sutton A, et al. Bayesian methods for evidence synthesis in cost-effectiveness analysis. *Pharmacoeconomics*. 2006;24:1-19.

48. Demiris N, Sharples LD. Bayesian evidence synthesis to extrapolate survival estimates in cost-effectiveness studies. *Stat Med*. 2006;25:1960-1975.

49. Weed M. 'Meta-interpretation': a method for the interpretive synthesis of qualitative research. *Forum: Qual Soc Res*. 2005;6:Art37.

50. Gardner C. Meta-interpretation and hypertext fiction: a critical response. *Comput Humanities*. 2003;37:33-56.

51. Harden A, Thomas J. Methodological issues in combining diverse study types in systematic reviews. *Int J Soc Res Methodol*. 2005;8:257-271.

52. Sutton AJ, Cooper NJ, Jones DR. Evidence synthesis as the key to more coherent and efficient research. *BMC Med Res Methodol*. 2009;9:29.

53. Ades AE, Claxton K, Sculpher M. Evidence synthesis, parameter correlation and probabilistic sensitivity analysis. *Health Econ*. 2006;15:373-381.

54. Khan KS, Riet GT, Popay J, Nixon J, Kleijnen J. Study quality assessment - (Stage II, Conducting the Review, Phase 5). In: Centre_for_Reviews_and_Dissemination, ed. *Systematic Reviews: CRD's Guidance for Undertaking Reviews in Healthcare*. York: Centre for Reviews and Dissemination; 2009:1–20. http://www.york.ac.uk/inst/crd/CRD_Reports/crdreport4_ph5.pdf.

55. Vandenbroucke JP. STREGA, STROBE, STARD, SQUIRE, MOOSE, PRISMA, GNOSIS, TREND, ORION, COREQ, QUOROM, REMARK... and CONSORT: for whom does the guideline toll? *J Clin Epidemiol*. 2009;62:594-596.

56. A drug-induced low. *Nature*. 2009;462:11–12.

57. Nutt D. Government vs science over drug and alcohol policy. *Lancet*. 2009;374:1731-1733.

58. Harvey S, Liddell A, McMahon L. *Windmill 2009: NHS Response to the Financial Storm*. London: King's Fund; 2009.

59. Harvey S, McMahon L, Liddell A. *Windmill 2007: The Future of Health Care Reforms in England*. London: King's Fund; 2007.

60. Schrage M. *Serious Play: How the World's Best Companies Simulate to Innovate*. Boston: Harvard Business Press; 1999.

61. O'Rourke K. An historical perspective on meta-analysis: dealing quantitatively with varying study results. *J R Soc Med*. 2007;100:579-582.

62. Shampo MA, Kyle RA. Blaise Pascal (1623–1662). *JAMA*. 1977;237:986.

63. Airy GB. *On the Algebraical and Numerical Theory of Errors of Observations and the Combination of Observations*. London: Macmillan & Company; 1861.

64. Pearson K. Report on certain enteric fever inoculation statistics. *BMJ*. 1904;3:1243-1246.

65. Fisher RA. *The Design of Experiments*. Edinburgh: Oliver and Boyd; 1935.

66. Cochran WG, Diaconis P, Donner AP, et al. Experiments in surgical treatments of duodenal ulcer. In: Bunker JP, Barnes BA, Mosteller F, eds. *Costs, Risks and Benefits of Surgery*. Oxford: Oxford University Press; 1977:176-197.

67. Neuhauser D. Ernest Amory Codman, M.D., and end results of medical care. *Int J Technol Assess Health Care*. 1990;6:307-325.

68. Pratt JG, Rhine JB, Smith BM, Stuart CE, Greenwood JA. *Extra-Sensory Perception after Sixty Years: A Critical Appraisal of the Research in Extra-Sensory Perception.* New York: Henry Holt; 1940.
69. Glass GV. Primary, secondary and meta-analysis of research. *Educ Res.* 1976;10:3-8.
70. Elwood PC, Cochrane AL, Burr ML, et al. A randomized controlled trial of acetyl salicylic acid in the secondary prevention of mortality from myocardial infarction. *BMJ.* 1974;1:436-440.
71. Aspirin after myocardial infarction. *Lancet.* 1980;1:1172–1173.
72. Peto R. Why do we need systematic overviews of randomized trials? *Stat Med.* 1987;6:233-244.
73. Last JM. *A Dictionary of Epidemiology.* Oxford: Oxford University Press; 2001.
74. Lok C. Literature mining: speed reading. *Nature.* 2010;463:416-418.
75. Salanti G, Higgins JP, Ades AE, Ioannidis JP. Evaluation of networks of randomized trials. *Stat Methods Med Res.* 2008;17:279-301.
76. Salanti G, Kavvoura FK, Ioannidis JP. Exploring the geometry of treatment networks. *Ann Intern Med.* 2008;148:544-553.
77. Fowler JH, Dawes CT, Christakis NA. Model of genetic variation in human social networks. *Proc Natl Acad Sci USA.* 2009;106:1720-1724.
78. Cochrane AL. *Effectiveness and Efficiency: Random Reflections on Health Services.* London: Nuffield Provincial Hospitals Trust; 1972.
79. Saad A. The evidence-based paradox and the question of the tree of knowledge. *J Eval Clin Pract.* 2008;14:650-652.
80. Miles A, Loughlin M, Polychronis A. Evidence-based healthcare, clinical knowledge and the rise of personalised medicine. *J Eval Clin Pract.* 2008;14:621-649.
81. Miles A, Loughlin M, Polychronis A. Medicine and evidence: knowledge and action in clinical practice. *J Eval Clin Pract.* 2007;13:481-503.
82. Henry SG. Recognizing tacit knowledge in medical epistemology. *Theor Med Bioeth.* 2006;27:187-213.
83. Loughlin M. Reason, reality and objectivity–shared dogmas and distortions in the way both 'scientistic' and 'postmodern' commentators frame the EBM debate. *J Eval Clin Pract.* 2008;14:665-671.
84. Murray SJ, Holmes D, Perron A, Rail G. No exit? Intellectual integrity under the regime of 'evidence' and 'best-practices'. *J Eval Clin Pract.* 2007;13:512-516.
85. Darzi A. *High Quality Care for All: NHS Next Stage Review Final Report.* London: Department of Health, United Kingdom; 2008.
86. Darzi A. Evidence-based medicine and the NHS: a commentary. *J R Soc Med.* 2008;101:342-344.
87. Darzi A. A time for revolutions–the role of clinicians in health care reform. *N Engl J Med.* 2009;361:e8.
88. Smith N, Mitton C, Peacock S. Qualitative methodologies in health-care priority setting research. *Health Econ.* 2009;18:1163-1175.
89. Chong CA, Chen IJ, Naglie G, Krahn MD. How well do guidelines incorporate evidence on patient preferences? *J Gen Intern Med.* 2009;24:977-982.
90. Floresco SB, St Onge JR, Ghods-Sharifi S, Winstanley CA. Cortico-limbic-striatal circuits subserving different forms of cost-benefit decision making. *Cogn Affect Behav Neurosci.* 2008;8:375-389.
91. Engelmann JB, Capra CM, Noussair C, Berns GS. Expert financial advice neurobiologically "Offloads" financial decision making under risk. *PLoS ONE.* 2009;4:e4957.
92. Livet P. Rational choice, neuroeconomy and mixed emotions. *Philos Trans R Soc Lond B Biol Sci.* 2010;365:259-269.
93. Hargreaves-Heap SP, Varoufakis Y. *Game Theory: A Critical Introduction.* London: Routledge; 2004.
94. Peters H. *Game Theory: A Multi-Leveled Approach.* Heidelberg: Springer; 2008.

95. Tarrant C, Stokes T, Colman AM. Models of the medical consultation: opportunities and limitations of a game theory perspective. *Qual Saf Health Care*. 2004;13:461-466.
96. Dowd SB. Applied game theory for the hospital manager. Three case studies. *Health Care Manag (Frederick)*. 2004;23:156-161.
97. De Jaegher K, Jegers M. The physician-patient relationship as a game of strategic information transmission. *Health Econ*. 2001;10:651-668.
98. Aumann RJ, Maschler M. Game theoretic analysis of a bankruptcy problem for the Talmud. *J Econ Theory*. 1985;36:195-213.
99. Skyrms B. *The Stag Hunt and the Evolution of Social Structure*. Cambridge: Cambridge University Press; 2003.
100. Dyer JS. MAUT – multiattribute utility theory. In: Figueira J, Greco S, Ehrgott M, eds. *Multiple Criteria Decision Analysis: State of the Art Surveys*. New York: Springer; 2005.
101. Ioannidis JP. Interpretation of tests of heterogeneity and bias in meta-analysis. *J Eval Clin Pract*. 2008;14:951-957.
102. van Valkengoed IG, Morre SA, van den Brule AJ, Meijer CJ, Bouter LM, Boeke AJ. Overestimation of complication rates in evaluations of *Chlamydia trachomatis* screening programmes–implications for cost-effectiveness analyses. *Int J Epidemiol*. 2004;33:416-425.
103. Ades AE. Commentary: evidence synthesis and evidence consistency. *Int J Epidemiol*. 2004;33:426-427.
104. Eddy DM. The confidence profile method: a Bayesian method for assessing health technologies. *Oper Res*. 1989;37:210-228.
105. Dakins ME, Toll JE, Small MJ, Brand KP. Risk-based environmental remediation: Bayesian Monte Carlo analysis and the expected value of sample information. *Risk Anal*. 1996;16:67-79.

Barriers to Evidence Synthesis

Kamran Ahmed, Nick Sevdalis, Ara Darzi, and Thanos Athanasiou

Abstract In the hierarchy of research designs, randomised controlled trials and meta-analyses of randomised controlled trials are considered to be the highest level of evidence. They have been established as essential areas of research since their introduction into clinical sciences. Research in the interventional disciplines such as surgery, rely mostly on observational studies. Therefore, the quality and quantity of randomised trials with regards to interventions remain limited. Researchers in these disciplines face various obstacles during building, assessment or implementation of evidence. This chapter aims to provide a critical overview of the obstacles to randomised trials and meta-analyses. It also proposes solution to these problems.

2.1
Introduction

In the hierarchy of research designs, randomised controlled trials (RCTs) are considered to be the highest level of evidence.[1] RCTs were introduced into clinical epidemiology after evaluation of streptomycin for management of tuberculosis.[2] Since then, RCTs have become the gold standard for assessing the effectiveness of therapeutic agents.

When various randomised studies are available on a same topic, a well-conducted meta-analysis of these randomised trials is regarded as the best level of evidence within evidence-based medicine (EBM). Meta-analyses statistically integrate the results of several independent studies considered to be combinable, thus allowing evaluation of the evidence within traditional studies that is at risk of being overlooked, and provide more precise estimates of treatment effects.[3,4]

K. Ahmed (✉)
Department of Surgery and Cancer, Imperial College London, St Mary's Hospital Campus, London, UK
e-mail: k.ahmed@imperial.ac.uk

T. Athanasiou and A. Darzi (eds.), *Evidence Synthesis in Healthcare*,
DOI: 10.1007/978-0-85729-206-3_2, © Springer-Verlag London Limited 2011

Meta-analyses offer an opportunity to test implicit assumptions about the hierarchy of research designs. Ideally, if associations between exposure and outcome were studied in both randomised controlled trials and cohort or case–control studies, and if these studies were then included in meta-analyses, the results could be compared according to study design.[1] However, RCTs may overlook clinically essential benefits because of poorly constructed design – for instance, inadequate attention to sample size.[5] Therefore, an amalgamation of studies using robust statistical methodologies can overcome some of the deficiencies within the primary studies.

Randomised trials and meta-analyses have been established as essential areas of research since their introduction into clinical sciences. Certain medical disciplines, such as surgical specialities primarily, use observational studies for identification of risk factors and prognostic indicators. In these disciplines, ethical issues related to type and timing of intervention may prevent clinicians from regularly conducing RCTs. Therefore, the quality and quantity of randomised trials with regards to interventions in specialties such as surgery remains limited.[6] Moreover, a number of other factors may limit conduct of good quality trials or meta-analyses. These factors are related to barriers due to building, assessment or implementation of evidence (Fig. 2.1).

This chapter aims to provide a critical overview of the obstacles to randomised trials and meta-analyses. It also proposes solution to these problems.

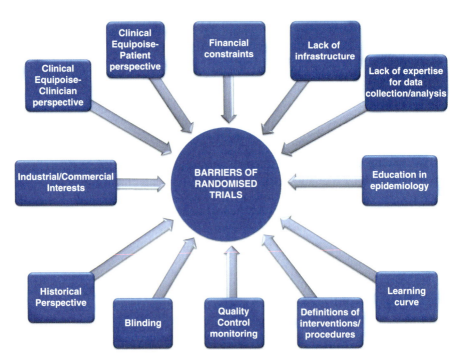

Fig. 2.1 Key determinants of successful building, assessment and implementation of evidence

2.2
Barriers to Randomised Trials

The purpose of a randomised trial is to provide the means by which the highest level of evidence from research can be judiciously and vigilantly applied to the prevention, detection, treatment and follow-up of health conditions. However, there are several obstacles to the successful conduct and application of RCTs. This section covers obstacles to the conduct of such trials (Fig. 2.2).

2.2.1
Historical Perspective

Validation of interventional procedures is generally not based on randomised trials. Conventionally, the steps in a procedure evolve with subtle changes over the passage of time. Once they are in practice, assessment of effectiveness against a placebo becomes difficult. The treatment benefit becomes so obvious that randomisation can be argued to be unethical.[7]

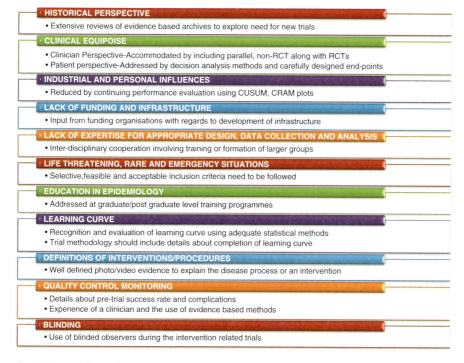

Fig. 2.2 Factors determining conduct and quality of randomised trials

Occasionally, developing therapeutic and diagnostic modalities may jeopardise the conduct of a clinical trial before its conclusion. For instance, an RCT needs to be stopped if novel surgical or technical developments render the results of the trial outdated before its completion.[8]

Moreover, an RCT cannot be conducted if a new technology or intervention is likely to undergo modifications in the near future or if this technology or technique is complex and has been developed only recently.

2.2.2
Clinical Equipoise: Clinician's Perspective

Clinical equipoise refers to uncertainty over whether a treatment will be beneficial or not. Shaw et al. argued that if a clinician has good reasons to believe that a new therapy is better than an existing therapy, he or she cannot take part in a comparative trial of the new versus old therapy. Under such circumstances, the clinician is ethically obligated to offer the new (and believed better) therapy to each new patient with a need for one of these therapies.[9] For this reason, clinicians who believe that they already practise the best option cannot participate into a trial.

On the other hand, uncertainty with regards to the best treatment option is beneficial for a patient. In this case, offering patients randomisation to equally preferred treatments is acceptable and does not violate ethical principles. This 'uncertainty principle' has been successfully used as a main eligibility criterion for large clinical trials.[10] Ambiguity on the part of all participants remains the moral and practical code of conduct that requires ethical justification of randomised trials.

2.2.3
Clinical Equipoise: Patient's Perspective

Equipoise is also important from the perspective of the patient. This is particularly true in RCTs of surgical interventions, where both trial and control arms are likely to have associated risks. Ethical principles dictate that patients should not consent to randomisation unless there is true uncertainty about the superiority of a treatment option.

Type III trials (comparing surgical and nonsurgical treatments) may pose some difficulties with the equipoise of patients.[11] Patients often refuse to take part in such RCTs as they prefer a firm decision on whether they will receive surgical or nonsurgical treatment, and not one left to be determined by chance.

2.2.4
Industrial and Personal Influences

Commercial and personal interests can interfere with the process of building or evaluating evidence, if this process is perceived to be potentially damaging to such interests.[11] For commonly available products, randomised studies can be threatening for the commercial organisations in terms of financial gains. Similarly, for widely practised procedures randomisation can be challenging to the objectivity and the practice of a surgeon.

Competition in a private sector may influence the clinicians.[11] For instance, in the initial 5 years after the introduction of cholecystectomy, only two randomised clinical trials were published.[12,13] This issue came to light after a number of reports were quoted with regards to increasing incidence of bile duct injuries.[14] Similarly, robotic-assisted procedures and single-incision laparoscopic approaches lack randomised studies to support their efficacy despite increasing clinical use of these approaches.[15]

In recent years, however, there is a progressing drift towards conduct of RCTs for newly developed treatment modalities. Different institutions are conducting RCTs worldwide for a variety of interventions.[16,17]

2.2.5
Lack of Funding and Infrastructure

Although randomised studies in interventional disciplines such as surgery are commonly performed across various regions, they are relatively few in number and lack standardised protocols compared to similar RCTs for non-interventional treatments. This may reflect a lack of expertise by participating clinicians in trials and shortage of funding for interventional trials.[18] It may also be due to the fact that funding bodies are reluctant to finance research in disciplines associated with previously poor research results.[19] Due to the lack of well-developed procedures, it has been shown that only a quarter of surgical trials report the randomisation process.[20]

2.2.6
Lack of Expertise for Appropriate Design, Data Collection and Analysis

Kelly et al. reported that many clinicians, especially surgeons, have an overambitious confidence in the ability of randomised trials to determine the practical value of interventions.[21] Consequently, energy is expended on data collection which can be fundamentally flawed due to inadequate power of the study.

Hall et al. explained why lack of focus on appropriate methodology and data analysis remain barriers to a good randomised trial.[20] It can be argued that there are primarily two types of clinical studies: explanatory and pragmatic.[22] Explanatory studies aim to assess whether a treatment has any efficacy in comparison with placebo under ideal, experimental conditions. Pragmatic studies aim to assess the effectiveness of a treatment in everyday clinical practice. Most trials attempt to address both explanatory and pragmatic types simultaneously. This practice, however, may result in findings that are not valid and that ultimately cannot provide a robust answer to either type of question.[20,22]

2.2.7
Life-Threatening and Emergency Situations

Emergency management occurs both during and out of the normal working hours. It makes consent and randomisation of the treatment or intervention difficult. Randomised trials, if conducted for emergency conditions, may miss clinically important benefits because of insufficient attention to patient selection and sample size. In order to conduct an RCT focused on an emergency condition, very selective inclusion criteria need to be followed.[23,24]

2.2.8
Dramatic Discoveries or Rare Clinical Conditions

In an incurable condition when survival is unlikely with or without treatment, an RCT is unnecessary if even one patient survives when a new treatment is administered. Similarly, if a new treatment modality, for instance appendicectomy for appendicitis, produces a rapid improvement in outcome in uncontrolled or nonrandomised controlled trials an RCT may be unnecessary or even unethical.[8] An RCT should be discontinued if a new intervention shows more than 70% absolute improvement in results compared with an established therapy.[8,11]

2.2.9
Education in Epidemiology

Detailed knowledge of epidemiology principles that are necessary for the competent conduct of an RCT remains rather poor in some groups of clinicians (e.g. surgeons).[11,25] However, there is no objective evidence that clinicians in surgical disciplines lack training of clinical epidemiology. Rather, surgical specialties tend to lack dedicated clinical teams with relevant epidemiological expertise who should be responsible for identification, design and conduct of randomised trials.

2.2.10
Learning Curve

Effective interventional techniques come into practice rapidly. Learning curve that represents average rate of learning is achieved after repeated practice. Various authors argue that RCTs should begin from the first report of a new procedure.[26] However, this approach is not ethically acceptable as the clinicians are in still at the beginning of their learning curves during the introduction phase of a new treatment.[27]

Surgical procedures are complex, and proficiency is achieved after frequent repetition. At early stages of the learning curve, errors and adverse events are likely to occur.[28,29] Randomising between a new and an established operation may introduce bias against the new methods.[30] Moreover, patient randomisation to surgeons, although an option, remains untested.[11]

2.2.11
Definitions of Interventions/Procedures

Procedural learning curves cause difficulty in timing and performing randomised trials. When comparing treatment modalities, clear definition of each treatment step is needed.

This leads to acceptance of limitations of variations for a certain procedure. Variations on an operation, however, are not uncommon and may influence outcomes. Moreover, it can be argued that definitions continue to change during the introductory phase of new interventions. Because of these issues with surgical treatments, non-standardised procedural definitions may lead to controversy whether a trial has truly investigated the intended treatment.[27] Definitions of treatment are overall more challenging for interventions than for drug trials, in which a 'treatment' is simpler to define.

2.2.12
Quality Control Monitoring

The methodology of a clinical trial and the technical quality of clinical interventions may have an impact on outcomes. The expertise of the clinicians who are carrying out the intervention is one of the determining factors of the quality of outcomes. Poor results fail to deliver intended treatment; therefore, effectiveness of the trial remains doubtful. Failure to maintain consistently high quality of procedures may narrow important technical differences and may have impact on outcomes.[31,32]

2.2.13
Blinding

Blinding is important to protect internal validity, and significant bias may result from unsuccessful blinding. Blinding, however, is particularly challenging in trials involving interventions. Examples where placebos are not possible or unethical include surgical interventions, as well as treatments where active participation of the patient is necessary (e.g. physical therapy). In fact, only about a third of published interventional trials have been reported to adequately address principles of blinding.[11,18]

2.3
Proposed Solutions to Overcome the Barriers of RCTs

To improve the quality of randomised trials, the barriers discussed above need to be addressed meticulously (Fig. 2.3). RCTs offer the highest level of evidence for assessing efficacy of treatments and direct relevant evidence from high-quality RCTs should be used wherever possible. Key problems with regard to conduct and quality of trials mainly affect trials in interventional disciplines, such as surgery and interventional radiology. For craft specialities (i.e. specialities that are dependent heavily on minor or major interventions), existing frameworks do not effectively address the range of potential problems, either conceptual or methodological.[8,11]

Figure 2.4 summarises a comprehensive framework that addresses a number of issues identified here through phased introduction of a trial, regular audit of data collection, and continuous evaluation of the quality of the trial. The framework identifies issues around learning curves, variations in technique or type of interventions, which need to be addressed

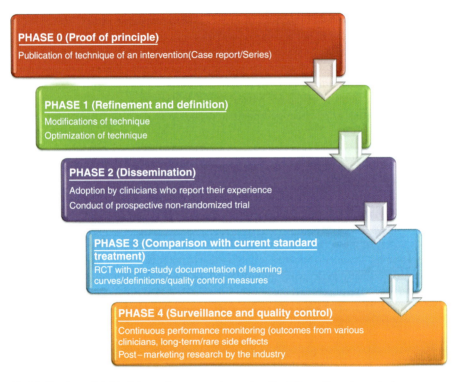

Fig. 2.3 Barriers related to intervention, researcher and methodology of a meta-analysis

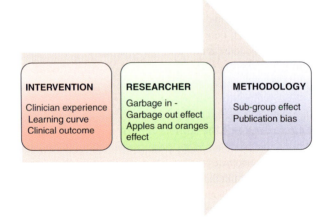

Fig. 2.4 Proposed framework for planning and conduct of RCTs in interventional specialities[27]

and documented appropriately to ensure adequate methodological quality. The framework also proposes an initial phase of non-randomised trials to be incorporated into RCTs in order to determine suitable end points.[11]

2.4
Barriers Specific to Meta-Analyses

The conduct of meta-analysis in case of rare conditions and interventions is particularly difficult and needs timely investigation, standardised definitions, availability of high-quality data (from RCTs and meticulously done observational studies) and statistical expertise.

This section delineates obstacles to meta-analyses and considers solutions to these problems (Fig. 2.5). The problems and their solutions fall into three distinct categories associated with: (1) the intervention, (2) the researcher and (3) the methodology.

2.4.1
Intervention-Related Barriers

The primary differences between meta-analyses in craft disciplines and those in other fields originate from the reproducibility of treatments and variations in practice that are difficult to compare. The outcomes of a surgical procedure principally depend on the level of experience of a clinician. This is not the case in other areas of research such as drug trials, where interventions tend to be significantly more consistent and drugs act in a uniform manner. Early meta-analytic assessment of a new procedure or technique may give a misleading picture of its efficacy due to lack of competence of the surgeons who are carrying out a new procedure. Factors determining whether an interventional procedure will

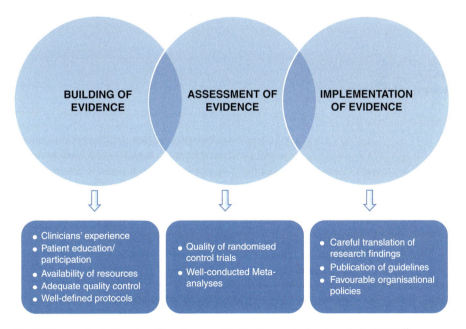

Fig. 2.5 Proposed solutions to address issues related to the conduct and control of RCTs[11]

be carried out competently include the clinician's experience, available equipment and time. Performance continues to improve until a plateau phase is reached as manifested by the 'learning curve'. The experience of a clinician is a key confounder during comparative trials involving interventions. Less experienced clinicians have relatively poorer outcomes,[33] which are less likely to be reported, thus adding further to publication bias.[3,34] These issues compromise the validity of a meta-analysis. For instance, with the advent of new interventions such as Natural orifice transluminal endoscopic surgery (NOTES) which are supported by lower levels of evidence,[35] caution must be exerted when the first meta-analysis of this procedure takes place. Small sample size in individual trials, year of publication and poor definitions need to be anticipated ahead of the analysis otherwise meta-analysis can be fraught with these issues.[36]

Meta-analyses may produce conflicting evidence when results are pooled from small trials with disparate outcomes. If the results are in conflict with large RCTs, the reliability of the evidence becomes debatable.[37,38] In a study comparing 19 meta-analyses and 12 large RCTs on the same topic, LeLorier et al. found that the results in 5 out of 40 outcomes were significantly different between the RCTs and those of the meta-analyses.[39] Meta-analysis cannot be a substitute for large clinical trials.[40] However, it may be a useful guide to clinical decision makers until explicit experimental evidence becomes available.

The year of publication of a study is also a strong confounder to the overall results revealed by a meta-analysis as population characteristics and outcome data may change over time. Furthermore, new developments in technology and changes in clinicians' technical expertise may translate into variable outcomes over time. All these factors need to be considered especially in surgical disciplines where new technologies and techniques are continuously developed and the learning curve is progressively overcome.[41] Increasing accumulation of evidence with time improves the robustness of results reported by a meta-analysis.[42]

2.4.2
Researcher-Related Barriers

A researcher may face several challenges whilst conducting meta-analysis. One of these is the *Garbage in, garbage out* effect: If a meta-analysis includes several low-quality studies, then basic errors in the primary studies will be translated across to the meta-analysis, where the errors may be difficult to identify. The quality of meta-analysis is determined by the quality and type of studies included. Because the nature of procedural interventions often makes it difficult to perform well-conducted RCTs, inclusion in meta-analyses of observational studies (cross-sectional, case series, case-control or cohort design) remains common yet controversial as they are vulnerable to bias by confounding factors.[43]

Another common problem is *the apple and oranges* effect, which results from combining different study designs in an analysis. This may lead to an erroneous result being produced (relative risk, odds ratio or weighted mean difference).[44] This apparent difference in effect across pooled studies is termed as 'heterogeneity'. In a meta-analysis, three principal sources of heterogeneity are clinical (e.g. baseline difference between patients from different studies), statistical (e.g. effects being estimated by individual studies in a meta-analysis are not identical) and methodological (e.g. design-related heterogeneity).[45] The ultimate aim of pooling data from different studies is to provide a single best estimate of treatment effect between two treatment groups. It, therefore, is vitally important to combine 'apples' with 'apples'.[46]

2.4.3
Methodology-Related Barriers

Several challenging aspects such as the subgroup effect and publication bias can compromise the methodology of a meta-analysis.

A meta-analysis aims to produce an estimate of the average effect seen in trials of a particular treatment termed as *subgroup effect*.[47] It is necessary to determine whether the overall effect applies to all participating individuals, or whether some subgroups have different effect than others.

Publication bias refers to the greater likelihood of studies with positive (i.e. statistically significant) results being published.[22] Exclusion of studies from the meta-analysis because they are small in size, found negative results or for other reasons can bias the results. This is termed as a 'file drawer problem'. It may be intentional or due to the results of a flawed and incomplete literature search.[48] This publication bias may render meta-analysis of published literature misleading, thus compromising patient safety.[49] Another problem is that of 'grey literature' which refers to the studies not published as formal, peer-reviewed journal articles (e.g. those found in conference abstracts, books, theses, government and company reports and other unpublished material). These can also potentially include studies that report negative results and are not published or lie dormant in a researcher's filing cabinet.

2.5
Proposed Solutions to Overcome the Barriers of Meta-Analysis

2.5.1
Solutions to Intervention-Related Problems

It is imperative to account for and wait for the learning curve to be achieved and differentiate between high-volume and low-volume centres. The individual trials should be conducted once the learning curve has been achieved, thereby having experts performing the procedures. Moreover, subgroup analyses between high-volume and low-volume centres should be performed to account for effect of case load, if any, on the results.

Quality control for the included studies should be assessed meticulously. A commonly used scoring method is that developed by Jadad et al. which assigns points based on the presence of randomisation, double blinding, and adequate description of withdrawals and dropouts.[50]

In case of a lack of adequate evidence, a meta-analysis is not an appropriate method of clinical appraisal, as the analysis will suffer from insufficient data and heterogeneous outcomes being reported. Such a scenario has been reported by Slim et al. in 2008 who tried to clarify the controversy surrounding the timing of elective surgery of colonic diverticulitis in young patients.[35] Out of 15 articles selected for inclusion in this study, only 3 papers reported information regarding the timing of surgery. The authors concluded that the researchers should no longer attempt to address this question by a meta-analysis.[35]

2.5.2
Solutions to Researcher-Related Problems

Several tools have been developed to assess the quality of individual meta-analyses.[51] Guidelines exist to assess the quality of both randomised (QUOROM statement) and observational studies (MOOSE statement).[52,53] A recent update to the QUOROM statement is PRISMA, which focuses on recognition of bias through meticulous quality assessment.[54] These tools can be an invaluable source to understand and quantify sources of variability across studies and should be encouraged.[53] Although several quality assessment tools (checklists) exist, there are discrepancies amongst them. The variability across different checklists suggests that each individual bias-reducing measure such as randomisation, concealment of allocation and blinding should be documented across studies.[55]

Identification of heterogeneity can highlight factors that influence outcomes that are not observable in individual trials. If performed before a new study, it may help the investigator improve the design by incorporating an understanding of the factors that contribute to heterogeneity. There are three ways to assess heterogeneity. First, through assessment of 'between-studies variance – τ^2'. This primarily depends on the particular effect size metric used. Second, 'Cochrane's Q test', which follows a chi-square distribution to make inferences about the null hypothesis of homogeneity. The problem with this test is that it has poor power to detect true heterogeneity when the number of studies is small. None of the above-mentioned methods have a standardised scale. Therefore, they are poorly equipped to make comparisons of the degree of homogeneity across meta-analyses.[56] Third method for quantifying inconsistency is '$I^2 = [(Q - df)/Q] \times 100\%$', where Q is the chi-squared statistic and df represents degrees of freedom.[57] This method is easier to utilise because it defines variability along a scale-free range as a percentage from 0% to 100%. This describes the percentage of the variability in effect estimates that is due to heterogeneity rather than sampling error (chance). Heterogeneity could be considered substantial when this value is greater than 50%.[57] It is worth noting that tests for assessment of heterogeneity lack power to reject the null hypothesis of homogeneous results and should be used even if substantial differences between the studies exist as they provide an opportunity for examining why treatment effects differ in different circumstances.[58]

Another way to account for heterogeneity is to make use of 'Random effects model' and 'fixed effects model'. If a test for homogeneity shows homogeneous results then the differences between studies are assumed to be a consequence of sampling variation, and a fixed effects model is appropriate. If, however, the test shows that significant heterogeneity exists between study results then a random effects model is advocated. If the heterogeneity is very high and not compensated by the random effects model, the viability of the meta-analysis becomes questionable.

Sensitivity analysis can also contribute to enhance the quality of the results by considering the extent of reporting of input parameters. It involves: (1) re-analysing the results by using all studies and then excluding poorer quality studies, (2) using both fixed and random effects meta-analyses to assess the robustness of the results to the method used and (3) repeating the meta-analysis by excluding any study that is an outlier to assess its influence.

2.5.3
Solutions to Methodology-Related Problems

Subgroup analysis delineates heterogeneity. However, if trials are split into too many groups, the probability of false-positive results increases (Type I error). Splitting a meta-analysis into subgroups should be subjected to a power analysis. There should also be a strong biological rationale for performing a subgroup analysis and care should be taken in the interpretation of any effects, which are likely to be composite.[59] Sub-group analyses may generate hypotheses which can assist decision-making between different treatment options.[60]

The presence of publication biases can be identified through stratifying the analysis by study size. Smaller effects can be significant in larger studies. If publication bias is present, larger studies are likely to report smaller effects. However, exclusion of the smallest studies has little effect on the overall estimate. Thus, sensitivity analysis is useful in that it assess whether the results from a meta-analysis are valid and not affected by the exclusion of trials of poorer quality or of studies stopped early. It also takes into account publication bias.[34] Because of the potential impact of publication bias, many meta-analyses now include a 'failsafe N' statistic that calculates the number of studies with null results that would need to be added to the meta-analysis in order for an effect to no longer be reliable.

Formal tests for publication bias exist, but in practice few meta-analyses have assessed or adjusted for the presence of this bias. Examination of a 'funnel plot' is one of the simplest and most commonly used methods to detect publication bias.[61] However, visual inspection of funnel plots might be subjective and so statistical tests for detecting plot asymmetry can also be used. Regression tests and rank correlation tests are some of the options available. In addition, various methods such as the 'trim and fill method' and 'weight modelling' could be undertaken to compensate for publication bias.[62] Other biases associated with time lag, English language, citation, duplication and outcome reporting should also be considered equally important when analyzing data.

2.6
Challenges to Implementation of Evidence from Randomised Trials and Meta-Analyses

In the previous sections, we detailed a range of potential barriers to evidence synthesis, either at the level of the randomised trial or at the level of the meta-analysis of such trials, and we also discussed solutions that could help overcome such barriers. Importantly, however, even well-conducted trails and meta-analysis that should, in theory, inform clinical practice are not taken up as much or as quickly as proponents of evidence-based medicine would expect.[63-66] In fact, lack of adequate uptake of the outcomes of such research work renders the previous discussion irrelevant: why care about the quality of evidence synthesis if the target audience (i.e. clinicians on the ground) will not implement the new findings? Reasons why high-level clinical evidence often does not change practice as much as should be expected are complex, and involve a range of factors. In what follows, three key categories of factors are discussed (the topic has been explored in great detail in numerous publications, to which we point the interested reader for further resources[6,67,68]).

A first category of reasons why novel evidence-based treatments are not implemented revolves around the *nature of the evidence* itself, as well as the processes of collecting and synthesising it. First of all, the rate of novel publications of RCTs and meta-analyses (as well as systematic reviews) exceeds the knowledge absorption rate of any clinician – even those working in academic environments. In 2006, the number of surgery-related RCTs in the Cochrane library was estimated near 35,000. This 'evidence flood' comes through an ever increasing number of journals, both specialty-specific and general medical journals.[69] No single person can possibly cope with this volume of new knowledge. To tackle this problem, it has been suggested that 'evidence filters' should be designed and applied, so that the relevant evidence does reach the intended audiences.[69] Information technology has also been implicated in attempts to make evidence more easily available.[68-70]

A second category of reasons underpinning lack of integration of evidence into practice relate to *clinicians* themselves. As discussed earlier, many clinicians are not familiar with the methodologies and techniques used in evidence synthesis and therefore they are not able to appraise the quality and importance of the work. In addition, searching through multiple databases using 'clever' keywords that are sensitive enough to select relevant papers but also not too inclusive so that hundreds or thousands of entries are retrieved is a skill.[71] Once a paper has been retrieved, appraising the quality of the reported study is an additional skill, necessary to be able to evaluate the robustness of the design and strength of the conclusions.[71] Current clinical training does not routinely equip clinicians with such skills – or at least it does not do so at the level required to routinely browse through databases to find reviews or RCTs that have the potential to change clinical practice. Keeping in touch with the ever-evolving evidence base and becoming informed of new techniques and approaches that can potentially benefit patients is part of clinicians' duty to robust continuing professional development.[72-75] As such, it ought to be recognised as a component of revalidation and recertification and actively encouraged within professional and regulatory networks (e.g. Royal Colleges).

Lack of knowledge or skills is often compounded by a disapproving attitude towards the methodology of RCTs, which reflects *philosophical/epistemological reasons* why evidence is not 'automatically' translated into practice. Clinicians often complain that RCTs report evidence derived from very carefully selected patients, who do not mirror those in their direct care.[76] A similar complaint arises in relation to the external validity of the procedure of the RCT, which is perceived to be carried out 'by ultraspecialists in quaternary care centres' – again not reflecting the 'average' clinician in an 'average' generalist hospital.[77] These questions are valid, and reflect the difficulty of safely extrapolating from a specific study population to a more general patient population. To some degree, these issues could be addressed at the design stages of the RCT. They should also be extensively addressed in the context of meta-analyses, where patient inclusion criteria should be scrutinised. Importantly, since patient populations will always differ, it should be remembered that direct replication of treatment benefits from a published RCT may not occur due to either random error (inevitable sample variations) or systematic error (which should trigger a new study), or specific subgroup analyses to establish whether treatment effects are uniform across different patient groups.[78]

Finally, it is important to note that *practicalities of the healthcare environment* as well as the prevailing *culture* in an organisation also affect evidence uptake. No matter how motivated to seek the newest, innovative treatment options for their patients, clinicians will not be able to do so if they are constantly working under time pressure to deliver service.[79] High pressure to increase patient throughput favours tried and tested approaches and also does not allow room for exploration of the evidence base. A key reason why junior trainees learn through observation, in addition to this being the traditional apprenticeship model of learning in medicine, is that this is the fastest way to learn how to treat a patient. Access to the evidence base that involves multiple trips to the medical library, or constant use of IT facilities is nearly impossible in an environment where consultations can only last a few minutes. Apart from practicalities, however, evidence-based medicine experts also discuss the issue of an 'EBM culture', which may or not be prevailing within a unit or organisation and which affects the willingness of clinicians to engage with evidence and make the most of it.[70] Taken together with the philosophical/epistemological issues mentioned above, although practicalities are often very demanding, care should be taken in the design of a clinician's job to allow time and 'mental space' for evidence review.

2.7
Conclusions

Randomised controlled trials and meta-analyses are valuable tools for effective evidence synthesis. If used judiciously and conducted with scientific rigor, they can guide clinical decisions and health policy towards improved patient outcomes. Overcoming barriers to robustly synthesising evidence and implementing it to everyday clinical practice can enhance the strength of evidence derived from research studies, and ultimately improve safety and quality of care. Future research should focus on developing refined protocols for the undertaking and reporting of randomised trials and meta-analyses, as well as on better understanding and sustainably overcoming barriers to implementing evidence.

References

1. Concato J, Shah N, Horwitz RI. Randomized, controlled trials, observational studies, and the hierarchy of research designs. *N Engl J Med*. 2000;342:1887-1892.

2. MRC_Investigation. Streptomycin treatment of pulmonary tuberculosis: a Medical Research Council investigation. *BMJ*. 1948;2:769-782.
3. Egger M, Smith GD, Phillips AN. Meta-analysis: principles and procedures. *BMJ*. 1997; 315:1533-1537.
4. Huque MF. Experiences with meta-analysis in NDA submissions. *Proc Biopharm Sect Am Stat Assoc*. 1988;2:28-33.
5. Sacks H, Chalmers TC, Smith H Jr. Randomized versus historical controls for clinical trials. *Am J Med*. 1982;72:233-240.
6. Farrokhyar F, Karanicolas PJ, Thoma A, et al. Randomized controlled trials of surgical interventions. *Ann Surg*. 2010;251:409-416.
7. Black N. Why we need observational studies to evaluate the effectiveness of health care. *BMJ*. 1996;312:1215-1218.
8. Solomon MJ, McLeod RS. Should we be performing more randomized controlled trials evaluating surgical operations? *Surgery*. 1995;118:459-467.
9. Shaw LW, Chalmers TC. Ethics in cooperative clinical trials. *Ann NY Acad Sci*. 1970;169: 487-495.
10. Weijer C, Shapiro SH, Cranley Glass K. For and against: clinical equipoise and not the uncertainty principle is the moral underpinning of the randomised controlled trial. *BMJ*. 2000; 321:756-758.
11. McCulloch P, Taylor I, Sasako M, Lovett B, Griffin D. Randomised trials in surgery: problems and possible solutions. *BMJ*. 2002;324:1448-1451.
12. Barkun JS, Barkun AN, Sampalis JS, et al. Randomised controlled trial of laparoscopic versus mini cholecystectomy. The McGill Gallstone Treatment Group. *Lancet*. 1992;340:1116-1119.
13. McMahon AJ, Russell IT, Baxter JN, et al. Laparoscopic versus minilaparotomy cholecystectomy: a randomised trial. *Lancet*. 1994;343:135-138.
14. Neugebauer E, Troidl H, Kum CK, Eypasch E, Miserez M, Paul A. The E.A.E.S. Consensus development conferences on laparoscopic cholecystectomy, appendectomy, and hernia repair. Consensus statements – September 1994. The Educational Committee of the European Association for Endoscopic Surgery. *Surg Endosc*. 1995;9:550-563.
15. Ahmed K, Khan MS, Vats A, et al. Current status of robotic assisted pelvic surgery and future developments. *Int J Surg*. 2009;7:431-440.
16. Nix J, Smith A, Kurpad R, Nielsen ME, Wallen EM, Pruthi RS. Prospective randomized controlled trial of robotic versus open radical cystectomy for bladder cancer: perioperative and pathologic results. *Eur Urol*. 2010;57:196-201.
17. Ouriel K. The PIVOTAL study: a randomized comparison of endovascular repair versus surveillance in patients with smaller abdominal aortic aneurysms. *J Vasc Surg*. 2009;49:266-269.
18. Solomon MJ, Laxamana A, Devore L, McLeod RS. Randomized controlled trials in surgery. *Surgery*. 1994;115:707-712.
19. Solomon MJ, McLeod RS. Surgery and the randomised controlled trial: past, present and future. *Med J Aust*. 1998;169:380-383.
20. Hall JC, Mills B, Nguyen H, Hall JL. Methodologic standards in surgical trials. *Surgery*. 1996;119:466-472.
21. Diamond GA, Forrester JS. Clinical trials and statistical verdicts: probable grounds for appeal. *Ann Intern Med*. 1983;98:385-394.
22. Easterbrook PJ, Berlin JA, Gopalan R, Matthews DR. Publication bias in clinical research. *Lancet*. 1991;337:867-872.
23. Hochman JS, Sleeper LA, Godfrey E, et al. Should we emergently revascularize Occluded Coronaries for cardiogenic shock: an international randomized trial of emergency PTCA/CABG-trial design. The SHOCK Trial Study Group. *Am Heart J*. 1999;137:313-321.
24. Hochman JS, Sleeper LA, White HD, et al. One-year survival following early revascularization for cardiogenic shock. *JAMA*. 2001;285:190-192.

25. van der Linden W. Pitfalls in randomized surgical trials. *Surgery*. 1980;87:258-262.
26. Chalmers TC, Celano P, Sacks HS, Smith H Jr. Bias in treatment assignment in controlled clinical trials. *N Engl J Med*. 1983;309:1358-1361.
27. McCulloch P. Developing appropriate methodology for the study of surgical techniques. *J R Soc Med*. 2009;102:51-55.
28. Parikh D, Johnson M, Chagla L, Lowe D, McCulloch P. D2 gastrectomy: lessons from a prospective audit of the learning curve. *Br J Surg*. 1996;83:1595-1599.
29. Testori A, Bartolomei M, Grana C, et al. Sentinel node localization in primary melanoma: learning curve and results. *Melanoma Res*. 1999;9:587-593.
30. Bonenkamp JJ, Songun I, Hermans J, et al. Randomised comparison of morbidity after D1 and D2 dissection for gastric cancer in 996 Dutch patients. *Lancet*. 1995;345:745-748.
31. Bonenkamp JJ, Hermans J, Sasako M, et al. Extended lymph-node dissection for gastric cancer. *N Engl J Med*. 1999;340:908-914.
32. McCulloch P. D1 versus D2 dissection for gastric cancer. *Lancet*. 1995;345:1516-1517. author reply 1517–1518.
33. Sauerland S, Seiler CM. Role of systematic reviews and meta-analysis in evidence-based medicine. *World J Surg*. 2005;29:582-587.
34. Egger M, Davey Smith G, Schneider M, Minder C. Bias in meta-analysis detected by a simple, graphical test. *BMJ*. 1997;315:629-634.
35. Slim K, Raspado O, Brugere C, Lanay-Savary MV, Chipponi J. Failure of a meta-analysis on the role of elective surgery for left colonic diverticulitis in young patients. *Int J Colorectal Dis*. 2008;23:665-667.
36. Hernandez AV, Walker E, Ioannidis JP, Kattan MW. Challenges in meta-analysis of randomized clinical trials for rare harmful cardiovascular events: the case of rosiglitazone. *Am Heart J*. 2008;156:23-30.
37. Borzak S, Ridker PM. Discordance between meta-analyses and large-scale randomized, controlled trials. Examples from the management of acute myocardial infarction. *Ann Intern Med*. 1995;123:873-877.
38. Cappelleri JC, Ioannidis JP, Schmid CH, et al. Large trials vs meta-analysis of smaller trials: how do their results compare? *JAMA*. 1996;276:1332-1338.
39. LeLorier J, Gregoire G, Benhaddad A, Lapierre J, Derderian F. Discrepancies between meta-analyses and subsequent large randomized, controlled trials. *N Engl J Med*. 1997;337:536-542.
40. Bailar JC 3rd. The promise and problems of meta-analysis. *N Engl J Med*. 1997;337:559-561.
41. Lau J, Ioannidis JP, Schmid CH. Summing up evidence: one answer is not always enough. *Lancet*. 1998;351:123-127.
42. Lau J, Antman EM, Jimenez-Silva J, Kupelnick B, Mosteller F, Chalmers TC. Cumulative meta-analysis of therapeutic trials for myocardial infarction. *N Engl J Med*. 1992;327:248-254.
43. Huston P, Naylor CD. Health services research: reporting on studies using secondary data sources. *CMAJ*. 1996;155:1697-1709.
44. Wachter KW. Disturbed by meta-analysis? *Science*. 1988;241:1407-1408.
45. Abrams KR, Gillies CL, Lambert PC. Meta-analysis of heterogeneously reported trials assessing change from baseline. *Stat Med*. 2005;24:3823-3844.
46. Ioannidis JP, Patsopoulos NA, Evangelou E. Uncertainty in heterogeneity estimates in meta-analyses. *BMJ*. 2007;335:914-916.
47. Davey Smith G, Egger M, Phillips AN. Meta-analysis. Beyond the grand mean? *BMJ*. 1997;315:1610-1614.
48. Rosenberg MS. The file-drawer problem revisited: a general weighted method for calculating fail-safe numbers in meta-analysis. *Evolution*. 2005;59:464-468.
49. Peters JL, Sutton AJ, Jones DR, Abrams KR, Rushton L. Comparison of two methods to detect publication bias in meta-analysis. *JAMA*. 2006;295:676-680.

50. Jadad AR, Moore RA, Carroll D, et al. Assessing the quality of reports of randomized clinical trials: is blinding necessary? *Control Clin Trials*. 1996;17:1-12.
51. Oxman AD. Checklists for review articles. *BMJ*. 1994;309:648-651.
52. Moher D, Cook DJ, Eastwood S, Olkin I, Rennie D, Stroup DF. Improving the quality of reports of meta-analyses of randomised controlled trials: the QUOROM statement. Quality of Reporting of Meta-analyses. *Lancet*. 1999;354:1896-1900.
53. Stroup DF, Berlin JA, Morton SC, et al. Meta-analysis of observational studies in epidemiology: a proposal for reporting. Meta-analysis Of Observational Studies in Epidemiology (MOOSE) group. *JAMA*. 2000;283:2008-2012.
54. Moher D, Liberati A, Tetzlaff J, Altman DG. Preferred reporting items for systematic reviews and meta-analyses: the PRISMA statement. *BMJ*. 2009;339:b2535.
55. Juni P, Witschi A, Bloch R, Egger M. The hazards of scoring the quality of clinical trials for meta-analysis. *JAMA*. 1999;282:1054-1060.
56. Huedo-Medina TB, Sanchez-Meca J, Marin-Martinez F, Botella J. Assessing heterogeneity in meta-analysis: Q statistic or I2 index? *Psychol Methods*. 2006;11:193-206.
57. Higgins JP, Thompson SG. Quantifying heterogeneity in a meta-analysis. *Stat Med*. 2002; 21:1539-1558.
58. Bailey KR. Inter-study differences: how should they influence the interpretation and analysis of results? *Stat Med*. 1987;6:351-360.
59. Sevdalis N, Jacklin R. Interaction effects and subgroup analyses in clinical trials: more than meets the eye? *J Eval Clin Pract*. 2008;14:919-922.
60. Cook DI, Gebski VJ, Keech AC. Subgroup analysis in clinical trials. *Med J Aust*. 2004;180: 289-291.
61. Mayer EK, Bottle A, Rao C, Darzi AW, Athanasiou T. Funnel plots and their emerging application in surgery. *Ann Surg*. 2009;249:376-383.
62. Duval S, Tweedie R. Trim and fill: a simple funnel-plot-based method of testing and adjusting for publication bias in meta-analysis. *Biometrics*. 2000;56:455-463.
63. Gray SM. Knowledge management: a core skill for surgeons who manage. *Surg Clin North Am*. 2006;86:17-39. vii-viii
64. Howes N, Chagla L, Thorpe M, McCulloch P. Surgical practice is evidence based. *Br J Surg*. 1997;84:1220-1223.
65. Kingston R, Barry M, Tierney S, Drumm J, Grace P. Treatment of surgical patients is evidence-based. *Eur J Surg*. 2001;167:324-330.
66. Meakins JL. Evidence-based surgery. *Surg Clin North Am*. 2006;86:1-16. vii.
67. Ergina PL, Cook JA, Blazeby JM, et al. Challenges in evaluating surgical innovation. *Lancet*. 2009;374:1097-1104.
68. Knight T, Brice A. Librarians, surgeons, and knowledge. *Surg Clin North Am*. 2006;86:71-90. viii–ix.
69. Glasziou P. Managing the evidence flood. *Surg Clin North Am*. 2006;86:193-199. xi.
70. Lee MJ. Evidence-based surgery: creating the culture. *Surg Clin North Am*. 2006;86: 91-100. ix.
71. McCulloch P, Badenoch D. Finding and appraising evidence. *Surg Clin North Am*. 2006;86: 41-57. viii.
72. Ahmed K, Ashrafian H. Life-long learning for physicians. *Science*. 2009;326:227.
73. Ahmed K, Jawad M, Dasgupta P, Darzi A, Athanasiou T, Khan MS. Assessment and maintenance of competence in urology. *Nat Rev Urol*. 2010;7:403-413.
74. Arora S, Sevdalis N, Suliman I, Athanasiou T, Kneebone R, Darzi A. What makes a competent surgeon?: experts' and trainees' perceptions of the roles of a surgeon. *Am J Surg*. 2009;198: 726-732.
75. Satava RM, Gallagher AG, Pellegrini CA. Surgical competence and surgical proficiency: definitions, taxonomy, and metrics. *J Am Coll Surg*. 2003;196:933-937.

76. Rothwell PM. Factors that can affect the external validity of randomised controlled trials. *PLoS Clin Trials*. 2006;1:e9.
77. Marshall JC. Surgical decision-making: integrating evidence, inference, and experience. *Surg Clin North Am*. 2006;86:201-215. xii.
78. Kraemer HC, Wilson GT, Fairburn CG, Agras WS. Mediators and moderators of treatment effects in randomized clinical trials. *Arch Gen Psychiatry*. 2002;59:877-883.
79. Sevdalis N, McCulloch P. Teaching evidence-based decision-making. *Surg Clin North Am*. 2006;86:59-70. viii.

Systematic Review and Meta-analysis in Clinical Practice

3

Srdjan Saso, Sukhmeet S. Panesar, Weiming Siow, and Thanos Athanasiou

Abstract Systematic review and meta-analysis provide a means to comprehensively analyse and objectively summarise and synthesize primary research. Prior to commencing, it is important to frame a specific question in a systematic review. Although such a review is ideal in many situations, it might not be possible to perform a meta-analysis due to the heterogeneity of summary statistics or nature of study design. Furthermore, it needs to be understood that performing a meta-analysis is a time-consuming, ordered process that needs to be well-planned in order to yield valid results.

The quality of the individual studies incorporated into the meta-analysis must be assessed. In addition, for clinicians interpreting a meta-analysis, its quality must also be assessed. The inclusion of negative trials and small studies might involve the inclusion of studies with suboptimal methodological quality leading to the inclusion of bias inherent in individual studies into the meta-analysis. As 'garbage-in' transliterates to 'garbage-out', this would lead to aberrant results. Publication bias and other forms of bias must be expected and accounted for via the utilisation of appropriate review methodology and statistical compensation in order to ensure the inclusion of the whole gamut of positive and negative trials available in a field of study. Meta-analysis in surgery warrant special attention as a greater degree of heterogeneity is expected when compared to meta-analysis of medical treatments. Generally, we note that the meta-analytic technique has limitations and detail should be paid to these when basing clinical decisions on the results of a meta-analysis. Nevertheless, well-conducted meta-analyses have the ability to inform and alter clinical practice.

S. Saso (✉)
Institute of Reproductive & Developmental Biology,
Imperial College London, Hammersmith Hospital Campus, London, UK
e-mail: srdjan.saso@imperial.ac.uk

T. Athanasiou and A. Darzi (eds.), *Evidence Synthesis in Healthcare*,
DOI: 10.1007/978-0-85729-206-3_3, © Springer-Verlag London Limited 2011

3.1
An Introduction to a Systematic Review

3.1.1
Rationale for 'Systematic Review'

Historically, clinical decisions were based on personal experience, unquestioned use of methods suggested by senior colleagues and recommendations from clinical authorities. The progress of absorbing higher forms of evidence into the clinical knowledge base has been slow. This is more evident in surgical practice where the proportion of systematic reviews and randomised controlled trials (RCTs) in leading surgical journals stands at 5%.[1]

The pressures of moral–ethical obligations, legal liability and health economic rationing have heralded the advent of evidence-based healthcare in the last few decades. To ensure the best possible outcomes for patients, clinicians are increasingly required to implement best practices and continuous quality improvement processes within the clinical environment. This inextricably involves the application of the best available knowledge, usually in the form of scientific research, to guide clinical decision making. Hence, the use of clinical research is no longer an option but a necessity. However, problems remain for a practising clinician as to what constitutes 'best available knowledge' and in particular which type of research should be used (Fig. 3.1).

3.1.2
Information Overload

With increasing pressures of being a practising clinician and the reduction in the number of working hours,[2] two problems remain. One is the ability to synthesise and apply the best evidence to improve patient care, bearing in mind that the average clinician would have to read 19 original articles each day in order to keep up with advances in his chosen field.[3] Furthermore, this problem is compounded by the recent information explosion in the biomedical field within the last quarter century as can be evidenced by the dense cornucopia of articles and journals which are now readily accessible and searchable through a variety of online web-based bibliographic databases such as PubMed and EMBASE. In addition to the huge volume of literature, its scattered nature poses further problems. Every time a new article appears, readers must compare new findings with the existing scope of evidence to come to a reframed overall clinical conclusion.

3.1.3
Conflicting Results

Moreover, the presence of conflicting results among individual research studies does not improve matters. Not only could inconsistent results and conclusions be attributed to the statistical play of chance but it might also be due to the presence of systematic

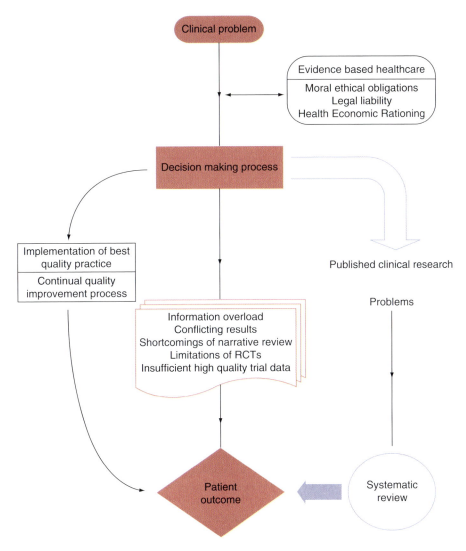

Fig. 3.1 Obstacles faced in reaching a favourable patient outcome

error from poorly designed study methodology. This would entail the need to critically analyse each individual trial for study quality, adding an extra dimension of burden to the clinician.

3.1.4
Narrative Review and Its Shortcomings

The narrative review partially resolves the problems above by providing a broad, updated and authoritative summary of research and opinion by key leaders in a field.

However, this type of review brings with it its own attendant problems where a number of review authors can provide differing viewpoints and anti-diametric conclusions from the very same source material used. This might be attributed to several factors like the use of an assorted mixture of ambiguous review methodologies, the lack of disclosure and transparency in techniques, the inability to statistically combine results and the inherent introduction of subjective bias present in the form of 'expert' opinion.[4]

3.1.5
Limitations of RCTs

Furthermore, although RCTs, when conducted properly, offer one of the more objective methods in determining the true relationship between treatment and outcome, the use of this particular type of study design also carries with it a number of limitations.

This includes the need for large numbers of participants in a trial, usually ranging from thousand to tens of thousands of subjects, in order to ensure sufficient statistical power. This is especially so if the treatment effects being studied are small in magnitude but are still deemed clinically useful. It is further compounded by the study of rare diseases of low incidence and prevalence where a randomised control trial might have to be conducted over a prolonged period of time in order to gather sufficient number of required subjects for any statistically significant result to be derived. The presence of a latency period between exposure, treatment and outcome will also necessitate the need for a longer-term follow-up. Hence, although this type of study design is objective and free from bias compared to other study designs, in certain situations it can prove to be costly in terms of time, manpower and money.

As all groups do not have such resources in excess at their disposal, compromises are reached whereby trials are conducted anyway in smaller discrete populations. These make the results from such smaller studies liable to be statistically insignificant or at best imprecise with larger degrees of uncertainty in result estimates. With that, the overall usefulness of such RCTs is reduced.

Moreover, the design of a randomised control trial mandates that a standardised population demographic be tested in a controlled environment. In comparison with the true multivariate nature of the 'real world' clinical setting, the presence of heterogeneity in ethnicity, age and geography might make any significant result from RCTs inapplicable.

3.1.6
Insufficient High-Quality Trial Data (in Surgical Research)

A problem more specific to surgical literature lies in the relatively small proportion of high-quality evidence in most surgical journals. The number of surgical RCTs is indeed small and case reports and series still are the predominant publication type. Even then, within surgical studies, there are also heterogeneous differences in study quality, such as insufficient sample size, unclear methodologies, and the use of non-clinical outcomes of interest.[5]

3.1.7
The Solution

It is evident that firstly there is a need for a more objective method of summarising primary research and secondly it is required to overcome the pitfalls in RCTs. Both these have spurred the development of a formalised set of processes and methodologies in the form of the systematic review and meta-analysis. In the clinical context, systematic reviews have become an important tool for finding important and valid studies while filtering out the large number of seriously flawed and irrelevant articles. By condensing the results of many trials, systematic reviews allow the readers to obtain a valid overview on a topic with substantially less effort involved.

3.1.8
Systematic Review Defined

A systematic review is defined as the objective, transparent and unbiased location and critical appraisal of the complete scope of research in a given topic and the eventual impartial synthesis and, if possible, meta-analysis of individual study findings. Therefore, in order to address a specific research aim, a systematic review collates all evidence that fits pre-specified eligibility criteria.

The aims of a systematic review are manifold and includes the following:

- Critical appraisal of individual studies
- Combination of individual results to create a useful summary statistic
- Analysis for presence of and reasons behind between-study variances
- Exposure of areas of research which might be methodologically inadequate and require further refinement
- Exposure of knowledge gaps and areas of potential future research possibilities

Every systematic review is composed of a discrete number of steps:

- Formulation of a specific question to be addressed with a clearly stated set of objectives
- Definition of eligibility (inclusion and exclusion) criteria for primary studies to be included
- Systematic search which identifies and locates all potentially eligible relevant studies whether published or unpublished
- Critical appraisal of each individual study via the use of explicit appraisal criteria
- Performance of a variety of statistical methods to assess for heterogeneity between studies
- Impartial unbiased analysis and assessment of the validity of the results
- Creation of a structured presentation, and synthesis to state and discuss upon findings and characteristics of collected information

3.1.9
Meta-analysis

In a systematic review, two types of synthesis can be performed: a qualitative synthesis where primary studies are summarised like in a narrative review and a quantitative synthesis

Fig. 3.2 A Venn diagram depicting a relationship between a systemic review and meta-analysis

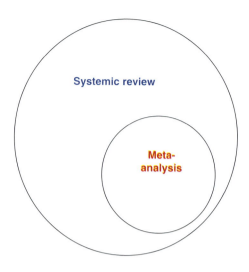

where primary studies are statistically combined. This quantitative synthetic component is termed a meta-analysis: *the statistical quantitative integration of individual study findings to get an overall summary result.*[6]

A common misunderstanding is that a meta-analysis is exactly identical to a systematic review and can be used interchangeably as synonyms. In truth, a meta-analysis is actually a subset component of a systematic review as illustrated in Fig. 3.2.

A meta-analysis is also not only limited to the summarisation of randomised controlled trial data. Different study designs, data types and follow-up spans as illustrated in Box 3.1

Box 3.1 List of Different Types of Meta-analysis

By types of study

- Meta-analysis of randomised controlled trials
- Meta-analysis of observational and epidemiological studies
- Meta-analysis of survival studies
- Meta-analysis using different study designs (Taleo-analysis)

By types of data

- Meta-analysis using aggregated trial summary data
- Meta-analysis using independent patient data

By follow-up period

- Meta-analysis at one point in time
- Meta-analysis cumulatively over time

could be also used in a meta-analysis. More details with regard to the usage of each type of meta-analysis together with its attendant pros and cons would be discussed later. For now, emphasis will be given to the meta-analysis of RCTs.

A meta-analysis can facilitate the synthesis of results for a number of scenarios where the findings of individual studies show the following:

- No effect because of a small sample size
- Varying directions of effect
- Effects versus no significant effects

All of these findings can be commonly encountered among surgical topics. A meta-analysis may serve to combine findings from similar studies to help increase the power to detect statistical differences.[7]

3.1.9.1
Advantages over Narrative Reviews

From the above, we conclude that the shortcomings of narrative reviews can be readily improved due to the following:

- Presence of explicit inclusion and exclusion criteria ensures the comprehensiveness of the review, while in the process minimising the inclusion of bias within individual studies.
- Presence of a meta-analysis can provide a quantitative summary of the overall effect estimate.
- Differences between study methodologies which affect results can be explored.
- Adherence to a strict scientific design with transparent methodology in analysis ensures objectivity and reproducibility of findings.

Narrative reviews by nature also tend to be generically broad and all-encompassing. The systematic review, in contrast, puts forward specific questions to answer which increases the applicability of such reviews in the clinical context.

3.1.9.2
Advantages over RCTs

The use of a meta-analysis for the purpose of conducting a systematic review enhances the statistical power of a group of RCTs since the pooling of data from individual studies would increase the study population. With an increase in statistical power comes an increase in the precision of findings and thereby, a reduction in both uncertainty and ambiguity. Systematic reviews can also enhance the applicability of a trial since the pooling and analysis of data from different RCTs with varied patient groups can reveal any heterogeneity or homogeneity of findings.

In conclusion, systematic reviews and meta-analyses have great importance in the summarisation and application of scientific surgical research. Their undertaking has become a cornerstone in forming clinical decisions and guidelines, and in the process has given us a better understanding of the areas in need of further research.

3.2
Conducting a Meta-analysis

3.2.1
Importance of Careful Planning

A common misconception exists that a meta-analysis is an easy study to undertake, performed with minimal effort. In reality, little attention is often paid to the details of design and implementation. A valid meta-analysis still requires the same careful planning as any other research study.[8]

Essentially, there are two goals to a meta-analysis. One is to summarise the available data and the other is to explain the variability between the studies. Ideally, all studies being meta-analysed should have similar patient characteristics and similar outcomes of interest. In reality, a certain degree of variability is expected between studies and this is the impetus for performing a meta-analysis.[8] Variability is assessed by subgroup analysis, heterogeneity assessment and sensitivity analysis all of which add 'flavour' to the meta-analysis.

As discussed previously, the steps involved in a detailed research protocol for a meta-analysis include (Fig. 3.3) the following:

- Definition of study objectives and formulation of problem
- Establishment of inclusion and exclusion criteria
- Collection and analysis of data
- Reporting of results

3.2.2
Defining the Objectives of the Study

The first step is to identify the problem. This includes specifying the disease, condition, treatment and population of interest, the specific treatments or exposures studied and the various clinical or biological outcomes investigated.

3.2.3
Defining the Population of Studies to be Included

In order to solve a distinct problem, a discrete and objective statement of inclusion and exclusion criteria for studies can be created. This is crucial in a meta-analysis, helping to eliminate selection bias. These criteria need to be specified in the meta-analysis protocol in advance. Any inclusion criteria must include the following:

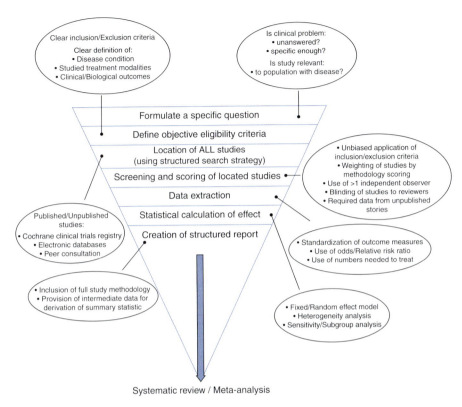

Fig. 3.3 Step-by-step approach for completing a systematic review/meta-analysis

Study type – It must be decided from the onset whether only RCTs or observational studies will be included, although there is constant debate and research with regards to this.[9,10] A hierarchy of evidence has been developed which allows for different types of studies to be included in the analysis. Naturally, the lower the level of evidence of a type of study, the lower the validity of the meta-analysis.[11] For more advanced types of meta-analysis, different study designs can also be included. This is termed a 'taleo-analysis' which although deemed a best of both worlds has its own limitations as detailed below and is out of scope for this work.

Patient characteristics – These include age, gender, and ethnicity, presenting condition, co-morbidities, duration of illness and method of diagnosis.

Treatment modalities – For the condition in question, the allowable treatment type, dosage, duration and conversion from one treatment to another should be addressed.

One must also remember to include only a single set of results from a particular study, even if multiple publications are available. For example, a study carried out in the year 2000 might be published as a 2-year follow-up in the year 2002. More data might be included in a 5-year follow-up in the year 2005, so for meta-analytical purposes, only the year 2002 or

2005 paper should be included so as to avoid duplication of the dataset. Thus, it is necessary to have a method for deciding which papers to include. Most often it is reasonable to specify that this will be the latest paper published, or the paper with the most complete data on the outcome measures of interest.[8]

3.2.4
Defining the Outcome Measures

Most studies have multiple outcome measures. The protocol for the meta-analysis should specify the outcomes that will be studied.[8] There are two schools of thought. The researcher can either focus on one or two primary outcomes or make it a 'fishing expedition' and assess as many outcomes as possible.

3.2.5
Locating All Relevant Studies

This is by far the most important, frustrating and time-consuming part of the meta-analysis. A structured search strategy must be used. This usually involves starting with databases such as NLH Medline, PubMed, EMBASE, CINAHL and even Google scholar. There are different search strategies for the various databases and effective use must be made of MeSH headings, synonyms and the 'related articles' function in PubMed. It is worth getting a tutorial with a librarian on how to obtain high yield searches that include most of the required (published) studies.

3.2.5.1
Screening, Evaluation and Data Abstraction

A rapid review of manuscript abstracts will eliminate those that are fit for exclusion because of inadequate study design, specific population and duration of treatment or study date. If the published material is just an abstract, there must be sufficient information to evaluate its quality. There must also be summary statistics to put into the meta-analysis, available either from the written material or in writing from the investigator. It is essential that when the available written information is insufficient for the meta-analysis, strenuous efforts be made to contact the principal investigator to obtain the information required in order to reduce the effect of publication bias. This becomes even more important for material that has not been formally published and which can only be obtained from the principal investigator.[8]

The next step is to collect the full papers. The data will then have to be extracted and added to a pre-designed data extraction form. It is useful if two independent observers extract the data, to avoid errors. Extraction of all patient demographics and baseline characteristics from the included studies and clinical outcomes of interest follows. A table incorporating all the extracted data can then be created which shows all the variables and their values from all the studies included in the meta-analysis. Furthermore, it is essential to ascertain how well matched the studies for various variables are. This is done by scoring them accordingly and noting the overall quality of the studies. No consensus on this issue exists in meta-analysis literature. Quality scores can be used in several ways: as a cut-off, with the meta-analysis including only studies above a pre-determined minimum score; as a weighing value, with studies with higher quality scores being given more weight in the analysis; or as a descriptive characteristic of the study, used in explaining study variability and heterogeneity.[12,13] Blinding observers to the names of the authors and their institutions, the names of the journals, sources of funding and acknowledgements can lead to more consistent scores.[12]

3.2.6
Choosing and Standardising the Measure Outcome

Individual results have to be expressed in a standardised format in order to compare the studies. If the end point is continuous such as the length of hospital stay after bypass surgery, the mean difference (weighted mean difference, WMD) between treatment and control groups is used.

These data are presented in a Forest plot as shown in Fig. 3.4. If the end point is binary or dichotomous, such as mortality or no mortality, then the odds ratio (OR) or relative risk or risk ratio (RR) is calculated.

The OR is the probability that a particular event will occur to the probability that it will not occur, and can be any number between zero and infinity. In gambling, the odds describe the ratio of the size of the potential winnings to the gambling stake; in health care, it is the ratio of the number of people with the event to the number without. Risk is the concept more familiar to patients and health professionals. Risk describes the probability with which a health outcome (usually an adverse event) will occur. Measures of relative effect express the outcome in one group relative to that in the other. Hence, RR is the ratio of the risk of an event in the two groups, whereas OR is the ratio of the odds of an event.

For treatments that increase the chances of events, OR will be greater than RR, so the tendency will be to misinterpret the findings in the form of an overestimation of treatment effect, especially when events are common (e.g., risks of events >20). For treatments that reduce the chances of events, OR will be smaller than RR, so again misinterpretation can possibly overestimate the effect of treatment. This error in interpretation is unfortunately quite common in published reports of individual studies and systematic reviews.[14]

Absolute measures, such as the absolute risk reduction or the number of patients needed to be treated (NNT) to prevent one event are more helpful when applying results in clinical practice.[15] The NNT can be calculated as 1/(absolute) risk difference (RD).

3.2.7
Statistical Methods for Calculating Overall Effect

The final step consists in calculating the overall effect by combining the data. Simply averaging the results from all the trials would give misleading results. This is what gives a meta-analysis 'impact' compared to a narrative review. The results from small studies are more subject to the play of chance and should therefore be given less weight. Methods used for meta-analysis use a weighted average of the results, in which the larger trials have more influence than the smaller ones.

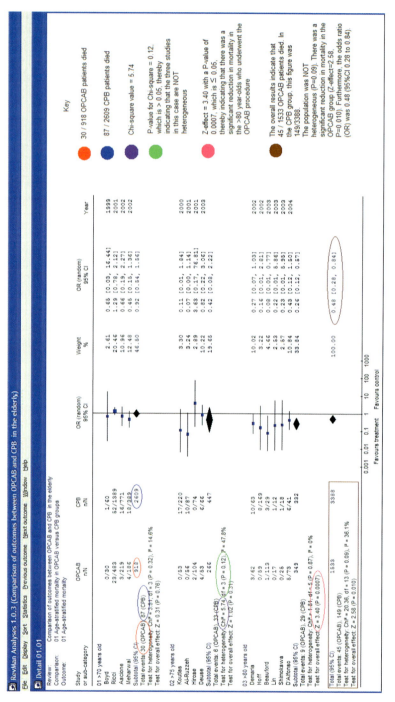

Fig. 3.4 Example of a Forest plot

3.2.7.1
Fixed and Random Effects Models

Two models can be used to assess the way in which the variability of results between studies is treated[16] The 'fixed effects' model considers that this variability is exclusively due to random variation. Therefore, if all the studies were infinitely large they would give identical results. The 'random effects' model assumes a different underlying effect for each study and takes this into consideration as an additional source of variation, which leads to somewhat wider confidence intervals than the fixed effects model.[17] Effects are assumed to be randomly distributed, and the central point of this distribution is the focus of the combined effect estimate. Both models have their limitations and a substantial difference in the combined effect calculated by the fixed and random effects models will be seen only if studies are markedly heterogeneous.[16]

Fixed Effect Meta-analysis

Methods of fixed-effect meta-analysis are based on the mathematical assumption that a single common (or 'fixed') effect underlies every study in the meta-analysis. In other words, if we were doing a meta-analysis of ORs, we would assume that every study is estimating the same OR. Under this assumption, if every study were infinitely large, every study would yield an identical result.[18] In a fixed effects analysis, the methods used to analyse binary outcomes are as follows:

(a) General inverse variance-based method
(b) Mantel–Haenszel method
(c) Peto's method

Each of these methods has certain advantages and disadvantages which will be discussed later.

Each study is assumed to be a random representative conducted on a homogenous population of patients. Thus, studies are in essence identical to one another and the study outcome should fluctuate around one common outcome or effect measure – hence the name 'fixed effects'. This is the same as assuming that there is no statistical heterogeneity among the studies. Hence, the summary measure is a simple weighted average and can be easily interpreted as an estimate of a single population outcome measure. The 95% Confidence Interval (CI) will reflect only the variability between patients; hence, with this class of methods, the 95% CI will be very narrow with more power to reject the null hypothesis. The fixed effects analysis may be justified when the test for heterogeneity is not significant, i.e., when there is no evidence of major differences among studies whether methodological, clinical or otherwise.

A very common and simple version of the meta-analysis procedure is commonly referred to as the 'inverse variance method'. The inverse variance method is so named because the weight given to each study is chosen to be the inverse of the variance of the effect estimate (i.e., one over the square of its standard error). Thus, larger studies that have smaller standard errors are given more weight than smaller studies that have larger standard errors. This choice of weight minimises the imprecision (uncertainty) of the pooled effect estimate.

A fixed effect meta-analysis using the inverse variance method calculates a weighted average as shown in Formula 3.1 below.

Formula 3.1 Generic Inverse Variance Weighted Average

$$\text{Generic inverse variance weighted average} = \frac{\Sigma\left(T_i / S_i^2\right)}{\Sigma\left(1 / S_i^2\right)}$$

Whereby T_i is the treatment effect estimated in study i, S_i is the standard error of that estimate and the summation is across all studies. The basic data required for the analysis are therefore an estimate of the treatment effect and its standard error from each study.

The Mantel–Haenszel method uses a different weighting scheme that depends upon which effect measure (e.g., RR, OR and risk difference) is being used. It has been shown to have better statistical properties when there are few events. The Mantel–Haenszel method is hence normally the default method of fixed effect analysis.[19,20]

The pooled estimate T_{MH} is calculated by Formula 3.2.

Formula 3.2 Pooled Estimate of OR (Mantel–Haenszel Method)

$$\overline{T}_{MH(OR)} = \frac{\sum_{i=1}^{k} \dfrac{a_i d_i}{n_i}}{\sum_{i=1}^{k} \dfrac{b_i c_i}{n_i}}$$

where a_i, b_i, c_i and d_i are the 4 cells of the 2×2 table for each study where $i = 1 \ldots k$ studies as shown in Formulas. 3.1 and 3.2 and n_i is the total number of people in the ith study (See Table 3.1).

Table 3.1 Outcome data from a single (a) randomised controlled trial (RCT) and (b) case control study

RCT	Failure (dead)	Success (alive)
New treatment	A	B
Control	C	D
Case control study	Diseased (cases)	Non-diseased (controls)
New treatment	A	B
Control	C	D

A variance estimate for the summary OR, T_{MH} is required to calculate a confidence interval around this point estimate. Formula 3.3 calculates a variance estimate for the log of $T_{MH(OR)}$ as follows:

Formula 3.3 Variance Estimate of Summary OR (Mantel–Haenszel Method)

$$v_{MH(\ln(OR))} = \frac{\sum_{i=1}^{k} P_i R_i}{2\left(\sum_{i=1}^{k} R_i\right)^2} + \frac{\sum_{i=1}^{k} (P_i S_i + Q_i R_i)}{2\left(\sum_{i=1}^{k} R_i\right)\left(\sum_{i=1}^{k} S_i\right)} + \frac{\sum_{i=1}^{k} Q_i S_i}{2\left(\sum_{i=1}^{k} S_i\right)^2}$$

where

$$P_i = \frac{(a_i + d_i)}{n_i}, \quad Q_i = \frac{(b_i + c_i)}{n_i}, \quad R_i = \frac{a_i d_i}{n_i} \text{ and } S_i = \frac{b_i c_i}{n_i}$$

A 100 $(1 - \alpha)$% confidence interval for the summary odds ratio θ, is calculated as follows (Formula 3.4):

Formula 3.4 100 $(1 - \alpha)$% Confidence Interval for the Summary Odds Ratio θ

$$\exp\left[\ln(\overline{T}_{MH(OR)}) - z_{\alpha/2}(v_{MH(OR)})^{1/2}\right] \leq \theta \leq \exp\left[\ln(\overline{T}_{MH(OR)}) + z_{\alpha/2}(v_{MH(OR)})^{1/2}\right]$$

Peto's method can only be used to pool ORs.[16] It uses an inverse variance approach but utilises an approximate method of estimating the log OR, and applies different weights. An alternative way of viewing the Peto method is as a sum of '$O - E$' statistics. Here, O is the observed number of events and E is an expected number of events in the experimental intervention group of each trial.

The approximation used in the computation of the log OR works well when treatment effects are small (ORs ~ 1), events are not particularly common and the trials have similar numbers in both experimental and control groups. In other situations, it has been shown to give biased answers. As these criteria are not always fulfilled, Peto's method is not recommended as a default approach for meta-analysis.

For k studies, the pooled estimate of the OR is given by (Formula 3.5):

Formula 3.5 Pooled Estimate of OR (Peto's Method)

$$\overline{T}_{PETO(OR)} = \exp\left[\frac{\sum_{i=1}^{k} (O_i - E_i)}{\sum_{i=1}^{k} v_i}\right]$$

where

$$v_i = E_i \left[(n_i - n_{ti}) / n_i\right] \left[(n_i - d_i) / (n_i - 1)\right]$$

Of note, n_i is the number of patients in the ith trial and n_{ti} is the number in the new treatment group of the ith trial, d_i is equal to the total number of events from both treatment and control groups and o_i is the number of events in the treatment group. E_i is the expected number of events in the treatment group (in the ith trial) and is calculated as

$$E_i = (n_{ti} / n_i) d_i \ .$$

For each study, two statistics are calculated. The first O-E is the difference between the observed and the number expected to have done so under the hypothesis that the treatment is no different from the control, E. The second, v, is the variance of the difference O-E. An estimate of the approximate variance of the natural log of the estimated pooled OR is given by (Formula 3.6):

Formula 3.6 Variance of Pooled Odds Ratio (Peto's Method)

$$\text{var}(\ln \overline{T}_{PETO(OR)}) = \left(\sum_{i=1}^{K} v_i \right)$$

A 100 $(1 - \alpha)$% non-symmetric confidence interval is given by (Formula 3.7):

Formula 3.7 100 $(1 - \alpha)$% Non-symmetric Confidence Interval (Peto's Method)

$$\exp \left[\frac{\sum_{i=1}^{k}(O_i - E_i) \pm z_{\alpha/2} \sqrt{\sum_{i=1}^{k} v_i}}{\sum_{i=1}^{k} v_i} \right]$$

All the methods discussed above have their merits and demerits which determine their use. Peto's method may produce biased ORs and standard errors when there is a mismatch in the numbers of the two groups being compared.[21] If the number of studies to be pooled is small, but the within-study sample sizes in each study are large, the inverse-weighted method should be used. Conversely, if the number of studies to be combined is large, but the within-study sample size in each study is small, the Mantel–Haenszel method is preferred.[22]

It is now recommended that a continuity correction be used (adding 0.5 to each cell) for sparse data except in cases where there is strong evidence suggesting that very little heterogeneity exists among component studies.[23]

Random Effects Meta-analysis

When there is some statistical heterogeneity, as detected by a statistically significant heterogeneity test, it will be implausible to assume that the 95% CI or imprecision of the summary outcome reflects only between-patient variability. Therefore, the fixed effects model will not fit the observed data well as the 95% CI will be too narrow. In the fixed effects analysis, each of the studies in the systematic review is assumed fundamentally identical and is simply an independent random experiment done on an identical population of patients. In the random effects analysis, it is assumed that all the studies are fundamentally different and that the outcome of a study will estimate its own unique outcome, which differs from that of the other studies. Hence, each study outcome is not assumed to fluctuate around a fixed, common population outcome but to fluctuate around its own true value. It is assumed, however, that each of these true values is drawn 'randomly' from some underlying probability distribution; i.e., that of a 'superpopulation', commonly assumed to be of Normal Distribution and, hence, the name 'random effects' analysis. That is, under a random effects assumption, not only is each study performed on a sample drawn from a different population of patients but that each of these populations is still taken randomly from a common 'superpopulation'. A random effects analysis makes the assumption that individual studies are estimating different treatment effects. Thus, the 95% CI in a random effects analysis, reflecting the overall variability in the data, will be wider than that of a fixed effects analysis because of both between-patient variability and between-study variability.[18]

The DerSimonian and Laird random effects method incorporates an assumption that different studies are estimating different but yet related treatment effects. This method is based on the inverse variance approach, making an adjustment to the study weights according to the extent of variation, or heterogeneity, among the varying treatment effects. The DerSimonian and Laird method and the inverse variance method will give identical results when there is no heterogeneity among the studies (and also give results similar to the Mantel–Haenszel method in many situations). Where there is heterogeneity, the confidence intervals for the average treatment effect will be wider if the DerSimonian and Laird method is used rather than a fixed effect method, and corresponding claims of statistical significance will be more conservative. It is also possible that the central estimate of the treatment effect will change if there are relationships between observed treatment effects and sample sizes.

Formula 3.8 expresses this point mathematically, where T_i is an estimate of the effect size and θ_i is the true effect size in the ith study:

Formula 3.8

$$T_i = \theta_i + e_i$$

where e_i is the error with which T_i estimates θ_i and

$$\mathrm{var}(T_i) = \tau_\theta^2 + v_i$$

where τ_θ^2 is the random effects variance and v_i is the variance due to sampling error in the ith study.

3.2.7.2
Heterogeneity Between Study Results

Sometimes, the variance between the overall effect sizes in each study might not be due to random sampling variation but instead could be due to the presence of other factors inherent within individual studies. This effect size variation due to slightly different study designs is termed heterogeneity. If the results of each study differ greatly from each other and are deemed to be largely due to heterogeneity, then it may not be appropriate to conduct a meta-analysis in the first place. If a test for homogeneity shows homogeneous results then the differences between studies are assumed to be a consequence of sampling variation, and a fixed effects model is appropriate. If, however, the test shows that significant heterogeneity exists between study results then a random effects model is advocated. If there is excess heterogeneity, then not even the random effects model could compensate for this and the viability of the meta-analysis should be questioned. A major limitation with heterogeneity tests is that these statistical tests will lack power to reject the null hypothesis of homogeneous results even if substantial differences between studies exist. This is because of a limited N number of studies available in each meta-analysis.

Although there is no statistical solution to this issue, heterogeneity tests should not be abandoned as heterogeneity between study results can also provide an opportunity for examining why treatment effects differ in different circumstances anyway. The causes and sources to explain for heterogeneity need to be explored in detail after heterogeneity and the degree of heterogeneity has been detailed.[24]

Assessing for the Presence of Heterogeneity

There are three ways to assess heterogeneity. First, one can assess the between-studies variance – τ^2. However, this depends mainly on the particular effect size metric used. The second is Cochrane's Q test, which follows a chi-square distribution to make inferences about the null hypothesis of homogeneity. The problem with Cochrane's Q test is that it has poor power to detect true heterogeneity when the number of studies is small. Because neither of the above-mentioned methods has a standardised scale, they are poorly equipped to make comparisons of the degree of homogeneity across meta-analyses.[25] A third more useful statistic for quantifying inconsistency is I^2 [$= [(Q-df)/Q] \times 100\%$], where Q is the chi-squared statistic and 'df' is its degrees of freedom.[26] This statistic is easier to utilise because it defines variability along a scale-free range as a percentage from 0% to 100%. This describes the percentage of the variability in effect estimates that is due to heterogeneity rather than sampling error (chance). Heterogeneity could be considered substantial when this value is greater than 50%.

Graphical Display: Forest Plot

Results from each trial, together with their confidence intervals, can be graphically displayed in a useful manner on a Forest plot (Fig. 3.5). Each study is represented by a black square and a horizontal line, which corresponds to the point estimate and the 95% confidence intervals of the outcome measure respectively. The dotted vertical line corresponds to no effect of treatment (e.g., OR or RR of 1.0). If CI includes 1, then the difference in the effect of experimental and control treatment is not significant at nominally tolerated levels ($p > 0.05$). The size (or area) of the black squares reflects the weight of the study in the meta-analysis while the diamond represents the combined OR, calculated using a fixed effects model, at its centre with the 95% confidence interval being represented by its horizontal line.[27]

Fig. 3.5 Graphical display of heterogeneity (Forest plot)

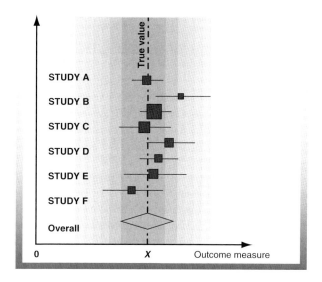

Most of the studies, if they are homogenous in design and population will have overlapping CIs. However, if CIs of two studies do not overlap at all, this is most likely because of existing variation between the two studies, as well as presence of heterogeneity and not likely due to chance. Other than graphically using a Forest plot, a numerical method could be achieved via use of the χ^2 (chi-squared test).[18]

Most statistical packages will give values for the Chi-square and its corresponding p-value. This is shown and explained in Fig. 3.4. This will help to assess how heterogeneous the results are. Furthermore, the combined outcome measure (OR/RR/WMD) will have an absolute value, its 95% CI and its corresponding p-value (Z-effect p-value) to see whether the results are statistically significant.

Sensitivity Analysis

The robustness of the findings of a meta-analysis needs to be assessed by performing a sensitivity analysis. Based on what was presented previously, both fixed and random effects modelling should be used. Secondly, the methodological quality of studies needs to be assessed by scoring the quality of the studies on an arbitrary scoring scale or using the scales mentioned above. The meta-analysis can be repeated for high-quality and low-quality studies. Thirdly, significant results are more likely to get published than non-significant findings and this can distort the findings of meta-analyses.[28] The presence of such publication bias can be identified by stratifying the analysis by study size: smaller effects can be significant in larger studies. If publication bias is present, it is expected that, of published studies, the larger ones will report the smallest effects. However, exclusion of smaller studies has little effect on the overall estimate. The sensitivity analysis thus shows that the results from a meta-analysis are valid and not affected by the exclusion of trials of poorer quality or of studies stopped early. It also takes into account publication bias.[27]

Subgroup Analysis

The principal aim of a meta-analysis is to produce an estimate of the average effect seen in trials of a particular treatment.[29] The clinician must make a decision as to whether his/her patient is comparable to the patient group used in the meta-analysis. For example, off-pump coronary artery bypass (OPCAB) surgery is shown to be more beneficial than on-pump coronary artery bypass (ONCAB) surgery in high-risk groups or subgroups such as the elderly and diabetics. Subgroup analysis shows a benefit whereas a meta-analysis comparing OPCAB to ONCAB technique in a general population may result in no superiority being shown by either technique.

However, this method can produce findings which are conflicting. One of the OPCAB RCTs used in the meta-analysis that primarily recruited females may show that OPCAB surgery is harmful in the female population, yet the overall message of the meta-analysis is that OPCAB surgery is superior to ONCAB in females. Stein's paradox must be invoked here.[30] Common sense suggests that gender has no bearing on the outcome so this RCT is discounted and should female patients come to the clinic, they would still be offered OPCAB surgery. The assumption is that inconsistent results are purely due to chance. But even if some real differences exist, the overall estimate may still provide the best estimate of the effect in that group.

Subgroup analysis could also be used to explain for heterogeneity by determining which component of the study design might be contributing to treatment effect.

Metaregression

Metaregression is an extension of subgroup analysis. It is the analysis of any significant effects between different subgroup populations of individual trials. Multiple continuous and categorical variables could be investigated simultaneously at the same time. Using metaregression, a better understanding of the causes for heterogeneity between study groups can be found. However, metaregression has a number of significant limitations. Firstly, the initial decision to perform a metaregression on a certain variable is entirely observer dependent and hence is also prone to selection bias. This is the case for a meta-analysis of RCTs. Furthermore, metaregression uses the aggregate outcome in each study as its source data and hence might fail to detect genuine relationships between individual variables or might not be able to ascertain the true effect size. Last but not least, metaregression requires many studies (>10) and there is a risk of obtaining a spurious correlation for a variable especially when many characteristics are studied.

3.2.8
Conducting a Meta-analysis in the Surgical Context

The main differences between meta-analysis in surgery and that in other fields originate from the reproducibility of treatments and variations in practice that are difficult to compare. The outcomes of a surgical procedure depend on the level of experience of an operating surgeon.

This is not the case in other areas of research such as drug trials where the intervention is consistent and the drug acts in a uniform manner. Moreover, standardisation and reproducibility in surgical techniques employed by the surgeons are not always consistent. Also, poor outcomes are less likely to be reported which further adds to publication bias.[31] The experience of a surgeon is one of the key confounders during comparative trials involving interventions. Less-experienced surgeons have been reported to have relatively poorer outcomes.[32] These issues have the propensity to add to study heterogeneity thus compromising the validity of a meta-analysis of clinical trials in surgery.

Similarly, early meta-analytical assessment of a new procedure or technique may give a misleading picture of its efficacy because issues such as lack of competence of surgeons. Competence is achieved after performing a set of repeated tasks. Factors determining competence include experience, equipment and time. Procedural performance continues to improve until a plateau phase is reached. This constitutes a traditional 'learning curve'.

Meta-analysis of trials comparing an established intervention (A) and a newly developed modality (B) may lead to a biased result favouring the latter. For instance, when a new developed intervention (A) is compared against a conventional method (B), the established modality will always be superior. This is because during the early years, surgeons learn how to practice A before they achieve competence. Similarly, once A has been adopted widely, it will be appear superior to B based on inadequate evidence such as lack of long-term outcomes during the earlier years.[33] The correlation is that a meta-analysis done too early comparing two interventions could be disastrous. Meta-analysis done once the newer technology has been accepted is also concerning. For example, in the use of beta-blockers versus placebo in the treatment of patients who had a myocardial infarction, from 1967 to 1980, most head-to-head trials did not show any significant benefit of beta-blockade. A meta-analysis done during these earlier years would probably have yielded negative results. A more recent meta-analysis that included studies from 1967 to 1997, has instead shown that beta-blockade reduces premature mortality after a myocardial infarction by 20%.[34]

The year of publication of a study is a significant determinant of heterogeneity as population characteristics and outcome data may change over time. Also the development in technology and technical expertise may translate into unfavourable outcomes over a defined period. All these factors need to be considered especially in surgical disciplines where new technologies and techniques are continuously developed and the learning curve is overcome progressively. Increasing accumulation of evidence with time improves the integrity of results reported by a meta-analysis.[35]

3.3
Assessing the Quality of a Meta-analysis

Two instruments are commonly used to assess the quality of meta-analysis: Overview Quality Assessment Questionnaire (OQAQ) scale and the Quality of Reporting of Meta-analyses (QUOROM) checklist.[36]

The OQAQ was selected because it has strong face validity, it provided data on several essential elements of its development, and had an available published assessment of its construct validity. The OQAQ scale measures across a continuum using nine questions (items 1–9) designed to assess various aspects of the methodological quality of systematic reviews and one overall assessment question (item 10). When the scale is applied to a systematic review, the first nine items are scored by selecting either 'yes', 'no' or 'partial/cannot tell'. The tenth item requires assessors to assign an overall quality score on a seven-point scale.[37]

The QUOROM statement was chosen for assessing reporting quality. Although, this checklist has not yet been fully validated, extensive work has been conducted and reported. The QUOROM statement is comprised of a checklist and flow diagram and was developed using a consensus process designed to strengthen the reliability of the estimates it yields when applied by different assessors. It estimates the overall reporting quality of systematic reviews. The checklist asks whether authors have provided readers with information on 18 items, including searches, selection, validity assessment, data abstraction, study characteristics, quantitative data syntheses and trial flow. It also asks whether authors have included a flow diagram with information about the number of RCTs identified, included and excluded, and the reasons for any exclusion. Individual checklist items included in this instrument are also answered in the same manner as above: 'yes', 'no' or 'partial/cannot tell'.[38]

3.4
Pitfalls in Conducting a Meta-analysis

Not only is the QUORUM used to assess for reporting quality but it also helps to mark out potential pitfalls in a meta-analysis. Although the aim of a meta-analysis is to reduce uncertainty, there are instances in which the opposite can be true. In the hierarchy of evidence, the systematic review is placed rightly at the top. However, similar systematic reviews with opposite conclusions or those which contradict well-powered high-quality double-blind RCTs are still possible.[39]

3.4.1
Conflicting Results Between Meta-analysis Compared to Large-Scale RCTs

Two important questions need to be answered. The first is whether meta-analyses of small trials agree with the results of large trials. No absolute definition exists of what constitutes a large trial, so separating small trials from large trials is not easy. Moreover, when considering the bigger picture, all trials add to the current base of evidence. The extent to which small trials agree or disagree with larger ones is a multifactorial process. Selection bias tends to skew the results. Large trials appearing in high-impact journals may have been selected as they provide new insight into the merits and demerits of a particular treatment. Furthermore, there may be less consistency for secondary end points than for primary end points in different trials.

The second important question is whether meta-analyses can in fact validly substitute large trials. It is known that meta-analyses and large trials tend to disagree 10–23% of the

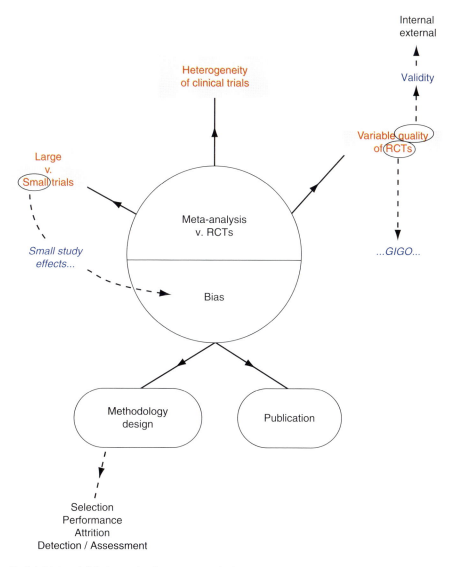

Fig. 3.6 Major pitfalls in conducting a meta-analysis

time, beyond chance. Clinical trials are likely to be heterogeneous, since they address different populations with different protocols. Patients, disease and treatments are likely to change over time. Future meta-analyses may find an important role in addressing potential sources of heterogeneity rather than always trying to fit a common estimate among diverse studies. With this, meta-analyses and RCTs must be scrutinised in detail for the presence of bias and diversity. Figure 3.6 summarises the above arguments.

3.4.2
Why Does Bias Exist in Meta-analysis?

Most of the factors responsible for bias are because of assumptions used when combining RCTs. The assumptions are as follows:

- Results of trials are true approximations to the actual true value of the outcome of study, and are different between trials due to the presence of random chance and not due to bias.
- Trials selected for combination are representative of all trials possible whether published or unpublished.
- Studies being combined are sufficiently homogenous in population and methodology such that they are combinable in the first place.

3.4.3
Types of Pitfalls in Conducting a Meta-analysis

With this, a list of problems faced by systematic reviews and meta-analyses becomes apparent:

- Publication bias and other forms of reporting bias
- Variable quality of included RCT studies
- Bias and skew due to the presence of small study effects
- Selection bias/personal bias in the selection of studies
- Heterogeneity between individual studies

3.5
Pitfalls: Variable Quality of Included Trials

3.5.1
Importance of 'Quality'

The quality of RCTs has a direct impact on the eventual quality and output produced by the meta-analysis. If not properly designed, flaws within RCTs can produce aberrant results which might not be a true reflection of the overall treatment effect. Hence, when incorporated into a meta-analysis, these flaws can trickle down to directly compromise and invalidate both meta-analysis results and subsequent findings. This dependency of RCT results in a meta-analysis is aptly termed: 'Garbage in – Garbage out' or GIGO effect.

3.5.2
So What is Quality in a RCT?

Quality is a multifaceted idea, which could relate to the design, conduct and analysis of a trial, its clinical relevance, or quality of reporting.[40] It is important to assess the validity of the included studies because of its huge bearing on the quality of the review. Two types of validity have been proposed, namely internal and external validity,[41] and have been shown to influence the analysis and conclusions of the review.

3.5.2.1
Internal Validity

Internal validity implies that the differences observed between groups of patients allocated to different interventions may, apart from random chance, truly be due to the treatments under investigation. It seeks to answer whether the research question is investigated in a manner free from bias. Assessments of internal validity are therefore termed 'assessments of methodological quality'.

3.5.2.2
Quality of Reporting

The assessment of the methodological quality of a trial and the quality of reporting go hand in hand. For meta-analysis researchers, it is a joy when a paper provides adequate information about the design, conduct and analysis of the study in question.[13] However, when inadequate information is provided, the difficulty lies in whether one should assume that the quality was inadequate or formally assess it by using different scales of quality.

3.5.3
Assessing the Quality of Reporting in RCTs

Many reviewers formally assess the quality of RCTs by using guidance from expert sources including the Cochrane collaboration. Recently in the last decade, the concepts discussed above have been ratified into the Consolidated Standards of Reporting Trials statement (CONSORT). The CONSORT statement is an important research tool that takes an evidence-based approach to improve the quality of reports in randomised trials. It offers a standard way for researchers to report trials and is composed of a standardised checklist and flow diagram for detailing the required conduct and reporting of methodology and results in individual randomised controlled trial reports.

The inclusion of the CONSORT guidelines into journal publication criteria has improved the quality of reporting in articles, made the peer review and editorial process more objective and has enabled systematic reviewers a greater ability in judging methodological quality for themselves.[42]

3.5.4
Dealing with 'Small Studies Effects'

In effect, the CONSORT guidelines would become a natural addition to inclusion and exclusion criteria and there should be no qualms in rigorously applying these criteria and dropping low-quality trials from a meta-analysis. This would help to reduce small studies effect in a trial. However, this action of rejection should be done in such a way that it can be assessed itself and it is recommended for a reject log to be kept for peer review if necessary. In some instances, one might need to declare the total exclusion of current research and express the need for better quality trials in the future in order to perform an adequate meta-analysis!

3.5.5
External Validity

External validity gives a measure of the applicability of the results of a study to other 'populations, settings, treatment variables, and measurement variables'.[13] It deals with situations where focus is on whether the results of a study can provide a correct basis for generalisations to other circumstances. It should be noted that internal validity is a requirement for external validity because when the results of a flawed trial become invalid, the question of its external validity automatically becomes redundant.[13,40]

In recent years, large meta-analyses based on data from individual patients have shown that important differences in treatment effects may exist between patient groups and settings. For example, antihypertensive treatment reduces total mortality in middle-aged patients with hypertension, but this may not be the case in an elderly population.[43] The baseline characteristics of studies included in the meta-analysis must be similar. It would only be appropriate to compare apples with apples and not apples with mangoes!

3.5.6
Why is Study Quality Important?

The quality of reporting and the methodological quality of meta-analysis must always be of high quality.[44] It is worth remembering that the inclusion of poorly conducted studies in the meta-analysis will result in poor results.

Full use must be made of quality scales, appreciation of the hierarchical structure of studies (RCTs or observational studies) and sensitivity analyses.

3.6
Pitfalls: Bias

3.6.1
What is Bias?

Bias primarily affects internal validity and is defined as 'any process at any stage of inference tending to produce results that differ systematically from [their] true values'.[41] It refers to 'systematic error', the effect of misleading conclusions from multiple replications of the same study. Sampling variation, however, leads to different effect estimates following above replications despite 'correct answers' on average. This is known as 'random error' and is because of imprecision, a term not to be confused with bias/risk of bias.

Therefore, bias can cause a systematic overestimation or underestimation in outcome which leads to a GIGO effect on meta-analytic results. Hence, in the conduct of a meta-analysis, a key assumption will be that any variability between individual RCTs is due to random variation and not from the presence of bias.

The presence of bias and the extent to which it affects a particular study is usually related to flaws in methodological analysis, conduct and design of clinical trials. It is more appropriate however to focus on 'risk of bias', a more suitable phrase, because results of a study can occasionally be unbiased despite methodological flaws. In addition, variation in the results of included studies can be explained more accurately by differences in risk of bias. These differences will highlight the more rigorous studies with more valid conclusions and will indirectly help us to avoid false-positive/negative conclusions.

Bias is especially of concern within small powered unpublished studies as the methodological quality in smaller trials might not be as vigorous as compared to larger ones where more time, effort and money might have been involved in the trial design. Moreover, as small studies might not be published, their underlying methodology might not be assessed with as much close scrutiny as during the editorial peer review process in journal publications.

Bias related to methodology design can be of five different kinds: selection, performance, detection, attrition and reporting bias (Fig. 3.7).

> *Selection bias*: Occurs when candidates in a study are preferentially selected into one group compared to another based on prior knowledge of their pre-existing medical condition.
> *Performance bias*: Occurs if additional treatment interventions are provided preferentially in one treatment group compared to another.
> *Detection/Assessment bias*: Arises if the knowledge of patient assignment influences the assessment of outcome. Yet again, blinding of the assessor/observer is the solution.
> *Attrition bias*: Arises where deviations from protocol and loss to follow-up lead to the exclusion of patients after they have been allocated to their treatment groups, causing a skew in aggregate treatment effect.
> *Reporting bias*: Occurs when systematic differences between reported and unreported variables are found. Several forms of reporting bias exist and will be dealt with in more detail in subsequent chapters: Publication bias, Time lag bias, English language bias, Citation bias, Duplication bias and Outcome reporting bias.

3.6.2
Assessing Potential Bias Inherent in RCTs

The use of high-quality trials in a meta-analysis, ideally prospective randomised double blind controlled trials with an intention to treat policy during results reporting, would eliminate many forms of bias.

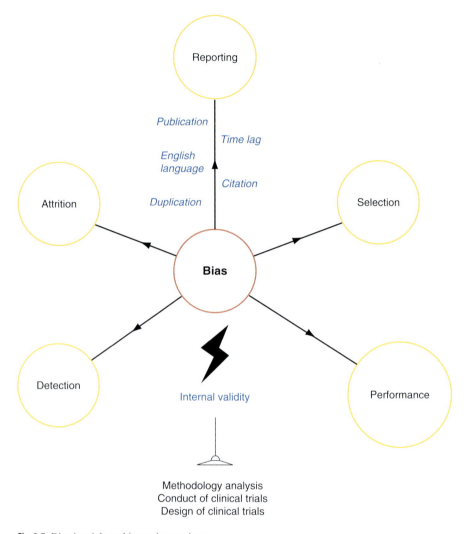

Fig. 3.7 Bias in trials and its various guises

The solution to selection bias is randomisation which will create groups that are equally comparable for any known or unknown potential confounding factors. Adequate randomisation in the use of pre-generated allocation sequences and concealment of allocation would ensure a standardised group of patients in both treatment and control. Ideally, randomisation should be instituted where neither the investigator nor the patient knows the allocation so that they are unable to guide which type of treatment should be used.

Randomisation, coupled with double blinding, where both patients and investigators are prevented from knowing which group each patient is allocated to, would prevent detection and performance bias. The use of objective compared to subjective measurable outcomes would also further make a trial less prone to assessment bias.[45]

To reduce attrition bias, an intention to treat or 'per protocol' policy could be used. An intention to treat policy dictates that all randomised patients should be included in the analysis and kept in their original groups, regardless of their adherence or non-compliance to the study protocol or loss to follow-up. Conversely, a 'per protocol' policy is where only patients who fulfil all protocol directives are included in the analysis.

As a 'per protocol', analysis tends to ignore patients who have ceased treatment due to possible adverse outcomes, an intention to treat policy is generally recommended. However, an intention to treat protocol also depends on the use of assumptions to determine the eventual outcome of patients' loss to follow-up. It has been recommended that the conduct of both forms of analysis and any underlying comparative differences between them would give the best level of available knowledge.[45]

Cochrane Handbook for Systematic Reviews of Interventions also describes various methods for assessing bias. It describes a tool titled a 'domain-based evaluation', in which critical assessments are made separately for different domains. Each type of domain, described below, assesses a specific type of bias.[46]

Sequence generation: A well-designed RCT incorporates and specifies a statistically sound rule for allocating a specific intervention to each patient. This rule has to be based on a chance (random) process (e.g., computer random number generator, coin tossing, shuffling envelopes) and must generate an allocation sequence, thereby allowing an assessment of whether it produces comparable groups. Both this and the next domain could only score positively when assessing RCTs.

Allocation concealment: Method employed to conceal the above allocation sequence in sufficient detail to determine whether allocations could have been predicted in advance, or during, enrolment. For example, using telephone or web-based randomisation or sequentially numbered, sealed envelopes.

Blinding of participants, personnel and outcome assessors: Measures used to remove prior knowledge of which type of intervention a patient received from the patient undergoing the surgery and from the surgeon performing the operation.

Incomplete outcome data: Lack of completeness of outcome data during the follow-up period.

Selective outcome reporting: Study protocol, including the main aims and outcomes of interest, is either incomplete or written with insufficient clarity. Not all of the pre-specified outcomes are reported in the pre-specified way.

Other potential threats to validity that can be considered: Of interest is a detailed description of the surgical methods employed, including whether patients were operated on by one or more surgeons and in one or more hospitals, and the diagnostic methods applied to calculate the necessary outcomes (i.e., techniques and personnel).

3.6.3
Publication Bias

So far, only bias related to actual gathering of data have been considered, i.e., methods involved in setting up the trial. Reporting bias is, on the other hand, related to the results' publication process. 'Publication bias' is the main subgroup, occurring when the publication of research is reliant upon the nature and direction of results. If the research that appears in the published literature is systematically unrepresentative of the population of completed studies, publication bias occurs. This leads to the preferential publication of certain types of trials compared to others resulting in a fraction of studies being published in an indexed journal, leaving a larger body of research in the form of incomplete draft manuscripts, presentations and abstracts unpublished. With this, a vast amount of research data could be omitted from indexed bibliographic databases, and thus, becoming difficult to locate. This data eventually is concealed away from systematic reviewers such that not all possible clinical trials could have been included within a meta-analysis of a topic. The end result is a meta-analysis which might not be truly representative of all valid studies undertaken ending in the development of spuriously precise but inaccurate summary findings.[10,47] Rather frustratingly, wrong conclusions can then be drawn by readers and reviewers with dangerous consequences (e.g., use of falsely deemed safe and effective treatment).

3.6.3.1
Why Does Publication Bias Exist?

Even though there is no consistent relationship between the publication of a study with study design, methodological quality, study size or number of study centres, the publication of a trial is more likely when it shows either a statistically significant large effect in the outcome for a new treatment (a positive trial) or when compared to existing treatments (a non-inferiority trial). The publication of a trial is less likely when there are non-significant findings, results with small effect sizes or negative findings (a negative trial).[10,47]

3.6.3.2
Reasons for Publication Bias in Negative Trials

Non-significant findings or negative findings are less likely to be published due to the following:

• Editorial censorship of uninteresting findings
• Subjective peer review
• Conflicts of interests
• Self-censorship dealing with publication bias

3.6.3.3
Grey Literature

The validity and reliability of a meta-analysis is dependent on the results of the trials it includes. To avoid publication bias, it is important to include trials found in the grey literature, i.e., those trials not published as a formal journal article (e.g., those found in conference abstracts, books, thesis, government and company reports and other unpublished material).

The most common type of grey literature is abstracts (55%). Unpublished data is the second largest type of grey literature (30%). The definition of what is classified as unpublished data is variable. It may include data from trial registers, file-drawer data and data from individual trialists. Book chapters are the third largest type of grey literature (9%), with unpublished reports, pharmaceutical company data, in press publications, letters and theses making up the small remainder.

Furthermore, it has been shown that published trials showed an overall greater treatment effect than grey trials. This may result in a more beneficial or detrimental effect if the meta-analysis only includes published data. This is particularly important for meta-analyses that contain only a few trials where the impact of excluding trials found in the grey literature has the greatest potential to introduce bias.

Nearly half of all abstracts presented at scientific meetings do not get published in full as journal articles or there is a time lag of about 3 years before they do. Consequently, when such abstract are identified, information about the trial, its methodological quality and its results should be obtained by contacting the trialist.[48]

3.6.3.4
Preventing Publication Bias and Other Forms of Reporting Bias

As put forward by the Quality of Reporting of Meta-analyses guidelines for systematic reviews in RCTs (QUORUM), a unified and an agreed-upon search strategy should be implemented which is comprehensive, transparent and repeatable.[38] There should be a reported list of used search keywords and strings in more than one centralised database which contains translated journal abstracts (e.g., Medline & Embase). This could be followed up by searches through non-English-based journals as much as possible.

There are several options for finding unpublished studies. Peer consultation, i.e., networking with professional colleagues and contacting specific investigators who are known to be active in the area can help identify additional studies and other investigators. Since abstracts are often not included in computer indexes, it is necessary to manually review special meeting issues of journals from the major professional organisations in the field. This normally manifests itself in a form of a supplementary issue which might not always be archived with the main bulk of journal issues in a library.

The National Institute of Health (NIH) and National Library of Medicine (NLM) also maintain registries of clinical trials for some diseases. Furthermore, public non-profit organisations can usually supply information about trials and other studies that they are sponsoring. The Cochrane Collaboration has contributed significantly in the manual searching and identification of controlled trials in English and non-English journals and indexes, culminating in the Cochrane Controlled Trials Registry which has become the quintessential database for trials. This registry contains a bibliography of controlled trials as well as abstracts of reviews of the effects of healthcare.[8]

The amnesty offered by journal editors for unpublished trials by authors has also helped to a degree and there is an increasing support for the publication of well-designed trials with non-significant results.[49]

Through the initiatives set about by the International Committee of Medical Journal Editors and the recently ratified Ottawa statement, a set of internationally recognised principles for the prospective registration of all clinical research projects has been established.[50,51] This involves the mandatory registration of trial type and methodology prior to commencement of the trial and the full disclosed reporting of results thereafter.

The Ottawa statement explicitly states:

> at a minimum, results for outcomes and analyses specified in the protocol (as approved by the institutional review boards/independent ethics committees), as well as data on harms, should be registered regardless of whether or not they are published.[50]

This statement is now becoming a prerequisite criterion for acceptance for publication. The implication for enforcement of study registration is that trials with results sponsored by pharmaceutical companies would no longer be published unless they are initially registered in a public database from the start; hence, reporting bias in all its forms could soon be minimised.

Currently, the Cochrane Controlled Trials Registry and the United States National Library Clinical Trials Registry are well poised to fill the requirement for prospective registration; newer registries pertaining to specific subjects of interest have also been established.[52]

It is also important to restrict the inclusion in systematic reviews of studies started before a certain date to allow for the delay in publication of studies with negative results in order to compensate for time lag bias.[47] The use of cumulative meta-analysis where re-analysis is performed whenever new publications surface, would also help in reducing this type of bias.

3.6.3.5
Assessing for Publication Bias

Even with the measures above, there is still a need to qualitatively and quantitatively assess the presence of reporting bias through the use of graphical and statistical methods.

Funnel Plots

Funnel plots aid graphically to reveal the presence of publication bias – being a scatter plot function of study effect size and estimated effect size.[53,54] The premise that larger studies will have result estimates more precise while the opposite applies for small studies is true. In an ideal setting where all possible published and unpublished trials are available, individual studies would form a symmetrical inverted funnel with more precise results from larger trials bunched up at the top and less precise results from smaller trials scattered symmetrically below.

An asymmetrical distribution can occur usually represented by a deficiency in a certain region of the funnel which can be attributed to the skewed distribution of studies created from publication or reporting bias.[53] This is shown in Fig. 3.8a, b.

Statistical Assessment and Correction Tools

The visual inspection of funnel plots might be subjective at times and so statistical tests for detecting plot asymmetry can also be used. Regression tests and rank correlation

Fig. 3.8 Funnel plots. (**a**) Ideal case involves a symmetrical distribution of studies. (**b**) Presence of asymmetry in funnel plot due to either publication bias or small studies effect

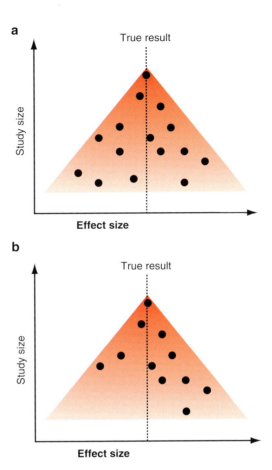

tests are some of the options available. Apart from this, various methods could be undertaken to compensate for publication bias including the 'trim and fill method', the 'fail safe N method' and 'weight modelling'.[55] Further discussion on how these statistical methods are performed to achieve these means is unfortunately out of the scope of this chapter.

However, funnel plot asymmetry might also be due to the presence of small study effects whereby a skew in results exists because of lower methodology inherent in smaller trials leading to spuriously larger treatment effects. The presence of heterogeneity whether clinical or methodological together with a low N number of trials in a systematic review can also contribute to asymmetry of results. One observational study on the use of funnel plot tests has shown that in most cases the use of funnel plots to detect bias was inappropriate and not meaningful.[56]

Rank Correlation Test

The rank correlation test is used to derive a quantitative association between the effect estimated and their variances. Smaller studies with larger variances will tend to have larger effect size estimates. This test is commonly used as an adjunct to the funnel plot.[57]

Linear Regression Test

To test the asymmetry of a funnel plot, a linear regression analysis of Galbraith's radical plot has been proposed. Further detailed evaluation of this test is required.[58]

3.6.3.6
Statistical Methods to Correct and Adjust Publication Bias

Once publication bias is suspected, several methods are available for correcting this. If a funnel plot looks skewed, it suggests that small negative studies are missing and one approach is to analyse only the large studies or high-quality studies and eliminate the rest. The second approach is to use 'Rosenthal's file-drawer method'. It aims to assess how many new studies averaging a null result are required to bring the overall treatment effect to being non-significant. In other words, it estimates the number of studies filed away by researchers without being published.

The 'Trim and Fill' method is a simple rank-based complementary technique to formalise the use of the funnel plot. Essentially, the number of 'asymmetric' studies on the right-hand side of the funnel plot is estimated – basically these are studies that have no left-hand counterparts. These studies are eliminated from the meta-analysis using standard meta-analytic techniques – the 'trim' method. The true centre of the funnel is calculated. The 'trimmed' studies are then replaced and their missing counterparts 'filled.' An adjusted confidence interval is then calculated.[59]

The methods above that are used to assess bias are depicted in Fig. 3.9.

3.7
Pitfalls: Biased Inclusion Criteria

Similar to selection bias in trials, bias could also occur inherently within a systematic review whereby systematic reviewers with foreknowledge of individual result studies can manipulate the inclusion and exclusion criteria in order to preferentially select or exclude positive or negative studies respectively leading to the shaping of an asymmetrical skewed sample of data. The introduction of subjectivity is dependent on the

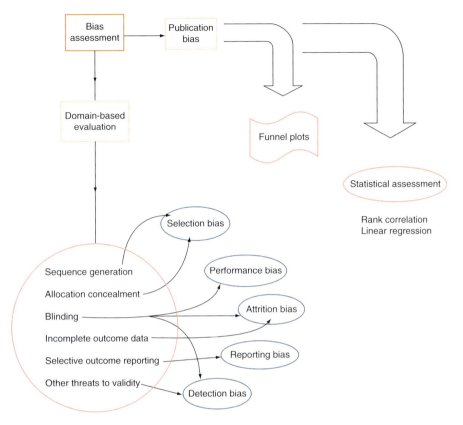

Fig. 3.9 Assessment of bias

investigators' familiarity with the subject, their own pre-existing opinions and experience and their conflicts of interest.

3.7.1
Dealing with Personal Bias and Inclusion Bias

A number of techniques in systematic review design could aid in the reduction of this form of bias. These can include the following:

- Prior agreement on selection criteria through consensus
- Pooling of search results between individual systematic reviewers
- Selection of results with use of distinct inclusion criteria by two individuals consisting of experts and non-experts in the field of study with a third one acting as an arbiter
- Use of a reject log for all excluded articles
- Blinding of systematic reviewers at the stage of selection criteria and critical appraisal

3.8
Which Meta-analysis Should be Published?

The investigation of heterogeneity between the different studies is the main task in each meta-analysis. A major limitation of formal heterogeneity tests is their low statistical power to detect any heterogeneity, if present. Both informal methods such as comparing results with different designs within different geographical regions and visual methods such as funnel and radial plots should be used. Authors must make every attempt to deal with heterogeneity. Failure to do so should be looked at unkindly by the editors of journals.

As discussed previously, the issue of publication bias is inherent to meta-analysis. Studies with non-significant or negative results get published less than those with positive results. Also 'replication studies' conducted in epidemiology tend to get published less in international journals as they do not add anything new to the literature.

Future research in the field of meta-analysis needs to focus on the deficiencies of various meta-analytic methods. The influence of different baseline risks, the different quality and type of exposure measurements made and the methods for pooling studies that have measured different confounding variables all need to be taken into account. There is a need for refined protocols for the undertaking and reporting of meta-analysis. The statistical methods used in complex meta-analysis also need to be refined. Rigorous standards must be deployed, as public health regulators will base their decision more and more on the results of meta-analyses.[60]

3.9
Systematic Review of Observational Studies

RCT results are the most objective form of evidence on the ladder of evidence available for a particular intervention. However, there are instances where RCTs are unfeasible and only observational studies like cross-sectional studies, case control studies and cohort studies are possible. This is especially so in studies which might involve small disease prevalence and incidence, moderate effect sizes or long latency periods. In observation studies, the aim is to confirm the association and quantitative assessment of degree of relation.

3.9.1
Use Cases for Observational Studies

An aetiological hypothesis generally cannot be tested in a randomised controlled setting. The aetiological risk contributing to a particular disease might be low but still clinically significant. When compounded with rare diseases of small incidences and prevalence, the resultant fraction of individuals with the disease in a study directly attributed to the aetiology risk might be extremely low. This makes the study of these individuals in a prospective randomised controlled trial very difficult due to costs in terms of monetary expenditure, manpower and time. Moreover, the ramifications of exposing individuals to risk factors make the randomisation of individuals to exposure and control groups unethical. In these circumstances, a cohort or case control studies could be a better study design.[31]

Even with the use of RCTs, observational studies would have to be undertaken in order to ensure comprehensive cover in medical effectiveness research. RCTs can only establish the efficacy of treatment and the more common adverse effects. This is because a randomised controlled trial can only be performed within a finite amount of time and hence less common adverse effects might not be picked up once the trial ends. Due to the lack of long-term follow-up, late onset adverse effects which have a long latency before presentation might not be identified. Once late onset adverse effects are discovered, ethical, political and moral obstacles would prevent the approval for a new prospective trial from being conducted. In these circumstances, either case control studies or post-marketing surveillance scheme analysis could aid in following up patients.[31]

The conclusions derived from RCTs might not be so applicable in clinical practice. The population enrolled into RCTs might differ from the average patient seen in clinical practice. Furthermore, the environment in which the trial is conducted might differ from clinical practice since most trials are conducted in a tertiary university hospital setting where more services and specialist advice could be attained. Demographically, a randomised controlled trial could have excluded women, elderly and minority ethnic groups which could prove to form a sizable bulk of patients in the real clinical setting. Observational studies could plug in the gaps left by trials in this case.

3.9.2
Problems in Systematic Reviews of Observational Studies

The meta-analysis of observational studies would aid in combining results allowing for increased power in the study of very rare exposures and risks. However, apart from the different forms of bias as described in the previous section (Sect. 3.6), there are further sources of bias in observational studies due to the nature of observational study designs. The potential for bias to affect results in the meta-analysis of observational studies is much greater than the one using RCTs such that even when meta-analysed, meta-analysis results could be implausible or worse, spuriously plausible.

The major forms of bias in observational studies include the following:

- Confounding bias
- Subject selection bias/recall bias
- Heterogeneity in methodology and study populations
- Misclassification bias

3.9.2.1
Confounding Bias

Confounding bias occurs when a factor which is related to both the exposure and the disease under study and its influence is not accounted for during analysis. It can be statistically removed by careful study design where individual variables thought to affect the exposure and disease outcome are well documented and measured and with the use of variance analysis methods, its influence can be removed from the findings. However, the correction for confounding bias is still dependent on the ability to measure with sufficient precision the magnitude of the confounding variable. If imprecise, residual confounding bias could still be present. Moreover, unless actively looked out for, the confounding variable might be overlooked entirely. This problem predominates in prospective and especially retrospective cohort studies.

3.9.2.2
Selection Bias and Other Forms of Bias

For case control studies, it is bias within the study which is more of a problem. In order to create the necessary study and control groups, selection criteria would need to be made. Since the selection process is a non-blinded one, there is a great possibility of selection bias. Furthermore, recall bias can occur whereby individuals in both study group and control group might preferentially or subconsciously remember or forget key factors in their individual recollections of exposure risk. This bias is dependent on knowledge of group allocation which cannot be blinded from either investigators or patients.

3.9.2.3
Heterogeneity in Study Methodology and Populations

Lastly, there is increased 'between-study' heterogeneity due to the usage of alternative methodologies in different observational study designs. This poses a more complex undertaking in the combination of individual summary results compared to RCTs. Moreover some types of studies, i.e., ecological studies only have data with regards to populations already exposed to the risk factor with no data for controls. This problem is in establishing comparable groups for combination of results between ecological, cohort and case control studies. The diversity of populations in epidemiology studies also makes useful summaries for a given population difficult.

3.9.3
Solutions to Problems in Observational Studies

In view of this, a number of strategies have been recommended.

Similar to CONSORT guidelines for RCTs, a set of guidelines have been established to allow for assessment of study quality of observational studies – Meta-analysis of Observational Studies in Epidemiology (MOOSE). As with other guidelines described above, it is also being established as criteria for publication in a variety of journals.

Egger et al. have advocated more detail in individual subject data versus overall study size. The collection of more detailed data on a smaller number of participants is a better strategy for obtaining accurate results than from a study that is collecting cruder data from a larger number of participants. More detail from individual subjects would allow for the easier identification and measurement of potential confounding factors and its statistical removal from the association between exposure and disease. If a precise measurement of the confounding variable is not possible, the use of other studies to derive external estimates of the confounding variable could be used in order to adjust for its influence.[31]

Quantitative statistical synthesis' should not be a prominent component of reviews of observational studies. To enable for combination of data, comparable groups must exist. Also consideration to possible sources of heterogeneity between observational study results must be made. Heterogeneity due to methodological quality like the composition of population under study, the level of exposure, the definition of disease in study, the presence of potential bias and confounding should be expected and accounted for. This can be achieved via the use of sensitivity analysis or by stratification or regression. In sensitivity analysis, the influence of different aspects of study methodology to meta-analysis results could be fully realised. However if heterogeneity is in excess, a meta-analysis is not recommended. Deciding on whether the differences are significant enough to warrant formal combination of results is dependent on both scientific necessity and statistical significance.[31]

The meta-analysis of observational studies via the use of independent patient data could allow for better focus on rarer conditions due to a larger available pool of subjects. Moreover, subject selection bias could be removed via the application of stricter inclusion and exclusion criteria. The standardisation of the removal of confounding factors is possible and with re-analysis, more valid and precise conclusions with regards to the exposure disease relationship could be obtained. Even then, this pooling of data allows for optimal subgroup analysis and sensitivity analysis to be undertaken. The meta-analysis of individual patient data in general is detailed in the next section.

3.10
Other Types of Meta-analysis

3.10.1
Meta-analysis of Individual Patient Data

In a typical meta-analysis, the summary data from individual studies are aggregated and combined together. If the required summary data is not present, it could either be derived from pre-existing published data or if inadequate, a request can be made directly to the original authors for this. Meta-analysis of individual patient data or 'pooled analysis' do not utilise summary results. Instead, the datasets of individual trials are directly requested from researchers, the data is standardised and merged together and overall summary overviews are calculated from this merged dataset (Fig. 3.10).

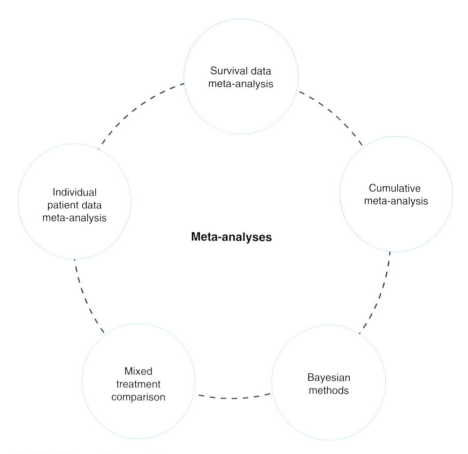

Fig. 3.10 Different 'silhouettes' of meta-analysis

3.10.1.1
Advantages

The advantages of this form of meta-analysis are legion including the ability to check and assess the implementation of trial methodology, the adequacy of randomisation, the demographics of individual test groups, the presence of gaps in data recording, the presence of loss from follow-up and how intention to treat policies are implemented. Further to this, the dataset could also be updated with a new round of follow-ups repeated with the aim to complete any incomplete data records and if not possible a standard intention to treat policy could be implemented across all study results. The use of stricter inclusion and exclusion criteria could also aid in standardisation. This is followed up by updated methods in the analysis and derivation of summary results where subgroup analysis, the charting of survival endpoints and survivorship studies could be performed. For all these features mentioned above, the meta-analysis of independent patient data is considered a gold standard to other forms of systematic reviews.

3.10.1.2
Disadvantages

In view of the need for patient datasets and follow-up of a large population of patients, the implementation and conduct of Individual Patient Data (IPD) studies could be very costly monetarily and time consuming. The provision of datasets is entirely dependent on cooperation of individual study authors and in some cases not all original data could have been kept, some could have been destroyed.

3.10.2
Meta-analysis of Survival Data

Survival study poses a unique problem with regards to a meta-analysis. In survivorship studies, the primary outcome of interest is the time from study initiation to an event occurrence (e.g., morbidity or mortality). Usually this data is plotted in a survivorship curve (Kaplan–Meier curve) and then a summary statistic describing the survival trend is derived (e.g., hazard ratio/log hazard ratio). A meta-analysis involves the combination of such summary measure of survivorship data. However, there are a variety of methods and different types of summary measures available. Unfortunately, not all trials report a log hazard ratio and hence this must be derived in order to allow for comparable results for combination. As most survivorship data is censored, the extraction of accurate data is difficult which can involve either estimations via mathematical conversions from the provided summary data or via direct measurement from a survival curve. There might not be enough summary data of sufficient quality in trial reports to derive out hazard ratios. Furthermore, the extraction information directly from Kaplan–Meier curves in papers introduces random measurement error and hence reduces the accuracy of results. In this case, the use of individual patient data is ideal as individual datasets could be merged fully to create a mega dataset and the summary statistic derived with far better precision.

3.10.3
Cumulative Meta-analysis

In comparison to a traditional meta-analysis which only covers a topic at a particular snapshot in time, cumulative meta-analysis encourages the process of performing a new or updated meta-analysis prospectively every time a new trial is published. An example of cumulative meta-analysis would be those present in the Cochrane Register of Systematic Reviews with each individual systematic review being revised either after new trials have been published or within a specified period of time (i.e., time to expiry).

The benefits of undertaking a cumulative meta-analysis are twofold. If done prospectively, it allows for the continual updating of overview estimates such that if there are any changes to estimates, it would be noticed earlier which leads to a faster, timelier response in changing clinical practice. This can potentially save more lives and resources. If done retrospectively, it allows for the exploration of effects of change in meta-analytical results when trials are added sequentially. When added by chronology, time lag bias and effect of temporal changes in current practice and population could be observed. If additions are undertaken by study size, influence of small study effects on the results of a meta-analysis could be elucidated.

3.10.4
Mixed-Treatment Comparison (MTC) Meta-analysis

A relatively new concept is that of MTCs or 'network' meta-analysis. This method is used where several treatment regimes e.g. A, B, C, D and E exist for a particular condition and the surgeon wants to rank the benefits and harms of each treatment modality so that the most superior one can be picked for patient care. The concept of heterogeneity is expanded in MTCs. There may be inconsistencies between direct and indirect comparisons of the same treatment. These may be due to sheer difference or bias.

There are several modelling methods used in MTCmeta-analysis. These methods are beyond the scope of this book. Use of hierarchical Bayesian meta-analysis and multi-parameter evidence synthesis methodology for MCTs allows the surgeon to incorporate all the available evidence as opposed to the best available evidence. Answers obtained from MCTs can be used to design new studies for which no direct evidence is yet available.[61]

3.10.5
Bayesian Methods of Meta-analysis

A Bayesian method signifies a unique method of analysis devoid of significance tests and confidence intervals. The emphasis lies on a continuous evidence update. A Bayesian analysis looks at uncertainty of quantities of interest and expresses them through a 'prior distribution'. 'Likelihood' seeks to explain the current data by addressing hypotheses as to how that data was obtained. These two terms are combined to give us a mathematical summary of the quantities of interest, termed 'posterior distribution', which very much resembles classical point estimates and confidence intervals. When conducting a meta-analysis, the 'prior distribution' principle and particularly its width reveals uncertainty behind odds ratio, risk ratio or mean difference calculations, i.e., any effect measure that is analysed as well as its size. If only little information can be gathered, a 'non-informative' prior distribution should be used thus ensuring that all values are equally likely.

Certain problems with Bayesian methods arise however. 'Prior distribution' creates a problem as its modus operandi is based on beliefs about effects and, therefore, subjective opinion. Automatically, one wonders how wise it is to combine the above with objective results. When one delves deeper into meta-analytical processes, a conclusion arises where non-informative prior distributions are required to reflect a position of prior ignorance. A way of remedying such a problem within meta-analysis is to use external evidence or carry out sensitivity analyses in order to demonstrate whether the conclusions actually rely on any such beliefs or assumptions.[46]

Despite this, further research into effects of Bayesian analysis is required, especially as it has demonstrated several advantages over classical methods of meta-analysis. Bayesian methods allow us to explore the relationship between treatment benefit and underlying risk and how influenced patients' beliefs are by the study results. It adds a deeper flavour to meta-analytical work by incorporating the idea of clinical outcome 'usefulness' as well as often-ignored evidence, such as study variation and intervention effects. Finally, it must be added that Bayesian calculations can only be carried out by WinBUGS software and not RevMan.[46]

3.11
What is the Use of a Meta-analysis?

A well-conducted systematic review and/or meta-analysis are invaluable for practitioners. Many of us feel overwhelmed by the volume of medical literature and, as a result, often prefer summaries of information to publications of original investigations. Thus, such types of evidence keep us abreast of the goings-on on a particular clinical topic. High-quality systematic reviews and meta-analyses can define the boundaries of what is known. They are extremely useful in health technology assessments and cost-effectiveness analysis.

Furthermore, they identify gaps in medical research and identify beneficial or harmful interventions. Investigators need systematic reviews and meta-analyses to summarise existing data, refine hypotheses, estimate sample sizes and help define future research agendas. Without these, researchers may miss promising leads or may embark on studies of questions that have been already answered. Industry is particularly interested in meta-analyses as it helps to direct resources to viable and beneficial health interventions.

Administrators and purchasers need integrative publications to help generate clinical policies that optimise clinical outcomes using available resources. For consumers and health policymakers who are interested in the bottom line of evidence, systematic reviews and meta-analyses can help harmonise conflicting results of research. They can be used as the basis for other integrative articles produced by policymakers, such as risk assessments, practice guidelines, economic analyses and decision analyses.

However, meta-analysis is only one of the pillars of 'evidence-based health care' that can be used to make clinical, professional and policy decisions.

3.12
Challenges of Conducting RCTs in Clinical Practice

Several problems of conducting RCTs in clinical practice especially in surgery have been reported as discussed previously. One solution of overcoming known biases in surgical trials is the 'expertise-based RCT'. In this type of trial, a surgeon with expertise in one of

the procedures being evaluated is paired with a surgeon with expertise in the other procedure who should ideally be from the same institution. Subjects are randomised to treatments and treated by a surgeon who is an 'expert' in the procedure. This study overcomes
some of the challenges associated with traditional orthopaedic RCTs including the caveat
that surgeons who wish to participate in traditional RCTs must be willing to perform both
techniques and that a lack of expertise or belief in one of the interventions under evaluation
may undermine the validity and applicability of the results.[62] A recent survey of orthopaedic surgeons found that most would consider this type of study design as it may decrease
the likelihood of procedural crossovers and enhance validity because unlike the conventional RCT, there is a low likelihood of differential expertise bias.[63] Furthermore, positive
steps are being made with the advent of larger multi-centre trials.[64]

A significant proportion of the surgical literature is in the form of 'observational studies'. It must be remembered that much of the research into the cause of diseases relies on
cohort, case control or cross-sectional studies. Also, observational studies can generate
significant hypotheses and have a role into delineating the harms and benefits of interventions. To ensure the robustness of reporting observational studies, the STROBE statement
was created. It aims to assist authors when writing up analytical observational studies, to
support editors and reviewers when considering such articles for publication, and to help
readers when critically appraising published articles.[65] All these steps will add to the quality of data that is used in future surgical meta-analyses.

3.13
Meta-analysis Software

The number of available packages has nearly doubled over the last decade. A detailed
cross comparison of all the available software to conduct meta-analysis is not within scope
of this book. However, a number of generalisations can be applied with choice of package
being dependent on use requirements. Pre-existing commercial general statistical programme suites like SAS, STATA and SPSS have been enhanced by the provision of add-on
third party macro programmes which provide a limited set of basic functions for meta-
analysis. Standalone packages are purpose built for meta-analysis and tend to have a
greater variety of functions available and have greater methods of input, processing and
output modes. Some software is free such as 'RevMan' provided by the Cochrane Centre.
Others are commercial.

3.14
Conclusion

Like primary research, meta-analysis involves a stepwise approach to arrive at statistically
justifiable conclusions. It has the potential to provide an accurate, quantitative appraisal of
the literature. It may objectively resolve controversies. The greatest challenge in conducting

a meta-analysis on a clinical topic is often the lack of available data on the subject, because there are few high-quality, published studies with an acceptable degree of heterogeneity.

If meta-analyses are to continue to have a role in surgical decision making, clinicians need to be able to perform, assess, compare and communicate the quality of meta-analyses, particularly in areas where several meta-analyses are available.

References

1. Panesar SS, Thakrar R, Athanasiou T, Sheikh A. Comparison of reports of RCTs and systematic reviews in surgical journals: literature review. *J R Soc Med*. 2006;99(9):470-472.
2. Royal College of Surgeons of England. Implementing the EWTD: College response. Available online at http://www.rcseng.ac.uk/publications/docs/ewtd_communicaion.html/attachment_download/pdffile. Last accessed on April 1, 2009.
3. Davidoff F, Haynes B, Sackett D, Smith R. Evidence based medicine: a new journal to help doctors identify the information they need. *BMJ*. 1995;310:1085-1086.
4. Williams CJ. The pitfalls of narrative reviews in clinical medicine. *Ann Oncol*. 1998;9(6): 601-605.
5. Sauerland S, Seiler CM. Role of systematic reviews and meta-analysis in evidence-based medicine. *World J Surg*. 2005;29(5):582-587.
6. Glass GV. Primary, secondary and meta-analysis of research. *Educ Res*. 1976;5:3-8.
7. Ng TT, McGory ML, Ko CY, et al. Meta-analysis in surgery: methods and limitations. *Arch Surg*. 2006;141(11):1125-1130.
8. Berman NG, Parker RA. Meta-analysis: neither quick nor easy. *BMC Med Res Methodol*. 2002;9(2):10.
9. Stroup DF, Berlin JA, Morton SC, et al. Meta-analysis of observational studies in epidemiology: a proposal for reporting. Meta-analysis of observational studies in epidemiology (MOOSE) group. *JAMA*. 2000;283(15):2008-2012.
10. Thompson SG, Pocock SJ. Can meta-analyses be trusted? *Lancet*. 1991;338(8775):1127-1130.
11. Olkin I. Meta-analysis: reconciling the results of independent studies. *Stat Med*. 1995; 14(5–7):457-472.
12. Jadad AR, Moore RA, Carroll D, et al. Assessing the quality of reports of randomized clinical trials: Is blinding necessary? *Control Clin Trials*. 1996;17(1):1-12.
13. Moher D, Jadad AR, Nichol G, et al. Assessing the quality of randomized controlled trials: an annotated bibliography of scales and checklists. *Control Clin Trials*. 1995;16(1):62-73.
14. The Cochrane Collaboration. Measures of relative effect: the risk ratio and odds ratio. In: *The Cochrane Handbook for Review Manager* 5. p. 111-113.
15. Laupacis A, Sackett DL, Roberts RS. An assessment of clinically useful measures of the consequences of treatment. *N Engl J Med*. 1998;318(26):1728-1733.
16. Berlin JA, Laird NM, Sacks HS, et al. A comparison of statistical methods for combining event rates from clinical trials. *Stat Med*. 1989;8(2):141-151.
17. DerSimonian R, Laird N. Meta-analysis in clinical trials. *Control Clin Trials*. 1986;7(3):177-188.
18. The Cochrane Collaboration. Diversity and heterogeneity: Identifying statistical heterogeneity. The Cochrane Collaboration open learning material 2002 cited; Available from: http://www.cochrane-net.org/openlearning/HTML/mod13-3.htm.
19. Mantel N, Hanezsel W. Statistical aspects of the analysis of data from retrospective studies of disease. *J Natl Cancer Inst*. 1959;22(4):719-748.
20. Greenland S, Robins JM. Estimation of a common effect parameter from sparse follow-up data. *Biometrics*. 1985;41(1):55-68.

21. Greenland S. Randomization, statistics, and causal inference. *Epidemiology*. 1990;1(6):421-429.
22. Fleiss JL. The statistical basis of meta-analysis. *Stat Meth Med Res*. 1993;2(2):121-145.
23. Sankey SS et al. An assessment of the use of the continuity correction for sparse data in meta-analysis. *Commun Stat Simul Comput*. 1996;25(4):1031-1056.
24. Bailey KR. Inter-study differences: how should they influence the interpretation and analysis of results? *Stat Med*. 1987;6(3):351-360.
25. Huedo-Medina TB, Sanchez-Meca J, Marin-Martinez F, et al. Assessing heterogeneity in meta-analysis: Q statistic or I2 index? *Psychol Meth*. 2006;11:193-206.
26. Higgins JP, Thompson SG, Deeks JJ, et al. Measuring inconsistency in meta-analyses. *BMJ*. 2003;327(7414):557-560.
27. Egger M, Smith GD, Phillips AN. Meta-analysis: principles and procedures. *BMJ*. 1997; 315(7121):1533-1537.
28. Easterbrook PJ, Berlin JA, Gopalan R, et al. Publication bias in clinical research. *Lancet*. 1991;337(8746):867-872.
29. Davey Smith G, Egger M, et al. Meta-analysis. Beyond the grand mean? *BMJ*. 1997; 315(7122):1610-1614.
30. Efron B, Morris C. Stein's paradox in statistics. *Sci Am*. 1977;236:119-127.
31. Egger M, Smith GD, Schneider M. Systematic reviews of observational studies. In: Egger M, Smith GD, Altman D, eds. *Systematic Reviews in Healthcare*. London: British Medical Association; 2001.
32. Krahn J, Sauerland S, Rixen D, Gregor S, Bouillon B, Neugebauer EA. Applying evidence-based surgery in daily clinical routine: a feasibility study. *Arch Orthop Trauma Surg*. 2006;126(2):88-92.
33. Ramsay CR, Grant AM, Wallace SA, et al. Statistical assessment of the learning curves of health technologies. *Health Technol Assess*. 2001;5(12):1-79.
34. Freemantle N, Cleland J, Young P, et al. beta Blockade after myocardial infarction: systematic review and metaregression analysis. *BMJ*. 1999;318(7200):1730-1737.
35. Lau J, Ioannidis JP, Schmid CH. Summing up evidence: one answer is not always enough. *Lancet*. 1998;351:123-127.
36. Shea B, Dube C, Moher D. Assessing the quality of reports of systematic reviews: QUOROM statement compared to other tools. In: Egger M, Smith G, Altman D, eds. *Systematic Reviews in Health Care: Meta-Analysis in Context*. London: BMJ Publishing; 2001:122-129.
37. Oxman AD. Checklists for review articles. *BMJ*. 1994;309(6955):648-651.
38. Moher D, Cook DJ, Eastwood S, et al. Improving the quality of reports of meta-analyses of randomised controlled trials: The QUOROM statement. Quality of Reporting of Meta-analyses. *Lancet*. 1999;354(9193):1896-1900.
39. Petticrew M. Why certain systematic reviews reach uncertain conclusions. *BMJ*. 2003; 326(7392):756-758.
40. Jüni P, Altman D, Egger M. Assessing the quality of controlled clinical trials. In: Egger M, Davey Smith G, Altman D, eds. *Systematic Reviews in Health Care: Meta-Analysis in context*. London: BMJ Books; 2001.
41. Campbell DT. Factors relevant to the validity of experiments in social settings. *Psychol Bull*. 1957;54(4):297-312.
42. Moher D, Jones A, Lepage L, CONSORT Group (Consolitdated Standards for Reporting of Trials). Use of the CONSORT statement and quality of reports of randomized trials: a comparative before-and-after evaluation. *JAMA*. 2001;285(15):1992-1995.
43. Gueyffier F, Bulpitt C, Boissel JP, et al. Antihypertensive drugs in very old people: a subgroup meta-analysis of randomised controlled trials. INDANA Group. *Lancet*. 1999;353(9155):793-796.
44. Shea B, Boers M, Grimshaw JM, et al. Does updating improve the methodological and reporting quality of systematic reviews? *BMC Med Res Methodol*. 2006;6:27.
45. Gluud LL. Bias in clinical intervention research. *Am J Epidemiol*. 2006;163(6):493-501.

46. Higgins J, Green S. *Cochrane Handbook for Systematic Reviews of Interventions.* Version 5.0.0 edn. Oxford: The Cochrane Collaboration; 2008.

47. Sterne JA, Egger M, Smith GD. Systematic reviews in health care: Investigating and dealing with publication and other biases in meta-analysis. *BMJ.* 2001;323(7304):101-105.

48. Hopewell S, McDonald S, Clarke M, et al. Grey literature in meta-analyses of randomized trials of health care interventions. *Cochrane Database Syst Rev.* 2007;18(2):MR000010.

49. Ezzo J. Should journals devote space to trials with no results? *J Altern Complement Med.* 2003;9(5):611-612.

50. Krleza-Jerić K, Chan AW, Dickersin K, et al. Principles for international registration of protocol information and results from human trials of health related interventions: Ottawa statement (part 1). *BMJ.* 2005;330(7497):956-958.

51. DeAngelis CD, Drazen JM, Frizelle FA, et al. International Committee of Medical Journal Editors. Clinical trial registration: a statement from the International Committee of Medical Journal Editors. *JAMA.* 2004;292(11):1363-1364.

52. McCray AT. Better access to information about clinical trials. *Ann Intern Med.* 2000;133(8): 609-614.

53. Egger M, Smith GD. Bias in location and selection of studies. *BMJ.* 1998;316(7124):61-66.

54. Stuck AE, Rubenstein LZ, Wieland D. Bias in meta-analysis detected by a simple, graphical test. Asymmetry detected in funnel plot was probably due to true heterogeneity. *BMJ.* 1998;316(7129):469.

55. Duval S, Tweedie R. A Nonparametric "Trim and Fill" Method of Accounting for Publication Bias in Meta-Analysis. *J Am Stat Assoc.* 2000;95:89-98.

56. Ioannidis JP, Trikalinos TA. The appropriateness of asymmetry tests for publication bias in meta-analyses: a large survey. *CMAJ.* 2007;176(8):1091-1096.

57. Begg CB, Mazumdar M. Operating characteristics of a rank correlation test for publication bias. *Biometrics.* 1994;50(4):1088-1101.

58. Egger M, Davey Smith G, et al. Bias in meta-analysis detected by a simple, graphical test. *BMJ.* 1997;315(7109):629-634.

59. Sutton A, et al. Publication bias. In: Sutton A, ed. *Methods for Meta-Analysis in Medical Research.* Chichester, UK: Wiley; 2000.

60. Blettner M, Sauerbrei W, Schlehofer B, et al. Traditional reviews, meta-analyses and pooled analyses in epidemiology. *Int J Epidemiol.* 1999;28(1):1-9.

61. Salanti G, Higgins J, Ades AE, et al. Evaluation of networks of randomized trials. *Stat Methods Med Res.* 2008;17:279-301.

62. Devereaux PJ, Bhandari M, Clarke M, et al. Need for expertise based randomised controlled trials. *BMJ.* 2005;330:88.

63. Bednarska E, Bryant D, Devereaux PJ, et al. Orthopaedic surgeons prefer to participate in expertise-based randomized trials. *Clin Orthop Relat Res.* 2008;466(7):1734-1744.

64. Sprague S, Matta JM, Bhandari M. Multicenter collaboration in observational research: Improving generalizability and efficiency. *J Bone Joint Surg Am.* 2009;91(Suppl 3):80-86.

65. von Elm E, Altman DG, Egger M, et al. The Strengthening the Reporting of Observational Studies in Epidemiology (STROBE) statement: guidelines for reporting observational studies. *Lancet.* 2007;370(9596):1453-1457.

Diagnostic Tests

4

Catherine M. Jones, Ara Darzi, and Thanos Athanasiou

Abstract This chapter explains the basic diagnostic statistics used in medicine, and outlines the most commonly used statistics for estimating the diagnostic accuracy of diagnostic tests. Principles of robust diagnostic study design are given to enhance both study design and critical appraisal of the literature. The methods used to collate multiple study results into a single diagnostic accuracy estimate through meta-analytical techniques are also given, with explanations and assessment of each method.

4.1
Introduction

The evidence base for diagnostic test accuracy is growing in line with the realisation that diagnostics are vital for effective treatment and high-quality patient care. The demands for diagnostic testing are increasing every year, as is the technology of radiological and pathological testing. Summary guidelines to incorporate clinical as well as financial impact are becoming increasingly available as the amount of diagnostic literature grows. It is apparent that whilst diagnostics has lagged behind the therapeutic specialties in evidence-based practice, it is rapidly catching up.

This chapter outlines the principles and basic theoretical framework of diagnostic test meta-analysis. For clinicians and researchers alike, an understanding of how to perform and interpret diagnostic accuracy tests will be increasingly useful over the foreseeable future.

C.M. Jones (✉)
Department of Surgery and Cancer, Imperial College London,
St Mary's Hospital Campus, London, UK
e-mail: cathjones78@yahoo.com.au

T. Athanasiou and A. Darzi (eds.), *Evidence Synthesis in Healthcare*,
DOI: 10.1007/978-0-85729-206-3_4, © Springer-Verlag London Limited 2011

4.2
What Is a Diagnostic Test?

In its broadest context, a medical diagnostic test is any discriminating question which, once answered, provides information about the status of the patient. Commonly used diagnostic tests include history and examination, laboratory investigations, radiological imaging, clinical scores derived from questionnaires, and operative findings. Each situation will be different, and the individual circumstances will determine which test, if any, is the most appropriate. Regardless of the situation, a diagnostic test should be performed only if patient benefit can be realistically expected.

Choosing a diagnostic test requires knowledge of its performance across different patient populations. There is no benefit in applying a test to a population in whom there is no evidence of diagnostic accuracy. Clinical experience and medical literature provide information on reliable interpretation of results. Screening programmes, such as cervical smears and mammograms, represent diagnostic tests on a grand scale.

4.3
How Do We Use Estimates of Diagnostic Accuracy?

Most clinicians are familiar with the concepts of sensitivity and specificity. Sensitivity is the pickup rate of a test amongst people who are positive for the disease. A sensitivity of 80% means that 80% of all patients who truly have the disease will be identified by the test. This means that on a test with high sensitivity, a negative result will rule out the disease. In particular, screening tests are targeted towards exclusion of disease, as they are applied on a grand scale to detect occult disease. If positive, the screening test is often followed by other investigations with higher overall accuracy. Specificity, on the other hand, measures the percentage of patients without the disease who are correctly identified as being negative on the test. A highly specific test, when positive, rules in the disease. Sensitivity and specificity are calculated by comparing the test results against the results from an accepted ('gold') standard.

Interpreting test results requires a threshold for the test to be positive. Dichotomous results where the answer is 'yes/no' are easy to interpret. Continuous results, like serum haemoglobin, require a diagnostic threshold for disease. For example, anaemia may be diagnosed when the haemoglobin is low enough to meet criteria for iron supplementation. Ordinal tests, with multiple ordered outcomes, require a decision about threshold to convert the result into 'yes/no'. Ventilation/perfusion scanning for pulmonary embolus is a good example of this – the result may be low, intermediate or high probability. Categorical variables with multiple non-ordered outcomes also require a definition of 'disease', for example in genetic testing.

Whether incorporated into the test or not, a diagnostic threshold is required for an effective test. This may be based on guidelines which are in turn based on results in the medical literature. Meta-analysis contributes significantly to evidence-based practice.

4.4
Estimating Diagnostic Accuracy

True positive (TP), true negative (TN), false positive (FP) and false negative (FN) outcomes are categorised according to concordance or discrepancy with the results from the reference standard (Fig. 4.1). 'True' outcomes on the index test are those which agree with the reference result for that subject. 'False' outcomes disagree with the reference result and are considered inaccurate. The reference standard may be flawed but for the purposes of diagnostic test accuracy is considered to produce accurate results in all patients. The ideal diagnostic test produces no false outcomes.

Sensitivity, specificity, negative predictive value and positive predictive value are commonly encountered in clinical practice. Statistically, sensitivity is $TP/(TP+FN)$ and specificity is $TN/(FP+TN)$. Sensitivity is also known as True Positive Rate (TPR), whilst $(1 - Specificity)$ is known as False Positive Rate (FPR). Sensitivity and specificity are useful when deciding whether to perform the test. Depending on the clinical scenario, high sensitivity or specificity may be more important and the best test can be chosen for the clinical situation.

Positive and negative predictive values (PPV and NPV) measure the usefulness of a result once the test has been performed. For example, a PPV of 80% indicates that 80% patients with a positive test result actually have the disease. A NPV of 40% indicates that only 40% of patients testing negative are truly healthy. PPV is $TP/(TP+FP)$ and NPV is $TN/(TN+FN)$. The ratios are calculated horizontally across the 2×2 table (Fig. 4.1).

Sensitivity and specificity are measures of the inherent accuracy of a diagnostic test and rely on the reference standard being correct. As a pair of figures, they represent the accuracy of a test and as such are used to compare different test accuracies. PPV and NPV are measures of clinical accuracy and provide the probability of a given result being correct. In practice, both types of summary measures are reported in the literature, and the difference between them should be clearly understood.

Likelihood ratios are different statistics altogether. They give an idea of how a test result will change the odds (rather than probability) of having a disease. The use of odds

		REFERENCE STANDARD		
		+	–	TOTAL
INDEX TEST	+	TP	FP	TP + FP
	–	FN	TN	TN + FN
	TOTAL	TP + FN	TN + FP	TP + FN + FP + TN

Fig. 4.1 Two-by-two table for calculating sensitivity, specificity, PPV and NPV

Odds	=	Probability / (1-Probability)
Probability	=	Odds / (1 + Odds)

Fig. 4.2 Formulas for converting odds into probability

Positive Likelihood ratio	(LR+)	=	Sensitivity / (1-Specificity)
Negative Likelihood ratio	(LR−)	=	(1-Sensitivity) / Specificity
Post-Test Odds		=	Pre-Test Odds x Likelihood Ratio
DOR		=	LR+ / LR−
		=	Sensitivity / (1-Specificity)
			(1-Sensitivity) / Specificity
		=	(TP x TN) / (FP x FN)
var {log(DOR)}		=	1/TP + 1/FP + 1/FN + 1/TN

Fig. 4.3 Formulas for commonly used measures of diagnostic accuracy

may be confusing to clinicians, and so it has not been as widely used as sensitivity and specificity. However, the conversion of probability into odds and back again is simple (Fig. 4.2). For example, a pre-test probability of 75% can be converted to odds of $0.75/0.25 = 3$. The odds are 3 to 1. The odds of having the disease after the test result is known (post-test odds) will depend on both the pre-test odds, and the likelihood ratios.

The positive likelihood ratio (LR+) indicates how the pre-test odds of the disease change when the test result is positive. A high LR + indicates that a positive result is likely to be correct. The negative likelihood ratio (LR-) indicates how the odds change with a negative test result. The pre-test odds must be estimated by the clinician before the post-test odds can be calculated. An overall measure of diagnostic accuracy is the diagnostic odds ratio (DOR), which is used to compare different diagnostic tests. The formulas for likelihood and diagnostic odds ratios are given in Fig. 4.3.

4.5
Traditional Diagnostic Meta-analysis Statistics

Meta-analysis aims to identify a clinical question and use the available data to produce a comprehensive answer. The collective data provides more reliable and credible conclusions than individual studies, provided that the methodology of the primary studies and meta-analysis is sound. Diagnostic meta-analysis focuses on the performance of a test across the range of studies in the literature. SROC analysis is the traditional method for combining the results from multiple studies.

The variation in results (heterogeneity) across different studies is due to random chance, errors in analytical methodology, differences in study design, protocol, inclusion and exclusion criteria, and threshold for calling a result positive. The underlying quality of the primary studies' methodology and reporting should be assessed for contribution to the heterogeneity of results.

4.5.1
Quality Analysis of Diagnostic Studies in Meta-analysis

Publication of poorly designed, implemented or reported studies leads to suboptimal application and interpretation of diagnostic tests. The importance of accurate and thorough reporting is now widely accepted, and published guidelines for diagnostic accuracy reporting are available. The QUADAS tool[1] for quality assessment of studies included in diagnostic test systematic reviews consists of fourteen items, each of which should be considered separately as possible contributors to heterogeneity of results. Sources of bias in diagnostic tests relate to flawed study design, population selection and investigator bias (Table 4.1).

The QUADAS tool is designed to identify aspects of primary study design that influence the accuracy results. Summary scores of study quality are inappropriate for assessment of study quality effect on meta-analysis results, as a summary score may mask an important source of bias.[2] Analysing each item in the QUADAS tool separately for effect on overall accuracy is thus a more robust approach. Westwood et al.[3] advocate univariate regression analysis of each item against logDOR, with subsequent multivariate modelling of influential items ($p < 0.10$ in the univariate model) to assess their combined influence on accuracy. The effect of each item in QUADAS (or covariate, for the process is the same) is expressed as the relative diagnostic odds ratio (RDOR). RDOR is calculated as the DOR when the covariate is positive, as a ratio to the DOR when the covariate is negative. The identification of design flaws, population characteristics, test characteristics and other case-specific parameters which affect the reported accuracy can explain the heterogeneity of results and sharpen the conclusions of the meta-analysis. A worked example is shown in Chap. 9.

4.5.2
Receiver Operating Characteristic (ROC) Analysis

The principles of diagnostic meta-analysis are based on receiver operating characteristic (ROC) and summary ROC (SROC) curves, so they shall be discussed first.

Tests which produce a continuous variable result rely on a choice of threshold to decide whether the overall result is positive or negative. The choice of threshold will necessarily determine the number of TP, TN, FP and FN when compared to a reference standard test, and so the sensitivity, specificity, PPV and NPV, likelihood ratios and DOR will all depend on the choice of diagnostic threshold. The threshold is usually chosen with advice from the literature or published guidelines.

The optimal threshold for overall accuracy is ascertained from the ROC curve. For each threshold, a test has a given sensitivity and specificity. In ROC analysis, sensitivity is also known as true positive rate (TPR), and (1 − specificity) is known as false positive rate (FPR). Once the TPR and FPR are calculated for a given threshold, another threshold is chosen, and calculations are performed again. Once all the (TPR, FPR) pairs for the test are calculated, TPR is plotted on the vertical axis, and FPR is plotted on the horizontal (Fig. 4.4). The range for TPR and FPR is zero to one, mapping the ROC curve over the unit square, [0, 0] to [1, 1].

Table 4.1 QUADAS tool for diagnostic meta-analysis quality assessment[1]

Item		Yes	No	Unclear
1	Was the spectrum of patients representative of the patients who will receive the test in practice?			
2	Were selection criteria clearly described?			
3	Is the reference standard likely to correctly classify the target condition?			
4	Is the time period between index test and reference standard short enough to be reasonably sure that the target condition did not change between the two tests?			
5	Did the whole sample, or a random selection of the sample, receive verification using a reference standard of diagnosis?			
6	Did patients receive the same reference standard regardless of the index test result?			
7	Was the reference standard independent of the index test (i.e. the index test did not form part of the reference standard)?			
8	Was the execution of the index test described in sufficient detail to permit replication of the test?			
9	Was the execution of the reference standard described in sufficient detail to permit its replication?			
10	Were the index test results interpreted without knowledge of the results of the reference standard?			
11	Were the reference standard results interpreted without knowledge of the results of the index test?			
12	Were the same clinical data available when test results were interpreted as would be available when the test is used in practice?			
13	Were uninterpretable/intermediate test results reported?			
14	Were withdrawals from the study explained?			

The ideal test threshold discriminates diseased from non-diseased subjects every time, having TPR of 1 and FPR of zero (top left corner of the ROC graph). Intuitively, a test which gives the incorrect diagnosis every time is simply the reverse of the ideal test, and whilst is not clinically useful, is actually a highly diagnostic test (once its flaws are known). The random test produces a TPR which always equals FPR, and the ROC curve is a straight

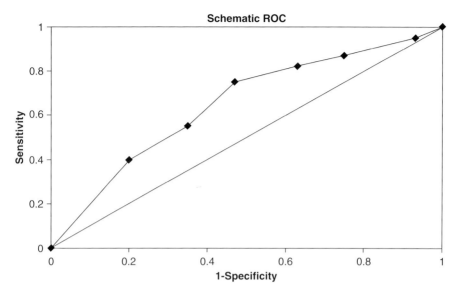

Fig. 4.4 Schematic ROC curve

diagonal line from [0, 0] to [1, 1] (Fig. 4.4). As the accuracy of the test improves, the curve moves closer to the top left hand corner of the graph.

The area under the ROC curve (AUC) is a summary measure of test performance which allows comparison between different tests. TPR and FPR values lie between zero and one inclusive, making the AUC for a perfect test equal to one. The random test has AUC of 0.5. An AUC closer to one (or zero) indicates a better test (with an AUC of zero corresponding to the test which is incorrect every time).

4.5.3
SROC Meta-analysis

Whether meta-analysis of pooled data can be conducted depends both on the number and methodological quality of the primary studies. Averaging the sensitivity and specificities across the studies is invalid because the test criteria, population and clinical setting have differed, leading to a relationship between sensitivity and specificity across the studies. Even weighted averages will not reflect the overall accuracy of the test, as extremes of threshold criteria can skew the distribution. Unfortunately for the meta-analyst, calculating sensitivity and specificity separately tends to underestimate test accuracy, as there is always interaction between them. DOR is a summary statistic which involves both sensitivity and specificity and is the statistic of choice to measure the overall diagnostic performance.

On axes similar to that of an ROC curve, a [TPR, FPR] pair from each study included in the meta-analysis can be plotted onto a pair of axes. The scatter-plot of data points formed from these results forms the basis for the summary ROC (SROC) curve. The curve is mapped over the data points, having been calculated through regression methods.

The principles of this regression are that logit (TPR) and logit (FPR) have a linear relationship when there is variety of thresholds in the primary studies, and that this relationship can be exploited with a line of best fit (regression techniques).[4] The calculations and regression equations are given in Fig. 4.5. Using linear combinations of the two variables as the dependent and independent variables in the regression equation solves the dilemma about the different 'least squares' solutions which would result from choosing one or the other logit.[4]

D is equivalent to log(DOR), or the diagnostic log odds ratio. S inversely measures the diagnostic threshold. High S values correspond to low diagnostic thresholds. D is mapped against S on a linear axis curve, and the least squares line of best fit is fitted to the data. The value of β reflects the interaction between accuracy and threshold. If β is zero, then the two are independent and α estimates logDOR, the global accuracy measure. If β does not equal zero, then there is significant interaction between threshold and accuracy, the curve is asymmetric and α is the estimated logDOR when sensitivity equals specificity. Once α and β are calculated from the intercept and slope of the D-S line respectively, the model is transformed back into the plane of (TPR, FPR), according to the equation given in Fig. 4.6. The Moses model often incorporates weighting into the analysis, using study size or inverse variance as the weights.

The SROC curve is plotted over the original (TPR, FPR) data points (Fig. 4.7), as both α and β are estimated from the line of best fit in the logit plane. Calculation of area under the curve is performed by integration of the above equation over the range (0, 1). If the range of raw FPR data points is small, it may be necessary to perform a partial AUC over the range of data. This is acceptable if the specificity of the test can be assumed to be similar in the target population which will receive the test in practice. Further information regarding calculations of the SROC curve can be found in Moses[4] or Walter.[5]

A big disadvantage of SROC is that summary estimates of sensitivity and specificity with their confidence intervals cannot be generated, as they are the independent and

Logit(TPR)	=	log {TPR/(1-TPR)}		
Logit(FPR)	=	log {FPR/(1-FPR)}		
(where log represents the natural logarithm)				
D	=	α	+	βS
D	=	logit(TPR) – logit(FPR)		
S	=	logit(TPR) + logit(FPR)		

where α is the intercept value, and β represents the dependence of test accuracy on threshold

Fig. 4.5 Logarithmic transformation equations for SROC analysis

$$TPR = \frac{\exp(\alpha/(1-\beta))-[FPR/(1-FPR)]^{(1+\beta)(1-\beta)}}{1+\exp(\alpha/(1-\beta))-[FPR/(1-FPR)]^{(1+\beta)(1-\beta)}}$$

Fig. 4.6 SROC curve calculations

Fig. 4.7 Example of a SROC curve

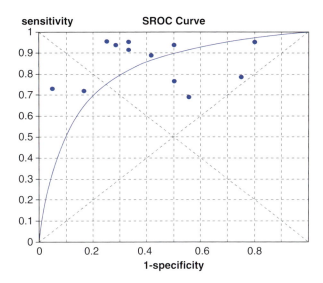

dependent variables in the model. This means that AUC is used as a summary value of overall accuracy, which is less than ideal as it is not well understood by clinicians. The clinical scenario may favour a test with high sensitivity or specificity, but not necessarily both. Additionally, the values of sensitivity and specificity vary with the diagnostic threshold, and so should one want to make inferences concerning average sensitivity and specificity, the analysis should be restricted to studies which have used the test at the same threshold. This may reduce the number of available studies to a point where analysis becomes unfeasible.

4.6
The Bivariate Approach to Diagnostic Meta-analysis

The bivariate approach, like the Moses model, acknowledges that sensitivity and specificity are codependent.[6] As well as keeping the two-dimensional principles of sensitivity and specificity intact, a single variable can be examined for effect on either sensitivity, specificity or both. Unlike the Moses SROC analysis, bivariate modelling produces estimates of sensitivity, specificity and their confidence intervals.

The bivariate model assumes that logit(sensitivity) and logit(specificity) are normally distributed across the primary studies and are correlated to each other. This creates a bivariate distribution (dependent normally distributed variables). Widely available software can be used, as the underlying distributions are assumed to be normal, and linear functions are used in the model. In addition, the use of random-effects makes estimating inter-study heterogeneity in either sensitivity or specificity straightforward. However, the bivariate model is more complex than the SROC model, and if further reading is desired, the papers by Reitsma et al.[6] and Harbord et al.[7] are recommended.

4.7
Hierarchical SROC Analysis

Hierarchical SROC (HSROC) is a multilevel approach to diagnostic meta-analysis that examines heterogeneity both within and between primary studies by modelling both accuracy and threshold as random-effects variables.[8] At the intra-study level, the number of positive results is assumed to be binomial. Threshold and accuracy are modelled as random effects, and the interaction between them as a fixed effect. If accuracy does not depend on threshold, this model is identical to the Moses approach. A second level of modelling generates a HSROC curve using the estimated accuracy and threshold (assuming a normal distribution). Estimates of sensitivity, specificity, likelihood ratios, DOR and other desirable endpoints like AUC can be produced at this stage.

The HSROC technique can also compare different tests from the same or separate studies. Study covariates (both intra- and inter-study) can be added into the model to investigate sources of heterogeneity.

4.8
Comparing the Bivariate and HSROC Models

The bivariate approach examines the influence of covariates on sensitivity and specificity (or both), whilst the HSROC model examines their influence on threshold or accuracy (or both). If there are no study-level covariates, or the covariate(s) are assumed to affect both variables in either model, the two models are identical. The HSROC method is more flexible in that variables can be omitted from the model, depending on the individual situation. The bivariate model, however, can be fitted using a variety of available software. Further information is available in Harbord et al.[7].

4.9
Final Remarks on Diagnostic Meta-analysis Techniques

Mastering the statistical techniques described above is an important (and necessary) step in producing robust conclusions. However, it is equally important to consider the value of performing the analysis, and carefully choose the clinical question which, once answered, will most improve patient care. The patient and study characteristics which influence the test accuracy will be known from experience and extensive reading; careful preparation and sound statistical methodology will result in useful and welcome conclusions. However, successful application of these conclusions to clinical practice ultimately relies on the ability of clinicians and health care managers to critique meta-analyses. Meta-analytical papers are becoming more stringently reviewed with the increasing acceptance of QUADAS and published guidelines for performance of diagnostic meta-analysis.

HSROC is now the standard technique for diagnostic meta-analysis. Although in the past it has been difficult to execute, Bayesian estimates have been shown to closely approximate the results from SAS,[9] making it more accessible. A worked example is shown in Chap. 9.

References

1. Whiting P, Rutjes AW, Reitsma JB, Bossuyt PM, Kleijnen J. The development of QUADAS: a tool for the quality assessment of studies of diagnostic accuracy included in systematic reviews. *BMC Med Res Methodol*. 2003;3:25.
2. Whiting P, Harbord R, Kleijnen J. No role for quality scores in systematic reviews of diagnostic accuracy studies. *BMC Med Res Methodol*. 2005;5:19.
3. Westwood ME, Whiting PF, Kleijnen J. How does study quality affect the results of a diagnostic meta-analysis? *BMC Med Res Methodol*. 2005;5:20.
4. Moses LE, Shapiro D, Littenberg B. Combining independent studies of a diagnostic test into a summary ROC curve: data-analytic approaches and some additional considerations. *Stat Med*. 1993;12:1293-1316.
5. Walter SD. Properties of the summary receiver operating characteristic (SROC) curve for diagnostic test data. *Stat Med*. 2002;21:1237-1256.
6. Reitsma JB, Glas AS, Rutjes AW, Scholten RJ, Bossuyt PM, Zwinderman AH. Bivariate analysis of sensitivity and specificity produces informative summary measures in diagnostic reviews. *J Clin Epidemiol*. 2005;58:982-990.
7. Harbord RM, Deeks JJ, Egger M, Whiting P, Sterne JA. A unification of models for meta-analysis of diagnostic accuracy studies. *Biostatistics*. 2007;8:239-251.
8. Rutter CM, Gatsonis CA. A hierarchical regression approach to meta-analysis of diagnostic test accuracy evaluations. *Stat Med*. 2001;20:2865-2884.
9. Macaskill P. Empirical Bayes estimates generated in a hierarchical summary ROC analysis agreed closely with those of a full Bayesian analysis. *J Clin Epidemiol*. 2004;57:925-932.

An Introduction to Decision Analysis

5

Christopher Rao, Ara Darzi, and Thanos Athanasiou

Abstract Clinicians learn to balance the intended benefits of alternative treatments against the risk of complications. Unfortunately, such implicit risk-benefit analysis is highly vulnerable to bias.

Decision analysis is a powerful tool that can be used to combine the best available evidence in order to aid clinicians in making rational decisions. It is most useful in complex clinical situations where there is uncertainty about model parameters or where many different outcomes can occur over different time scales. It can also be used as a tool to incorporate patient preference for the desirability of different outcomes into the decision-making process.

In this chapter, we explain the fundamental methodology and techniques used in decision analysis. We describe the potential applications of decision analysis in healthcare. We also discuss the more advanced decision analytical techniques that may also be encountered within the literature.

Abbreviations

CABG   Coronary Artery Bypass Graft
IHD   Ischaemic Heart Disease
PTCA   Percutaneous Transluminal Coronary Angiogram

C. Rao (✉)
Department of Surgery and Cancer, Imperial College London,
St Mary's Hospital Campus, London, UK
e-mail: christopher.rao@imperial.ac.uk

T. Athanasiou and A. Darzi (eds.), *Evidence Synthesis in Healthcare*,
DOI: 10.1007/978-0-85729-206-3_5, © Springer-Verlag London Limited 2011

5.1
Introduction

Decision making is inherent to clinical practice. Clinicians learn to intuitively balance the risk of negative outcomes resulting from alternative management strategies against the intended benefits. Unfortunately, such implicit risk-benefit analysis is highly vulnerable to bias for a number of reasons[1] and is problematic when decisions are complex and information is uncertain.[2]

"Decision Analysis is a formalization of the decision making process"[3] and can be used to overcome many of the weaknesses of intuitive decision making. It uses analytical tools to combine information from several sources, synthesise data when empirical data is absent or scarce, and explicitly explore the uncertainty associated with a decision.[4]

Decision analysis has its theoretical foundations in statistical decision theory,[5,6] a derivative of game theory described by von Neumann in the 1920s[7] and shares common theoretical origins with expected utility theory.[8] It also has very close associations with Bayesian statistical analysis, which is often applied to decision making.[9] It has been widely used in economics since the 1940s[2]; however, it was not used in healthcare until the late 1960s, when decision analysis was used to evaluate the outcomes of patients undergoing surgery for oral cancer.[10] Whilst decision analysis has not been widely used in healthcare research in the past,[11] it is increasing being used to estimate the long-term outcomes of healthcare interventions[12,13] and has become an important element of cost-effectiveness analysis (Chap. 6).[4]

In this chapter, we explain the fundamental methodology and techniques used in decision analysis. We describe the potential applications of decision analysis in healthcare. We also discuss the more advanced decision analytical techniques that may be encountered within the literature.

5.2
The Role of Decision Analysis in Healthcare Evaluation

Healthcare evaluation has two facets.[8] The first is the process of measurement. The process of measurement focuses on estimation and hypothesis testing using experimental studies, focusing on relatively few parameters and the relationships between these parameters. Often measured parameters are not of direct clinical importance, but are used as proxies for more clinically relevant outcomes which are more difficult to measure. For example, the effect of hypertension therapy on blood pressure is often measured rather than the effect of the therapy on myocardial infarction or mortality as larger studies would be required to detect statistically significant differences in these outcomes.

The second facet of clinical evaluation, decision analysis, involves using measured information on current practice from multiple sources to inform future practice. Optimal decision making requires identification of each possible strategy, knowledge of the likelihood of future events, and an analytical framework for balancing future risk and benefits.

Decisions are then based on the expected outcomes of each course of action. There should be an acceptance that there will always be some degree of uncertainty associated with a decision because of variation between individual patients, uncertainty associated with measured parameters, and uncertainty associated with analytical assumptions.[4,8]

5.3
The Principles of Decision Analysis

It is often helpful to divide the process of decision analysis into five sequential components[3]:

1. Identifying and bounding the problem
2. Structuring the problem, often using a *decision analytical model*
3. Acquiring necessary information or *populating the model*
4. Analysing the problem
5. Investigating the uncertainty associated with results of the analysis (*sensitivity analysis and alternative analysis*)

5.3.1
Identifying and Bounding the Problem

The first step is *identifying* the problem and breaking it down into manageable sections (often referred to as *bounding the problem*). All alternative courses of action, events that follow the initial courses of action, and relevant outcome measures should be identified.[2]

5.3.2
Structuring the Problem

In order to structure the problem, a decision analytical model is often constructed. This frequently takes the form of a *Decision Tree*. The decision tree is used to link actions with outcomes. It can then be used to calculate the probability and the value of outcomes. It is a useful tool as it forces the clinician to consider all possible outcomes, their desirability and the likelihood that they will happen.

Figure 5.1 illustrates a simple decision tree that was used to combine information on mortality and complications following deployment of different types of stents for the palliation of oesophageal cancer.[14] The decision tree is governed by a number of conventions; it is constructed from left to right, earlier events and choices are depicted on the left, later ones are depicted on the right. The decision tree consists of *nodes* and the lines that join the nodes are called *branches*. The squares, or decisions nodes, represent clinical decisions (e.g. whether a patient is treated with a metal or plastic stent). The circles represent chance occurrences (e.g. whether a patient may suffer complications or require re-intervention following stent insertion). Each possible chance occurrence has a probability assigned to

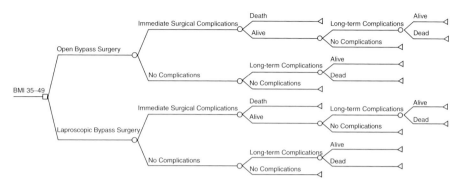

Fig. 5.1 A decision tree (Adapted from Siddiqui et al.[14])

it, called a *path probability* that represents the likelihood that the particular event will occur. The triangles or terminal nodes represent final outcomes such as death or a permanent cure. All terminal nodes have "*payoffs*" associated with them (e.g. improved quality of life or reduction in mortality). The payoffs and path probabilities are collectively called *model parameters*.

5.3.3
Acquiring the Model Parameters

Model parameters should be based on the highest quality, most relevant evidence. Strategies for searching and acquiring information should be explicit and comprehensive as models can easily be biased by a failure to include important evidence. When evidence has been synthesised, the methodology should be robust (Chap. 3).[11] The same rigour should be applied to ensure primary experimental or observational data is of a good quality. If data is used from randomised controlled trials, its relevance in a "real-world" setting should be examined. Data from observational trials should be examined for sources of potential bias.[4,8]

Often it is necessary to use expert estimation as there is an absence of information from other sources. Methods most commonly used to formalise the process of expert estimation such as the *Modified Nominal Group (NG)* and *Delphi method* focus on achieving consensus and do not explore the uncertainty associated with estimates.[15] This can limit the value of estimates obtained using these methods in decision analysis which focuses on exploring the uncertainty associated with a problem. If expert estimation is used, the reasons for doing so, the values of the estimations and the uncertainty associated with those values should be clearly justified.

5.3.4
Determine the Value of Each Alternative Strategy

To calculate the expected value for alternative courses of action, the values associated with each outcome, weighted by the likelihood that each outcome will occur, are added together. This is often called *rolling-back* the decision tree.

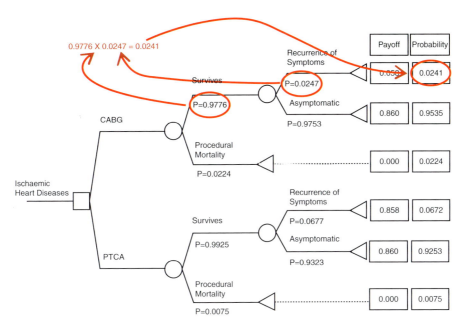

Fig. 5.2 "Rolling back the tree" – Stage 1. A hypothetical example comparing coronary artery bypass grafting (CABG) and percutaneous transluminal coronary angiogioplasty (PTCA) for the treatment of stable ischaemic heart disease (IHD)

This is achieved by first calculating the probability that each outcome will occur. As all chance nodes theoretically represent independent events, this is achieved by multiplying all probabilities between the decision node and the terminal node (Fig. 5.2). The expected value of each outcome is the product of the probability that the outcome will occur and the value or *payoff* associated with that outcome. The expected value associated with every outcome that could result from a course of action is then summed to calculate the expected value of that course of action (Fig. 5.3). Depending on whether a payoff has negative implications (such as a monetary cost that must be incurred) or positive implications (such as an improvement in quality of life), either a low or high expected value may be considered desirable.

5.3.5
Investigating Uncertainty

The explicit exploration of uncertainty is fundamental to decision analysis as there will always be some degree of uncertainty associated with the results.[2,4] This occurs for several reasons. Firstly, there will be uncertainty associated with the true values of parameters used to calculate input cost and effects (often called parameter or second-order uncertainty).[4,8] This often occurs because of practical problems in obtaining sufficient information to compare interventions; in particular, valuing health states and obtaining detailed costing data for newer interventions or interventions when long-term follow-up costs and

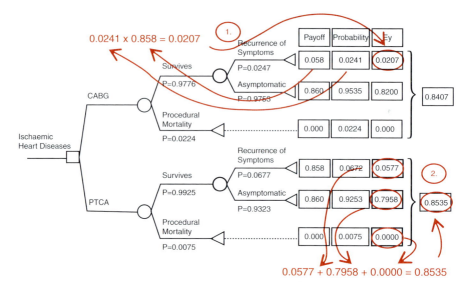

Fig. 5.3 "Rolling back the tree" – Stage 2. A hypothetical example comparing coronary artery bypass grafting (CABG) and percutaneous transluminal coronary angiogioplasty (PTCA) for the treatment of stable ischaemic heart disease (IHD)

outcomes need to be considered.[2,4,8] Secondly, there will be uncertainty because of individual patient variation (often called first-order uncertainty, or heterogeneity when explained and variability when unexplained). Finally, there will be uncertainty associated with the study design. For example, in studies based on decision analytical models, there will also be uncertainty associated with the model structure (see Chap. 6) whilst in experimental studies, there will be uncertainty associated with sources of potential bias.[11,16-18]

Different methods are commonly used to explore different sources of uncertainty. The effect of modelling assumptions and heterogeneity can be explored by adopting a reference case and conducting alternative analysis in which the effect of alternative modelling assumptions is explored. Parameter uncertainty is explored by conducting sensitivity analysis.

Sensitivity analysis can take the form of *univariate* (in which uncertainty associated with the value of one input parameter is explored), *multivariate* (in which the combined uncertainty associated with two or more parameters is explored) or *probabilistic* sensitivity analysis (in which the combined uncertainty of all model parameters is explored).[8]

5.3.5.1
Univariate Sensitivity Analysis

The simplest form of sensitivity analysis is *univariate* sensitivity analysis. In univariate sensitivity analysis, a single input parameter is varied from its highest value to its lowest value. The expected value of each alternative course of action is recalculated as the value of the input parameter is varied. If the optimum decision changes as the input parameter varies, the result is said to be *sensitive* to the uncertainty associated with this input parameter. This process can then be repeated for all the input parameters.

5.3.5.2
Multivariate Sensitivity Analysis

Often the combined uncertainty associated with two or more variables can cause the optimum decision to change when the uncertainty associated with either of these variables individually would not.

In order to explore the combined uncertainty associated with two input parameters, *two-way* or *bivariate* sensitivity analysis is performed. Both input parameters are varied from their highest to lowest value, and the model is recalculated for every combination of values. Figure 5.4 shows how this can be represented graphically. The different shaded areas represent the most effective strategy for different combinations of the two input parameters. Two-way sensitivity analysis is most useful when the result is not sensitive to either input parameters being investigated individually.

It is possible to perform three or four-way sensitivity analysis; however, it is time-consuming, difficult to interpret the results and difficult to represent the results graphically. Unless there are relatively few model parameters with associated uncertainty, then three or four-way sensitivity analysis is of questionable value.

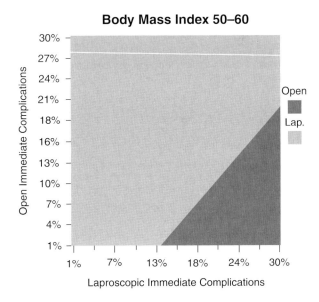

Fig. 5.4 Graphical representations of the results of bivariate sensitivity analysis (Adapted from Siddiqui et al.[14])

5.3.5.3
Probabilistic Sensitivity Analysis

In probabilistic sensitivity analysis, each parameter is assigned a probability distribution that reflects the uncertainty associated with that parameter. The expected value of each course of action is then recalculated several times (often 1,000 or even 10,000 times) with each of the parameters randomly sampled from the probability distributions every recalculation.[19] Many authors argue that this represents the most robust method for exploring and quantifying the uncertainty associated with a decision.[20]

The results of probabilistic sensitivity analysis can be presented as probability density distributions of the expected value of alternative courses of action, or the incremental expected value of one course of action compared to another. Figure 5.5a shows the distribution of the incremental expected value (measured in *Quality Adjusted Life Years*) adapted from a published decision analytical model.[13] Figure 5.5b shows the corresponding cumulative probability distribution, suggesting that bypass surgery can be said to be the optimum intervention with approximately 80% certainty.

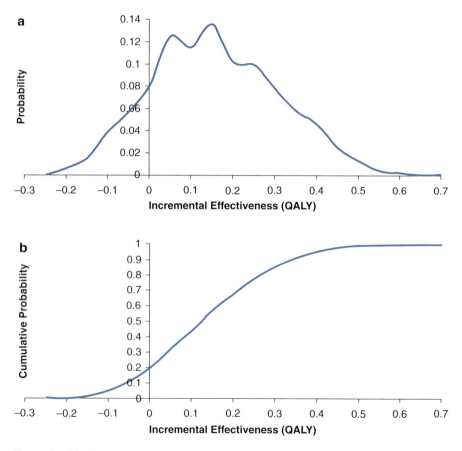

Fig. 5.5 Graphical representations of the results of probabilistic sensitivity analysis. (**a**) Probability density function. (**b**) Cumulative probability density function (Adapted from Rao et al.[13])

5.3.5.4
Alternative Analysis

The uncertainty associated with model structure and variables such as population demographics cannot easily be investigated in sensitivity analysis. Consequently, several *alternative analyses* are performed to investigate the uncertainty associated with these factors. For example, alternative analysis could be performed for male and female cohorts of differing ages, with appropriate morbidity and mortality.

5.4
Introducing Time Dependence

Whilst decision trees are powerful tools for analysing clinical decisions, they are cumbersome when the effects of a clinical decision must be examined over several years.[4] In an example from the literature, outcomes following two surgical techniques for replacing the mitral valve are compared.[12] Figure 5.6a shows a simple decision analytical model, designed to compare outcomes after mitral valve replacement, with and without preservation of the sub-valvular apparatus over a one-year time horizon. Figure 5.6b, by contrast, demonstrates that even when a relatively simple clinical problem is addressed over a longer time horizon, the tree becomes complex and analysis becomes difficult. An easier way to deal with the problem of modelling the long-term consequences of a health care intervention is to use *Markov modelling* or *simulation.*[2]

5.4.1
Constructing a Markov Model

In a Markov model (Fig. 5.7), a theoretical patient can exist in one of the several mutually exclusive health states. At the end of a defined period (a year or 6 months for example) called a *cycle*, a patient can continue to exist in that state, or can move to another state. The likelihood that a patient will change states is called a *transition probability*. There are two sorts of Markov model: a *Markov-Chain Simulation*, where the transition probabilities remain constant in all cycles; and a *Markov Process*, where the transition probabilities can vary as the cycles vary. For example, the baseline population mortality may increase with

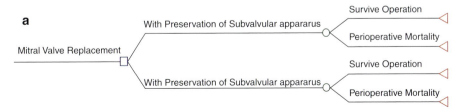

Fig. 5.6 Decision tree to investigate outcomes following mitral valve replacement. (**a**) One-year time horizon. (**b**) Ten-year time horizon

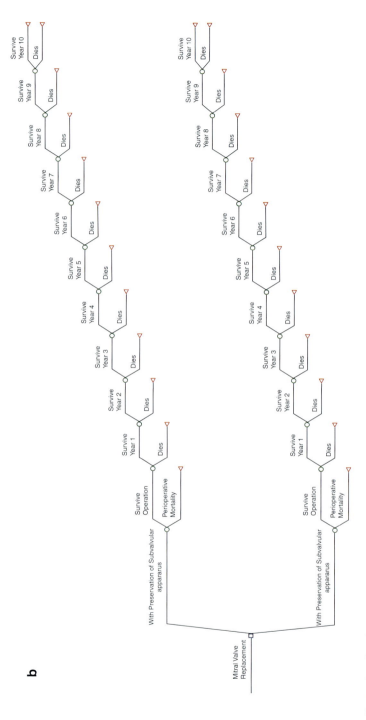

Fig. 5.6 (continued)

Fig. 5.7 A simple Markov model (Adapted from Rao et al.[12])

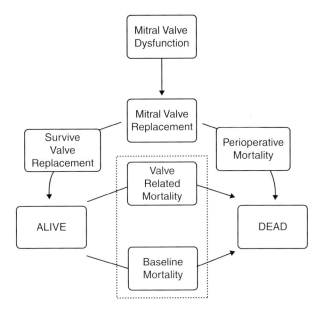

increasing patient age. To calculate transition probabilities from incidence obtained from experimental, observational or meta-analytical data, the following formulas are used:

$$R = -1 \,/\, P x ln(1 - I)$$

$$T = 1 - exp^{-RxC}$$

Where I = the incidence of the event of interest in the study population, P = the period over which the data was collected, R = rate at which the event of interest occurs, T = the transition probability, C = the cycle length.

Some states, are called *absorbing states*, as when a patient enters this state, they cannot leave, for example death. The simulation continues until the patient enters an absorbing state or other defined criteria are fulfilled. For example, one of the termination conditions could be that the simulation should terminate after ten cycles. If each cycle were 1 year in duration, the time horizon would then be said to be 10 years. As a patient passes through health states, in each cycle they accumulate benefits, or incur costs depending on which states they pass through. The rewards that the hypothetical patient has accumulated during the simulation are then added together to calculate the payoff of the intervention or course of action for that particular patient.[4,8,21]

5.4.2
Analysing a Markov Model

The Markov simulation is run several thousand times. The rewards that the hypothetical patients have accumulated during the simulations are averaged to obtain results for a

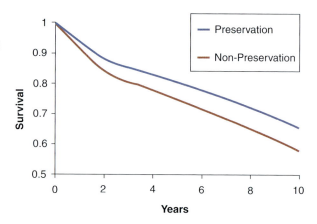

Fig. 5.8 Survival curves constructed using the results of a Markov model (Adapted from Rao et al.[12])

hypothetical cohort of patients. This is called *microsimulation*. It is an important approach when evaluating interventions for infectious diseases as it can be adapted to model the interaction between individual patients. A more computationally efficient method is to sample expected values for all model input parameters and calculate the payoffs for a whole patient cohort. In both cases, new values of the model input parameters are then re-sampled and the process is repeated several hundred or several thousand times in order to perform probabilistic sensitivity analysis, similar to the way a decision tree is analysed.[4]

It is also possible to calculate the proportion of patients who where in each of the Markov states during each cycle. This information can be used to construct survival curves for patient cohorts following each intervention (Fig. 5.8).

5.5
Limitations of Decision Analysis

The challenges faced by those seeking to use decision analysis can be thought of as either relating to *populating the model* or *structuring the model*.

- Many of the challenges faced by those seeking to undertake decision analysis relate to the difficulty in acquiring estimates of model parameters. This is a particular problem for new diagnostic tests, procedures or treatments where long-term data may be limited and interventions may not have been directly compared. It is important to ensure the model is generalisable and avoids bias when estimating model input parameters; consequently, a robust search strategy for estimates of model parameters is essential. Particularly, care must be taken when evidence is synthesised or expert estimation is used to ensure that the methodology is robust and explicit.[16,20,22]
- Decision analysis is a powerful tool that can be used to simplify or structure complex clinical problems in order to assist decision makers. However, sometimes clinical problems are so complex that they cannot easily be reduced to a simple list of outcomes. In

complicated decision problems, it is also often exceedingly laborious and computationally demanding to analyse the model.[2] Validating and exploring the uncertainty associated with model structure present a further problem, especially when there is limited empirical evidence about the new intervention, or emerging disease that is being modelled.[22]

Whilst structuring and populating decision analytical models are challenging, decision makers have always faced challenges relating to the synthesis and interpretation of clinical evidence. Arguably, the explicit structuring of clinical problems, synthesis and weighting of evidence inherent in decision analysis is an improvement on the implicit and opaque criteria previously used by decision makers previously.[16,22] In the words of the twentieth century statistician George Box, '*all models are wrong, but some are useful*'.[4]

5.6
Conclusion

Decision analysis is a powerful tool that can be used to combine the best available evidence in order to aid clinicians in making rational decisions. It is most useful in complex clinical situations where there is uncertainty about model parameters or where many different outcomes can occur over different time scales. It can also be used as a tool to incorporate patient preference for the desirability of different outcomes into the decision-making process.[11]

Decision analytical modelling has been widely and successfully applied in the corporate world and defence sector for a number of years and research currently focuses on how analytical techniques can be expanded to evaluate more complex strategic problems.[1] However, it is not applied in many clinical situations in which it could prove most useful, arguably because many within the medical profession and clinical research are unfamiliar or even resistant to decision analytical techniques.[17] The potential of decision analytical modelling is being explored by the Medical Research Council, one of the largest funding bodies in the UK. It is already fundamental to the National Institute for Health and Clinical Excellence and National Coordinating Centre for Health Technology Assessment programmes[17,23]; and given its increasingly frequent appearance in the medical literature,[2] it is likely that it will become more widely applied in clinical practice.

References

1. Edwards W, Miles RF Jr, von Winterfeldt D. *Advances in Decision Analysis: From Foundations to Applications*. New York: Cambridge University Press; 2007.
2. Petitti DB. *Meta-Analysis, Decision Analysis and Cost-Effectiveness Analysis: Methods for Quantitative Synthesis in Medicine*. New York: Oxford University Press; 2000.
3. Weinstein MC, Fineberg HV. *Clinical Decision Analysis*. Philadelphia: Saunders; 1980.
4. Briggs A, Sculpher M, Claxton K. *Decision Modelling for Health Economic Evaluation*. Oxford: Oxford University Press; 2006.

5. Raiffa H, Schlaifer R. *Probability and Statistics for Business Decisions*. New York: McGaw-Hill; 1959.

6. Raiffa H. *Decision Analysis: Introductory Lectures on Choices Under Uncertainty*. Reading: Addison-Wesley; 1968.

7. Von Neumann J, Morgenstern O. *Theory of Games and Economic Theory*. New York: Wiley; 1947.

8. Drummond MF, Sculpher MJ, Torrance GW, O'Brien BJ, Stoddart GL. *Methods for the Economic Evaluation of Health Care Programmes*. Oxford: Oxford University Press; 2005.

9. Spiegelhalter DJ, Abrahams KR, Myles JP. *Bayesian Approaches to Clinical Trials and Health Care Evaluation*. Chichester: Wiley; 2003.

10. Henschke UK, Flehinger BJ. Decision theory in cancer therapy. *Cancer*. 1967;20:1819-1826.

11. Friedland DJ, Go AS, Davoren JB, et al. *Evidence-Based Medicine: A Framework for Clinical Practice*. Stamford: Conn Appleton & Lange; 1998.

12. Rao C, Hart J, Chow A, et al. Does preservation of the sub-valvular apparatus during mitral valve replacement affect long-term survival and quality of life? A microsimulation study. *J Cardiothorac Surg*. 2008;3:17.

13. Rao C, Stanbridge RL, Chikwe J, et al. Does previous percutaneous coronary stenting compromise the long-term efficacy of subsequent coronary artery bypass surgery? A microsimulation study. *Ann Thorac Surg*. 2008;85:501-507.

14. Siddiqui A, Livingston E, Huerta S. A comparison of open and laparoscopic Roux-en-Y gastric bypass surgery for morbid and super obesity: A decision-analysis model. *Am J Surg*. 2006;192:e1-7.

15. Hutchings A, Raine R, Sanderson C, Black N. A comparison of formal consensus methods used for developing clinical guidelines. *J Health Serv Res Policy*. 2006;11:218-224.

16. Claxton K, Cohen JT, Neumann PJ. When is evidence sufficient? *Health Aff (Millwood)*. 2005;24:93-101.

17. Claxton K, Eggington S, Ginnelly L, et al. *A Pilot Study of Value of Information Analysis to Support Research Recommendations for the National Institute for Health and Clinical Excellence York*. University of York: Centre for Health Economics; 2005.

18. Guide to the Methods of Technology Appraisal. London: National Institute for Clinical Excellence (NICE); 2004.

19. Gold MR, Siegel JE, Russell LB, Weinstein MC. *Cost-Effectiveness in Health and Medicine*. New York: Oxford University Press; 1996.

20. Philips Z, Ginnelly L, Sculpher M, et al. Review of guidelines for good practice in decision-analytic modelling in health technology assessment. *Health Technol Assess*. 2004;8:iii-v. ix–xi, 1–158.

21. Muennig P. *Designing and Conducting Cost-Effectiveness Analysis in Health and Medicine*. San Francisco: Jossey-Bass; 2002.

22. Brennan A, Kharroubi S, O'Hagan A, Chilcott J. Calculating partial expected value of perfect information via Monte Carlo sampling algorithms. *Med Decis Making*. 2007;27:448-470.

23. Claxton K, Ginnelly L, Sculpher M, Philips Z, Palmer S. *A Pilot Study on the Use of Decision Theory and Value of Information Analysis as Part of the NHS Health Technology Assessment Programme*. 2004:1-103. iii.

An Introduction to Cost-Effectiveness Analysis

6

Christopher Rao, Kathie A. Wong, and Thanos Athanasiou

Abstract Cost-effectiveness analysis is now widely used to evaluate whether the effect of a healthcare intervention justifies additional expenditure. In this chapter, we outline the principles of cost-effectiveness analysis and compare different types of cost-effectiveness analysis. We discuss interpretation of cost-effectiveness analyses, graphical representations of the results of cost-effectiveness data, the benefits and limitations of cost-effectiveness analysis.

Abbreviations

CET   Cost-effectiveness Threshold
HRQoL   Health-related quality of life
ICER   Incremental cost-effectiveness ratio
NHS   National Health Service
NICE   National Institute of Clinical Excellence
NMB   Net monetary benefit
QALY   Quality-adjusted life years
WTP   Willingness to pay

6.1 Introduction

Cost-effectiveness or *Economic Analysis* was developed to evaluate whether the effect of a healthcare intervention justifies additional expenditure. It has been used by insurance companies, governmental organisations and agencies,[1] manufacturers and clinicians to justify

C. Rao (✉)
Department of Surgery and Cancer, Imperial College London,
St Mary's Hospital Campus, London, UK
e-mail: christopher.rao@imperial.ac.uk

T. Athanasiou and A. Darzi (eds.), *Evidence Synthesis in Healthcare*,
DOI: 10.1007/978-0-85729-206-3_6, © Springer-Verlag London Limited 2011

investing or withholding resources.[2-4] The term *cost-effective* is often mistakenly applied to an intervention which has been demonstrated to be effective without consideration of its cost, or cost-saving in the absence of information about its effectiveness; however, both costs and effects must be considered. Frequent misuse of the term undoubtedly contributes to widespread confusion about its meaning.[5]

In this chapter, we outline the principles of cost-effectiveness analysis and compare different types of cost-effectiveness analysis. We discuss the interpretation of cost-effectiveness data and the graphical representations of the results of cost-effectiveness analysis. Finally, we discuss the strengths, limitations and applications of cost-effectiveness analysis.

6.2
Perspective

When only costs and benefits relevant to a particular organisation or group are considered, the analysis is said to have been performed from the *perspective* of that particular organisation or group. For example, a *patient perspective* when all the costs incurred by individual patients are included; a *third-party payer perspective* (either *private* such as an insurance company, or *public* such as a government health programme) when all the costs incurred by that organisation are considered; or a *societal perspective* when all costs and consequences to all stakeholders within the borders of a country are considered.[6]

The perspective adopted for cost-effectiveness analysis significantly affects estimates of the costs and benefits associated with an intervention. For example, if we consider the total cost of a hernia repair to a *third-party payer*, such as the government, we must include the cost of pre-operative care, the cost of the procedure itself, the cost of outpatient follow-up, the costs incurred in primary healthcare, and the potential costs of treating recurrence of the hernia or complications of the procedure. If we consider the cost incurred by the patient for the same procedure, all of the previous costs would be irrelevant and we would only need to consider the cost of travel expenses and loss of earnings.

A standard perspective or "*reference case*" has been advocated by some authors[2]; however, there is no consensus on what perspective should be used in cost-effectiveness analysis. In the UK, the *National Institute for Health and Clinical Excellence (NICE)* recommends a *National Health Service (NHS)* (third-party payer) perspective[1]; however others favour a societal perspective.[2] Ultimately, whatever perspective is adopted, it is important that it is explicitly stated, as interpretation of cost-effectiveness data is impossible when the perspective is unclear.[7]

6.3
Measures of Effect

Cost-effectiveness analyses can be classified according to how outcomes (or effects) of the interventions are measured. In this section, we will discuss the most frequently used methods.

6.3.1
Cost-Minimisation Analysis

In cost-minimisation analysis, it is assumed that alternative interventions are equally effective. Interventions are compared simply on the basis of cost. This method does not facilitate examination of uncertainty associated with the relative effectiveness of interventions. As we can rarely be sure that two interventions are equally effective on every occasion in all patients, cost-minimisation analysis is not an appropriate study design in most cases, and is no-longer widely used.[8]

6.3.2
Cost-Effectiveness Analysis

The term *cost-effectiveness analysis* is confusingly also commonly applied to a subset of economic analysis in which the effect can be any non-monetary parameter that relates to the effect of the interventions, for example "cost per episode free day" for chronic diseases,[9] or "cost per case detected" for a diagnostic tests.[10] This allows comparison of alternative interventions for the same disease within the same field, for example surgical management and conservative therapy for peripheral vascular disease. It is not, however, possible to compare the cost-effectiveness of interventions for different diseases.[7]

6.3.3
Cost-Benefit Analysis

In cost-benefit analysis, both the costs and effects are expressed in monetary units. This has significant advantages and disadvantages. Unlike other forms of analysis cost-benefit analysis evaluates the absolute benefit of a programme without reference to other interventions, and if the costs (inputs) are less than the effects (outputs), than the programme can be considered cost-effective.[7] The other significant advantage of cost-benefit analysis is that it facilitates comparison of healthcare interventions with other public spending, for educational or infrastructure projects.[6]

The disadvantages of cost-benefit analysis are related to the ethical and practical problems associated with valuing morbidity and mortality. Many authors object to cost-benefit analysis, arguing that valuing health in monetary terms implicitly favours health-interventions for diseases of the affluent. Others find valuing human life distasteful. For these reasons, cost-benefit analysis is rarely used in healthcare.[5-7]

6.3.4
Cost-Utility Analysis

Whereas cost-effectiveness analysis uses natural, programme-specific, measures of effect such as symptom-free day,[9] cost-utility analysis uses quality-adjusted measures of effect, for example Quality-Adjusted Life Years (QALY), Health-Adjusted Life Years (HALY) or Disability-Adjusted Life Years (DALY).[6] Many authors either make no distinction between cost-effectiveness and cost-utility analysis[2] or argue that cost-utility analysis is a subtype of cost-effectiveness analysis.[5]

Cost-utility analysis has several advantages: it allows consideration of both mortality and morbidity from all causes when evaluating the effectiveness of an intervention, it facilitates comparison of cost-effectiveness between healthcare disciplines, and allows values to be attached to outcomes which are considered good or bad.[6,7] As QALY are perhaps the most commonly used measures of effect in cost-effectiveness analysis, we will discuss them in more detail in the following section.

6.4
The Quality-Adjusted Life Year

The concept of the QALY was first introduced in 1968,[11] and the term "QALY" had become widely used by the late 1970s.[12] QALY account for the effect an intervention on either the length or quality of life by multiplying the change in *Health-Related Quality of Life (HRQoL)* (quantified using a *utility* score) by the change in the length of life, as follows[5]:

$$\Delta QALYs = \Delta Utility\ of\ Health\ State \times \Delta Length\ of\ Life$$

Utility scoring can be thought of as a method of quantifying the strength of a patient's preference for a particular health sate or outcome. Conventionally, a utility of 1 is deemed to be equivalent to perfect health and 0 is deemed to be equivalent to death. Most health states are assigned utility values that are between 1 and 0, with health states considered worse than death assigned negative values. There are several methods for determining utility values such as interval scaling, the standard gamble and the time trade-off methods. Unfortunately, these methods are time consuming and conceptually difficult for the patient. Alternatively, pre-scored multi-attribute health status classification systems such as the EQ-5D system formulated by the EuroQol Group (www.euroqol.org), the Quality of Well-Being (QWB) questionnaire, the Health utilities Index (HUI) and the Short form 6D (SF-6D) can be used. These consist of questionnaires with scoring systems that have been validated in large population groups.[2,5,7]

As all methods for quantifying utility are grounded in economic decision theory, their validity and consequently the validity of QALY are dependent on important assumptions. It is assumed that patients will behave rationally to maximise their personal satisfaction or utility, that they are willing to trade years of life in a given health state for fewer years in a better health state, and that patients are risk neutral.[7] Several authors suggest that these assumptions may not be valid in clinical practice. In particular, studies have suggested that not only is there considerable variation between participants in their attitude to risk, but the same participants often have different attitudes to risk in different circumstances or even in the same circumstance when questioned differently.[13]

It has also been argued that QALY do not reflect societal preferences. For example, implicit in cost-effectiveness analysis is the assumption that QALY are equally valuable no matter at what age and to whom they are assigned. Whilst this may appear egalitarian, society may prefer to assign QALY to a patient who is very ill rather than to a patient who is comparatively well; or to a patient who has been ill most of their life, rather than to a patient who has been well most of their life.[7]

It is argued that the QALY represent a close enough approximation of individual and societal preference to justify their use, despite the weaknesses described,[2] and in the absence of functional and robust alternatives, they are widely used in cost-effectiveness analysis.

6.5
Discounting

Most people would rather have $100 now rather than $100 in 10 years time, even when the $100 is adjusted for inflation. This is called "*positive time preference*" and occurs for several of reasons. Firstly, future financial gains are less valuable than current gains as society is becoming wealthier. Secondly, individuals are generally risk averse, often preferring definite returns now to possible returns in the future. Finally, there is no opportunity to use or invest future financial gains (so-called opportunity cost).[7]

For these reasons, future costs are devalued, or *discounted*, in cost-effectiveness analysis using the following formula:

$$X = C_y / (1 + r)^y$$

Where X=the discounted future cost, C_y=the future cost, incurred at year=y and r=the annual discount rate.

Discounting outcomes is more controversial. The current convention is to discount all benefits of an intervention even when they are not monetary as most people would prefer to have a year of perfect health now rather than a year of perfect health at the end of their life. Critics argue, however, that health benefits are not transferable like monetary benefits.

In the UK, the discount rate is currently set by the treasury at 3.5% for all public service projects and NICE recommend using the limits of 0–6% in sensitivity analysis.[1,7] The United States Panel on the Cost-effectiveness of Medicine recommended a discount rate of 3% (0–5% for sensitivity analysis),[2] whilst the World Health Organisation recommends 3% (0–6% for sensitivity analysis).[14] However, many authors continue to use 5% in order to facilitate comparison with the large body of published data based on a discount rate of 5%. Most cost-effectiveness analyses do not account for inflation as it is assumed that all costs will inflate at the same rate.[7]

6.6
Interpreting the Results of Economic Analysis

6.6.1
The Incremental Cost-Effectiveness Ratio

When an intervention is both less costly and more effective than the alternative, it is clearly more cost-effective and is said to be *dominant*. However, it is more problematic when the more effective intervention is also more costly: which intervention should the decision maker choose? As this situation commonly accompanies innovation in healthcare, the results of cost-effectiveness analysis are often expressed using an *Incremental Cost-Effectiveness Ratio (ICER)*. The ICER represents the ratio of the difference in costs between interventions, to the difference in effectiveness between interventions. It is calculated as follows:

$$ICER = \frac{C_x - C_y}{E_x - E_y}$$

Where C_x = the cost of intervention X, C_y = the cost of intervention Y, E_x = the effectiveness of interventions X and E_y = the effectiveness of interventions Y.[5]

There are two ways in which to interpret the ICER. It can be compared to the ICER of other interventions or it can be compared to a *Cost-Effectiveness Threshold (CET)*.[7]

6.6.2
Ranking Cost-Effectiveness Ratios

There was a trend to rank cost-effectiveness ratios to allow readers to put them into perspective (Table 6.1). Cost-effectiveness ratios are now rarely ranked in this way as in order to interpret "league tables," there must be methodological homogeneity between studies.[7] This seldom occurs.[1,2,15] Ranking cost-effectiveness ratios is also criticised because it does not account for the uncertainty associated with the ratios.[7]

6.6.3
The Cost-Effectiveness Threshold

Inherent to the cost-effectiveness "league table" as a tool to inform decision makers is the idea that, going down the table, at some point, the interventions will cease to be cost-effective. The cost-effectiveness ratio at this point could be termed the *Cost-Effectiveness Threshold (CET)*. If the ICER of an intervention is less than the CET, it can be said to be

Table 6.1 Cost-effectiveness league table

Intervention	ICER (£/QALY)
Cholesterol testing and diet therapy only (all adults, aged 40–69)	220
Pacemaker implantation	1,100
Cholesterol testing and treatment	1,480
Kidney transplant	4,710
Neurosurgical intervention for malignant intracranial tumours	107,780

Source: Adapted from Drummond et al.[7]

cost-effective. The CET represents the amount that the healthcare provider is prepared to pay for an improvement of one QALY.[7]

Anecdotal evidence that different CETs are applied in different areas of healthcare in the UK[16] suggests that decision makers consider socio-economic factors as well as cost-effectiveness when determining research allocation. Critics of a universal CET argue that it fails to account for social priorities such as equity or disease burden. It is also argued that the amount that a healthcare provider is willing to pay for health improvement cannot be independent of the cost of implementing health improvement programmes.[7] For example, a healthcare provider may not be able to afford to implement the most cost-effective and expensive intervention and might instead be compelled to choose a cheaper and less cost-effective alternative. Whilst decision analytical tools are being developed to maximise benefits within the constraints of a finite budget,[13] their complexity currently makes widespread application in healthcare problematic and the details of these modelling techniques lie outside the scope of this book.

Other critics of the universal CET argue that it has no place in cost-effectiveness analysis as researchers, who have no expertise in policy making, should not state whether an intervention is cost-effective and should simply provide decision makers with the facts.[6] The desire by researchers to put their results into context is however natural and legitimate.[7] Furthermore, the distinction between researcher and policy maker is often not clearly demarcated, and often the adoption of new technology is driven by clinicians and not policy makers.

Despite these criticisms of the CET, it is a useful tool which is widely used and accepted in the published literature and by national healthcare intervention assessment programmes. The CET of US$50,000/QALY is often used in the published literature. A study of the decisions of the Australian Pharmaceutical Benefit Advisory Committee suggests that they are unlikely to accept interventions with an ICER in excess of AUS $76,000/QALY and unlikely to reject an intervention with an ICER of less than AUS $42,000/QALY. In the UK, NICE loosely apply CET of £30,000/QALY in cases where efficacy is proven and £20,000/QALY in cases where clinical effectiveness is more controversial.[7]

When the incremental cost is plotted against the incremental effect, this is called the *cost-effectiveness plane*.[6] The CET and ICER can be plotted on the cost-effectiveness plane (Fig. 6.1). The quadrants of the cost-effectiveness plane are often numbered from I to IV, starting in the top right-hand quadrant. If we plot the incremental cost against the incremental effect for an intervention and it lies in quadrant II, the intervention is cost-effective and said to be *dominant*, as it is both cheaper and more effective. If it lies in quadrant IV, it is said to be *dominated* as the alternative intervention is both cheaper and more effective than the intervention. If it is in quadrant I above the CET, then the intervention, despite being more effective, is said to be too expensive. Conversely, if it is below the CET, greater effectiveness is thought to justify the extra costs and the intervention is cost-effective.[6,7] It is more problematic if the plot lies in quadrant III as it has been suggested that the compensation that patients expect when they forego a more effective intervention is considerably more than they are prepared to pay for the same programme. Consequently, the CET would probably look more like the solid grey line in quadrant III.[17]

Fig. 6.1 The cost-effectiveness plane

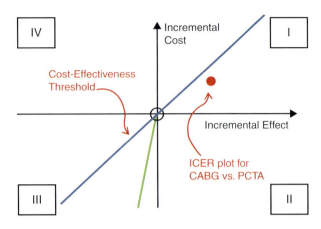

6.6.4
The Willingness-to-Pay Threshold

The notion that an intervention is cost-effective if the ICER is less than the CET can be expressed as follows:

$$\Delta C / \Delta E < T$$

Where ΔC = the incremental cost, ΔE = the incremental effect and T = the cost-effectiveness threshold.

This can be rearranged to:

$$T\Delta E - \Delta C > 0$$

"$T\Delta E - \Delta C$" is called the *Net Monetary Benefit (NMB)*.

As it represents the amount a healthcare provider is willing to pay for an increase in effectiveness of ΔE, minus the associated increase in costs, ΔC, an intervention can be said to be cost-effective if:

$$NMB = T\Delta E - \Delta C > 0$$

As the *willingness-to-pay threshold* (WTP) (which is analogous to the CET) is generally unknown, the results of cost-effectiveness analyses can be presented graphically in the following way (Fig. 6.2). The advantage of presenting the results in the form of a linear function of the WTP and NMB is that it is easier to manipulate and interpret than a ratio of incremental costs and effects.[7,18]

6.7
Handling Uncertainty

The explicit exploration of uncertainty is important in cost-effectiveness analysis as there will always be some degree of uncertainty associated with parameter and individual patient variation (see Chap. 5). There will also be uncertainty associated with the study design.

Fig. 6.2 Threshold analysis

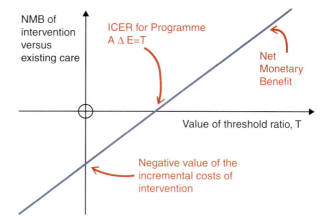

For example, in studies based on decision analytical models, there will also be uncertainty associated with the model structure (see Chap. 5) whilst in experimental studies, there will be uncertainty associated with sources of potential bias.[2,6,7,18]

Different methods are commonly used to explore different sources of uncertainty. The effect of modelling assumptions and different patient populations on the cost-effectiveness of an intervention can be explored by adopting a reference case and conducting *alternative analysis* in which the effect of alternative modelling assumptions is explored. Parameter uncertainty is explored by conducting *sensitivity analysis*.

6.7.1
Sensitivity Analysis

Sensitivity analysis can take the form of *univariate, bivariate* or *probabilistic* sensitivity analysis (see Chap. 5).[6] Probabilistic is recommended in several guidelines for economic analysis, and consequently now appears more frequently in the literature than univariate and bivariate sensitivity analysis.[1]

Probabilistic sensitivity analysis in a cost-effectiveness study is performed using a similar method to probabilistic sensitivity analysis of decision analytical data. Each parameter is assigned a probability distribution that reflects the uncertainty associated with that parameter. The incremental cost and effect is then recalculated several times (often 1,000 or even 10,000 times) with each of the parameters randomly sampled from the probability distributions every recalculation.[18] The ICER can then be calculated from the mean incremental cost and effect.

6.7.2
Interpreting the Results of Probabilistic Sensitivity Analysis

It is conceptually difficult to quantify the uncertainty associated with the ICER using conventional statistical tools, such as the mean and standard deviation, as a negative ICER could result from the incremental cost being negative and the incremental effect being positive (i.e. the intervention is dominant) or the incremental cost being positive and the incremental effect being negative (i.e. the intervention is dominated).

This problem is often overcome in the literature by plotting the results of each model recalculation from the probabilistic sensitivity analysis on to the cost-effectiveness plane (Fig. 6.3). This allows the reader to make rough approximations of the proportion of points that fall into each quadrant or lie below the cost-effectiveness plane. The number and density of plots, however, make it impossible for the reader to quantify the results of sensitivity analysis. This method is also problematic because the CET is rarely known, and as Fig. 6.4 illustrates, if the position of the CET on the plane changes, the proportion of plots that lie below the cost-effectiveness plane will also change.[7,18]

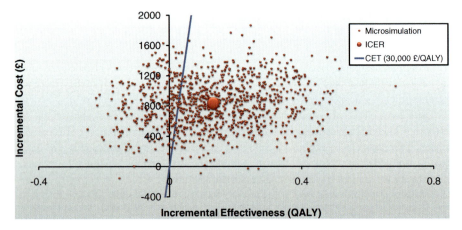

Fig. 6.3 The Cost-effectiveness plane showing the results of probabilistic sensitivity analysis (Adapted from Rao[4])

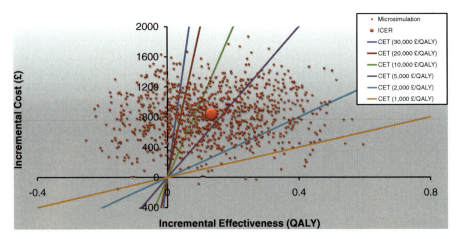

Fig. 6.4 The Cost-effectiveness plane showing the effect of different cost-effectiveness thresholds (Adapted from Rao[4])

The *willingness-to-pay* or *cost-effectiveness acceptability curve* (Fig. 6.5) is a useful alternative to the cost-effectiveness plane for presenting the results of a probabilistic sensitivity analysis. For each WTP, the proportion of the model recalculations that are below the CET are plotted. The willingness-to-pay curve represents a more intuitive representation of the uncertainty associated with the cost-effectiveness of an intervention. It is usually interpreted in a Bayesian fashion; thus, for every WTP, the curve represents the probability that the intervention is most cost-effective. The willingness-to-pay curve can be plotted for several competing healthcare interventions in order to illustrate to decision makers how the cost-effectiveness and associated uncertainty are affected by the amount they are willing to pay for health improvement (Fig. 6.6).[7,18] The WTP curve represents a robust analytical framework to explicitly explore the effect of uncertainty which can be extended to assess the need and value of further research.[18]

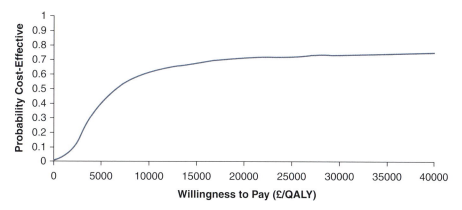

Fig. 6.5 Willingness-to-pay curve (Adapted from Rao[4])

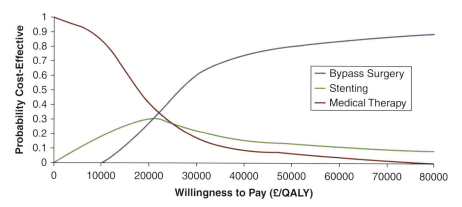

Fig. 6.6 Willingness-to-pay curve illustrating the cost-effectiveness of several interventions (Adapted from Griffin[3])

6.8
Limitations of Cost-Effectiveness Analysis

The adoption of a new healthcare intervention is not purely an economic decision as social, political, ethical and moral considerations are also important. For example, a decision maker who is concerned with alleviating health inequality may feel an intervention is important as it targets a disease associated with social deprivation, or a risk adverse decision maker may be more reluctant to adopt new or unproven technology.[5,7] Cost-effectiveness analysis is criticised as it cannot account for such considerations. Furthermore, it is suggested that cost-effectiveness analysis does not account for all important economic considerations, such as the effect of a programme's size on a decision maker's threshold for adopting it.[7]

Even the most ardent advocate of cost-effectiveness analysis would argue, however, that the results of cost-effectiveness analysis are not intended to be applied in a mechanistic fashion: that it is merely a tool for decision makers and not a replacement.[2,5,7]

6.9
Conclusion

Cost-effectiveness analysis in healthcare is a relatively new field of healthcare research. Many of the concepts may be unfamiliar and poorly understood by clinicians and researchers. There may also be some reluctance to accept that clinical practice should be influenced by external factors like cost. Consequently, cost-effectiveness analysis has not historically been applied in situations when it would most impact on patient care.[5,6,19]

In the western world, however, aging populations, increasing expectations of healthcare and the cost of modern medical practice stretch the finite resources available for healthcare and exert considerable pressure to rationalise health resources allocation.[2,20,21] Whilst cost-effectiveness analysis is currently a challenging field for many clinicians and researchers, as the methods and concepts become more widely understood, the range of clinical situations where cost-effectiveness analysis is applied will increase. Furthermore, the potential population health benefits of resource optimisation arguably place an ethical responsibility on clinicians and researchers to consider these issues.

References

1. National Institute for Clinical Excellence (NICE). *Guide to the Methods of Technology Appraisal*. London: NICE; 2004.
2. Gold MR, Siegel JE, Russell LB, Weinstein MC. *Cost-Effectiveness in Health and Medicine*. New York: Oxford University Press; 1996.
3. Griffin SC, Barber JA, Manca A, et al. Cost effectiveness of clinically appropriate decisions on alternative treatments for angina pectoris: prospective observational study. *BMJ*. 2007; 334:624.

4. Rao C, Aziz O, Panesar SS, et al. Cost effectiveness analysis of minimally invasive internal thoracic artery bypass versus percutaneous revascularisation for isolated lesions of the left anterior descending artery. *BMJ*. 2007;334:621.

5. Petitti DB. *Meta-Analysis, Decision Analysis and Cost-Effectiveness Analysis: Methods for Quantitative Synthesis in Medicine*. New York: Oxford University Press; 2000.

6. Muennig P. *Designing and Conducting Cost-Effectiveness Analysis in Health and Medicine*. San Francisco: Jossey-Bass; 2002.

7. Drummond MF, Sculpher MJ, Torrance GW, O'Brien BJ, Stoddart GL. *Methods for the Economic Evaluation of Health Care Programmes*. Oxford: Oxford University Press; 2005.

8. Briggs AH, O'Brien BJ. The death of cost-minimization analysis? *Health Econ*. 2001;10: 179-184.

9. Sculpher MJ, Buxton MJ. The episode-free day as a composite measure of effectiveness: an illustrative economic evaluation of formoterol versus salbutamol in asthma therapy. *Pharmacoeconomics*. 1993;4:345-352.

10. Hull R, Hirsh J, Sackett DL, Stoddart G. Cost effectiveness of clinical diagnosis, venography, and noninvasive testing in patients with symptomatic deep-vein thrombosis. *N Engl J Med*. 1981;304:1561-1567.

11. Klarman H, Francis J, Rosenthal G. Cost-effectiveness analysis applied to the treatment of chronic renal disease. *Med Care*. 1968;6:48-54.

12. Weinstein MC, Stason WB. Foundations of cost-effectiveness analysis for health and medical practices. *N Engl J Med*. 1977;296:716-721.

13. Edwards W, Miles RF Jr, von Winterfeldt D. *Advances in Decision Analysis: From Foundations to Applications*. New York: Cambridge University Press; 2007.

14. Tan Torres T, Baltussen RM, Adam T, et al. *Making Choices in Health: WHO Guide to Cost-effectiveness Analysis*. Geneva: World Health Organization; 2003.

15. Drummond M, Torrance G, Mason J. Cost-effectiveness league tables: more harm than good? *Soc Sci Med*. 1993;37:33-40.

16. Appleby J, Devlin N, Parkin D. NICE's cost effectiveness threshold. *BMJ*. 2007;335:358-359.

17. O'Brien BJ, Gertsen K, Willan AR, Faulkner LA. Is there a kink in consumers' threshold value for cost-effectiveness in health care? *Health Econ*. 2002;11:175-180.

18. Briggs A, Sculpher M, Claxton K. *Decision Modelling for Health Economic Evaluation*. Oxford: Oxford University Press; 2006.

19. Friedland DJ, Go AS, Davoren JB, et al. *Evidence-Based Medicine: A Framework for Clinical Practice*. Stamford: Conn Appleton & Lange; 1998.

20. Ham C. *Health Policy in Britain: The Politics and Organisation of the National Health Service*. London: Palgrave Macmillan; 2004.

21. Talbot-Smith A, Pollock AM. *The New NHS: A Guide*. Abingdon: Routlage; 2006.

Evidence Synthesis Using Bayesian Belief Networks

7

Zhifang Ni, Lawrence D. Phillips, and George B. Hanna

Abstract Bayesian belief networks (BBNs) are graphical tools for reasoning with uncertainties. In BBNs, uncertain events are represented as nodes and their relationships as links, with missing links indicating conditional independence. BBNs perform belief updating when new information becomes available; they can handle incomplete information and capture expert judgments along with data. BBNs provide a normative framework for synthesizing uncertain evidence.

Abbreviations

BBN   Bayesian belief network
NPV   Negative predictive value
PPV   Positive predictive value

7.1
Introduction

Evidence-based medicine (EBM) is the process of systematically reviewing, appraising and using clinical research findings to aid the delivery of optimum clinical care to patients.[1] This approach places emphasis on the strength of evidence. Box 7.1 shows the evidence grading used by the Scottish Intercollegiate Guidelines Network[2] for developing medical guidelines.

As shown, the more rigorous the design, the higher the grading is. Fully randomised controlled trials (RCTs) are regarded as the highest level of evidence whereas expert opinions the lowest. However, even RCTs, which are commonly regarded as the 'gold

Z. Ni (✉)

Department of Surgery and Cancer, Imperial College London,
St Mary's Hospital Campus, London, UK
e-mail: z.ni@imperial.ac.uk

T. Athanasiou and A. Darzi (eds.), *Evidence Synthesis in Healthcare*,
DOI: 10.1007/978-0-85729-206-3_7, © Springer-Verlag London Limited 2011

Box 7.1   Levels of Evidence

1++   High-quality meta-analyses, systematic reviews of RCTs, or RCTs with a very
       low risk of bias
1+   Well-conducted meta-analyses, systematic reviews, or RCTs with a low risk of bias
1−   Meta-analyses, systematic reviews, or RCTs with a high risk of bias
2++   High-quality systematic reviews of case control or cohort or studies
       High-quality case control or cohort studies with a very low risk of confounding or
       bias and a high probability that the relationship is causal
2+   Well-conducted case control or cohort studies with a low risk of confounding or
       bias and a moderate probability that the relationship is causal
2−   Case control or cohort studies with a high risk of confounding or bias and a
       significant risk that the relationship is not causal
3   Non-analytic studies, e.g. case reports, case series
4   Expert opinion

---

standard' for testing the benefits of a particular intervention, could produce misleading results. For instance, the GREAT trial [3] compared the effectiveness of thrombolysis given by general practitioners in the patients' own homes with later treatment once the patients reached their local hospital. At 3 months, patients who received home treatment had 49% ($p=0.04$) fewer deaths than those who received hospital treatment (23/148 versus 13/163). Larger experiments done earlier, however, presented a far more conservative picture – home therapy led to only about 20% reduction in mortality. How do we make sense of the seemingly incongruent results? The rational method for answering this type of question is to apply a probability theorem, namely *Bayes' theorem.*[4]

7.2
Bayes' Theorem

Bayes' theorem prescribes how one should update his/her beliefs in light of new information. To illustrate, imagine a patient of yours has just been inserted a nasogastric feeding tube. According to your experience, there is a good chance, that is seven out of ten times (or 70%) that the tube is correctly inserted into the stomach but the tube can also end up in the intestine (30%). You know from the literature that stomach pH is most likely below 6 (85%) whereas intestine pH is most likely above 6 (80%). To maximize the chance of safe feeding, you test the pH of tube aspirate, which turns out to be 5. How likely is the tube in the stomach instead of in the intestine?

Let H_i denote one of n mutually exclusive events (hypotheses) and D some diagnostic datum (evidence). Bayes' theorem can be written as Fig. 7.1:

$$P(H_i|D) = \frac{P(H_i)P(D|H_i)}{\sum\limits_{i=1}^{n} P(H_i)P(D|H_i)}$$

Fig. 7.1 Bayes' theorem

Table 7.1 Belief updating after the observation of a pH equal to 5

Tube site	Prior $P(H_i)$	Likelihood $P(D|H_i)$	Joint probability $P(H_i) \times P(D|H_i)$	Posterior $P(H_i|D)$
Stomach	0.70	0.85	0.595	0.91
Intestine	0.30	0.20	0.060	0.09
		Sum $= P(D) = 0.655$		

In Fig. 7.1, $P(H_i)$ is the *prior probability* of H_i before knowing D. $P(H_i | D)$, read as 'H_i given D', is the *posterior probability* of H_i given D; $P(D | H_i)$ is the *conditional probability* (*likelihood*) of D given H_i. The nominator at the right-hand side of the equation, that is the product of $P(H_i)$ and $P(D|H_i)$, is the *joint probability* of H_i and D occurring at the same time, or $P(H_i, D)$. Summing up all joint probabilities across the hypotheses, as in the denominator at the right-hand side of Fig. 7.1, yields $P(D)$, or the probability of D.

Return to our tube-feeding example. We test the hypothesis that whether the tube is in the stomach (H_1) or in the intestine (H_2). We have some idea about it (*a priori*) but have also done a pH test to provide further evidence, which can be summarised in the following *conditional probability matrix*:

To assess the posterior probability of stomach intubation given a pH of 5, we apply Bayes' theorem (Fig. 7.1). As shown in Table 7.1, this probability is 91%, or about nine in ten chance, which is a substantial increase from the original seven in ten chance that the tube is in the stomach.

Pocock and Spiegelhalter[5] performed a Bayesian reanalysis of the results of the GREAT trial. Results from two previous trials formed the basis of the prior distribution and the results of the GREAT trial constituted the likelihood function. The updated relative risk of home therapy, as captured in the posterior distribution, indeed showed a positive shift. The change was, however, mild and the halving of mortality found in the GREAT trial was most likely a chance event.

The belief updating process embodied in Bayes' theorem is inherent in many medical decisions. However, even our somehow simplistic example allows a glimpse of how cumbersome the computation of Bayes' theorem could become. Computation complexity was one reason for the slow uptake of Bayesian applications, e.g.[6] The solution only came recently, with the development of Bayesian belief networks.

7.3
Bayesian Belief Networks

Bayesian belief networks (BBNs)[7,8] are the modern form of Bayesian applications. Also known as Bayesian networks, belief networks and probabilistic causal networks, BBNs are capable of handling problems with great complexity while maintaining a succinct and explicit representation. In recent years, BBNs have become increasingly popular in medicine, e.g.[9] A two-node BBN representation for the tube-feeding example is shown in Fig. 7.2.

In BBNs, nodes represent uncertain events (hypotheses, risk factors, diseases, symptoms, signs, test results, etc.), connected by links that indicate the dependence between the

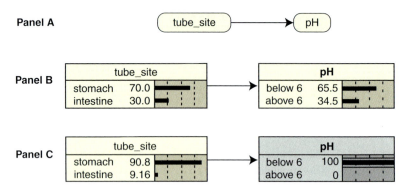

Fig. 7.2 BBNs for the tube-feeding example. The BBN in Panel A illustrates the structure of the problem. The BBNs in Panel B and C show respectively one's beliefs before the pH evidence becomes available (70% chance of stomach) and after (90.8% chance of stomach)

Table 7.2 A conditional probability matrix

Tube site	pH below 6	pH above 6
Stomach	0.85	0.15
Intestine	0.20	0.80

parent node (tube site) and the child node (pH level). Conditional probability matrices (e.g., Table 7.2) describe the strength of such dependence. Once information of one event enters the network, it is transmitted across the entire network via the links. Uncertainties are updated even for events without direct observations.

BBNs have many advantages over early Bayesian applications, including a graphical representation that is intuitive, compact and explicit, as well as enhanced computational efficiency. A key to this lies in a property of the tool. That is, in BBNs, missing links indicate *conditional independence*, meaning the states of one event have no influences on the states of another event given the states of a third event.

7.4
Conditional Dependence/Independence

The BBN in Fig. 7.3 shows three tests, each capable of providing evidence about the location of a feeding tube. The tests are not linked to each other but share the same parent node 'tube_site'. With the observation of a low pH, not only the chance of stomach intubation increases, so is the chance of observing *non-bile stained* aspirates with an appearance consistent with *stomach aspirates*. That is, the information of pH is transmitted to the other two tests via the shared parent. However, once the tube site is known, the three tests

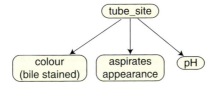

Fig. 7.3 Conditional independence for events sharing the same parent

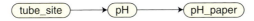

Fig. 7.4 Conditional independence for events in a chained relationship

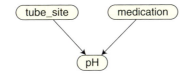

Fig. 7.5 Conditional dependence for events sharing the same child

become conditionally independent of each other and whatever information about one test can no longer affect the results of other tests.

Conditional independence also applies to events in a chained relationship (Fig. 7.4), such as the location of a feeding tube ('tube_site'), the pH of tube aspirate ('pH') and the reading from Baxter paper ('pH_paper'). In this case, knowing the tube in the stomach increases the chance of a lower aspirate pH, which in turn makes acidity reading from the Baxter paper more likely. However, once (the real) pH is known, the dependence between 'tube_site' and 'pH_paper' no longer exists.

A symmetric concept is *conditional dependence* when events only become related given the knowledge of a third event. This happens to events that share the same child node, such as 'tube_site' and 'medication' in Fig. 7.5.

As shown, aspirate pH depends not only on the location of the tube but also on whether or not the patient receives acid inhibitor ('medication'), which potentially increases stomach pH. Knowing nothing about the pH, tube site and medication exert no mutual influences, that is, the two are conditionally independent. The situation however changes with the full knowledge of the pH. To see why this happens, imagine a low pH is observed. This leads to an increase in the probabilities of congruent states, that is *stomach* intubation and *no* acid inhibitor. Now suppose we know for certain that the patient *is* receiving acid inhibitor. This leads to a further *increase* in the chance of stomach intubation because one of the two reasons for the acidity has been removed. By contrast, if we know for certain the patient is *not* receiving acid inhibitor, the chance of stomach intubation will *decrease* because the acidity has been *explained away*. Note that although explaining away is an intuitive concept, it is hard to capture in stochastic modelling, with the exception of Bayesian networks.

7.4.1
Why Is Conditional Independence Important?

The assumption of conditional independence makes BBNs computationally frugal. We no longer need the entire set of joint probabilities to specify any probability distributions but only the subset for the nodes that are directly linked. To illustrate, consider the BBN in Fig. 7.6.

Without the assumption of conditional independence, we compute the joint probabilities of these four nodes, T (tube_site), M (medication), C (colour), P (pH), by Eq. 7.1:

$$P(T,M,P,C) = P(T)P(M \mid T)P(P \mid T,M)P(C \mid P,T,M)$$

(7.1)

The assessment of $P(C|P,T,M)$ requires consideration of aspirates of all different colours being observed when pH, tube site and medication take all possible combinations – there are at least $8(=2^3)$ such combinations. If the judgment comes from experts, this task is extremely difficult if not impossible. However, the built-in conditional independence in BBNs renders this task unnecessary. This is because missing links between 'medication' and 'tube_site' as well as between 'medication' and 'colour' imply $P(M|T) = P(M)$ and $P(C|P,T,M) = P(C|T)$. Eq. 7.1 therefore becomes Eq. 7.2:

$$P(T,M,C,P) = P(T)P(M)P(P \mid T,M)P(C \mid T)$$

(7.2)

For a problem containing hundreds or thousands of nodes, conditional independence leads to enormous savings in computation. It is this capacity of BBNs for incorporating hierarchical representation of complex diagnostic problems, using only conditional probability matrices of linked events that alleviated the combinatorial explosion problem experienced in earlier Bayesian applications.

7.5
What Type of Data Can BBNs Handle?

In BBNs, uncertainties are expressed as probabilities. Whether these probabilities come from expert (human) judgments, published literature, clinical databases, etc, BBNs do not discriminate one type of data or the other. The BBN of the tube-feeding example (Fig. 7.2) was created using our understanding of the problem, including the relationship between the events, the direction and the strength of their dependences. In other words, the model incorporates subjective judgments. Although not shown, a BBN that represents the

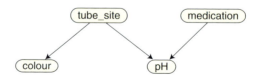

Fig. 7.6 A Bayesian network with four events

Bayesian analysis performed by Pocock and Spieglehalter would have a likelihood function based on an RCT and a prior distribution based on subjective assessment of multiple RCTs (For handling continuous rather than discrete variables, AgenaRisk (http://www.agenarisk.com/) is a powerful alternative to Netica).

Different types of data however have different characteristics. Data in the published literature are probably the most rigorously collected, which means they are also most reliable. But such data suffer from publication biases, including a significance level of 5%. Published data may also be less applicable to a particular clinical setting, for example data from US studies for clinical decisions in the UK. By contrast, clinical databases offer a rich source of information that is often site-specific, highly relevant and highly informative. One danger is however incomplete and inconsistent data collection. The sheer volume of information stored in a database can also be a challenge. Fortunately, algorithms have been developed to automatically extract Bayesian networks from databases.[10]

Different from the other two, expert judgments are rooted in individual experiences, and may encompass all sorts of information accumulated over the years, shaped by salient memory of recent and memorable experiences, vivid anecdotes, literature, etc. The role of expert judgments is controversial.[11] Decades-long behavioural studies show that people make systematic errors of judgement in assessing uncertainty,[12] reflected in discrepancies between the true value of the uncertain quantity and the average of assessors. The greater the bias, the less well any method based on aggregating individual judgements performs. This insight leads to the development of structured group solicitation process, e.g.[13] One notable example is *decision conferencing*,[14] which is a series of intensive working meetings, called decision conferences, attended by stakeholders concerned about some complex issues. One reason decision conferencing works is the presence of an impartial facilitator.[15] With skilled facilitation, no one person is allowed to dominate the group, and an atmosphere is created in which information is treated as a neutral commodity, to be shared by all. Natural adversarial processes can then emerge, helping to minimise bias, to correct for the inappropriate use of heuristics, and to provide a breadth of perspective.

Expert judgments play an important role even when models are directly extracted from databases. Gevaert et al (2006) built a BBN for predicting pregnancy with unknown locations.[16] They elicited expert judgments about parameter values and structural relationship between variables. To examine the impact of expert priors, they derived BBN models from the same database but under four different levels of prior information: no priors, parameter prior, structure prior and both priors. The results showed that the best performance was achieved using parameter prior or using both parameter and structure priors. In both cases, the area under the ROC curve (see below) was 0.87 out of the maximum 1.

Gevaert et al argued that expert priors had several advantages. When data were scarce, structure prior allowed the model to learn the dependence more efficiently. When the data were abundant, parameter priors improved the fitness of the model. Interestingly, the networks had different structures depending on whether they were built from the parameter prior versus from the parameter *and* structure prior. This suggested discrepancies between the knowledge perceived by the experts and the one contained in the database.

Gevaert et al also tested performance of a previously developed logistic regression model on the same data set. They showed that the BBNs performed slightly better than the traditional logistic regression analysis and the findings of BBNs were easier to interpret.

Fig. 7.7 A non-linear relationship between age and cancer. The *solid line* depicts the real non-linear relationship, and the *dotted line* is the best fitting line from a linear regression

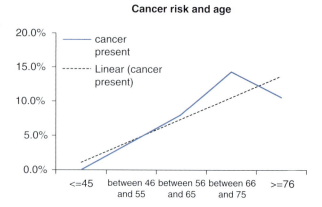

One reason is BBNs' capacity to handle non-linear relationships. For instance, Fig. 7.7 shows a hypothetical relationship between age and risk of colorectal cancer. As age increases, the risk of cancer also increases – but only for patients 75 years or younger. Beyond that the risk starts to fall. Linear regression is commonly used to capture the relationship between age group and cancer risk. However, predictions from such models (the dashed line in Fig. 7.7) fail to capture non-linearity, as easily incorporated as conditional probabilities.

When information from different sources are available, the discussion suggests it is best to use them from different sources in complementary to each other – retrieving conditional probabilities from published literature or well-maintained databases, soliciting expert knowledge to inform the structure of the model and to provide quantitative input especially in the absence of 'hard evidence', while testing model predictions against experts' intuitions as well as clinical databases for model applicability, e.g.[9] It is worth noting that BBNs can function even with incomplete information, making inferences and predictions based on whatever information is available, and making assumptions about what is not, for example a flat prior distribution.

7.6
Interpret Bayesian Belief Networks

A complete Bayesian network model contains a structural part and a parametric part. One advantage of BBNs, especially when used with a group of experts, lies in the need to specify these two different types of information, thus rendering the hidden logic and assumptions available for analysis and communication. For example, Fig. 7.8 shows a BBN called 'Asia', part of a larger network that can actually be used to make diagnoses.[8]

As can be seen, the network contains eight interlinked events, arranged in a hierarchy, reflecting the belief that the lower-level events (conditionally) depend on the higher-level ones. From top to bottom, nodes at each level represent respectively the risk factors ('Visit

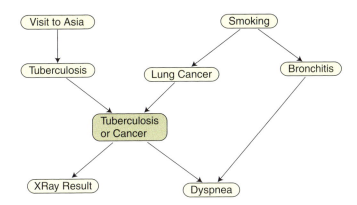

Fig. 7.8 Bayesian network 'Asia'

To Asia', 'Smoking'), the diseases ('Tuberculosis', 'Lung Cancer', 'Bronchitis', 'Tuberculosis or Cancer'), and the evidence ('Dyspnea', 'XRay Result').

Using 'Asia' to make diagnoses, we assume that a new patient presented to the chest clinic has certain combination of the three diseases, that is tuberculosis, or lung cancer and bronchitis. The chance that the patient has these diseases depends on the risk factors as well as on the prevalence of the diseases, which, in a complete BBN, needs to be specified as the prior probabilities of the diseases in the target population. Beyond the prevalence and the risk factors, diagnoses are informed by results from an x-ray or the symptom of dyspnea. The dependences between the linked variables, such as how likely a cancer patient has abnormal x-ray results or dyspnea, are captured by conditional probabilities, which are hidden from the user in this case.

One interesting aspect of network 'Asia' is event 'Tuberculosis or Cancer'. It seems redundant, as its relationships with its two parent nodes are self-evident, that is *absent* when both tuberculosis and cancer are absent and *present* otherwise. However, the presence of this event reveals an important hidden message. That is, the two diseases, tuberculosis and lung cancer, have *exactly* the same influences on the evidence (x-ray result and dyspnea). In other words, neither the test nor the symptom is useful in further differentiating between the two diseases.

In summary, the qualitative and quantitative information contained in a Bayesian network can be used to aid clinical decisions, teaching, learning and training..

7.6.1
A Real-Life Example

One notable example of BBN-powered decision support system is the Computer-aided diagnosis of Acute Abdominal Pain (AAP, University of Leeds & Media Innovations Ltd, Leeds, UK) developed by Tim de Dombal and his team in 1972[17] and still in use today. Adams et al.[18] reported a multi-centre study that examined the validity of the system in over 16,700 patients and including 250 doctors. Initial diagnostic accuracy rose from 45.6% to 65.3%; the negative laparotomy rate fell by almost 50%, as did the perforation rate among patients with appendicitis (from 23.7% to 11.5%). The management error rate fell from 0.9% to 0.2%, and the observed mortality fell by 22%. These improvements can be translated into reduction of 278 unnecessary laparotomies and 8,516 bed nights. The system created a positive learning environment – junior doctors were stimulated and motivated to do the work correctly.

7.7
Measuring Performance

Routine measures of test diagnosticity include *sensitivity, specificity, positive* and *negative predictive values*. For instance, suppose the task is to determine whether or not the tube is in the stomach, using pH of tube aspirate as the test. Sensitivity and specificity examine diagnosticity from the point of view of the true state of the *hypothesis*. A sensitive test captures true stomach intubation with few false negatives and a specific test captures true non-stomach intubation with few false positives. By contrasts, positive and negative predictive values examine diagnosticity from the point of view of the *test*. A higher positive/negative predictive value indicates a higher proportion of true stomach/non-stomach intubation among all the observed positive/negative test results. The indices are obtained by comparing the predictions against the information supplied by the best test available, or the *gold standard*. To illustrate, suppose after blind insertion of nasogastric feeding tubes, we first test and record pH of tube aspirates and then apply x-rays to verify the location for a total number of 220 patients. The results are shown in Table 7.3. Using this information, we can compute that the pH test has a sensitivity of 83.6% (= 102/122), a specificity of 81.6% (= 80/98), a PPV of 85% (102/120) and an NPV of 80% (80/100).

The indices, however, only work for tests with binary outcomes, that is, whether or not the pH is below 6 suggests whether or not the tube is in the stomach. Since BBNs make predictions in the form of probability distributions, for example 60% chance of stomach intubation, we set up cut-offs that convert continuous predictions to binary ones. A high versus low cut-off produces different combinations of sensitivity and specificity. To illustrate, compare using 60% versus 30% as the cut-off for stomach intubation, which means all (predicted) posterior probabilities above/below this threshold are taken as evidence for stomach/non-stomach intubation. The higher the cut-off, the less sensitive but the more specific the pH test becomes. To capture the trade-off between sensitivity and specificity, we construct a *Receiver Operating Characteristic* (ROC) curve (Fig. 7.9). The overall diagnosticity of the test determines the *Area under the ROC curve*, which has a maximum value of 1, the larger it is, the more diagnostic the test.

Table 7.3 Diagnosticity of a pH test of tube sites

Tube site	pH below 6	pH above 6	Sum
Stomach	102	18	120
Intestine	20	80	100
Sum	122	98	

Fig. 7.9 A Receiver Operating Characteristic (ROC) curve

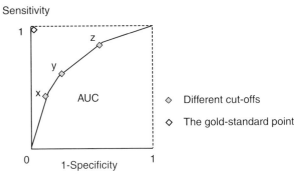

Selecting cut-offs is no easy task – it entails an assessment of the consequences. In the tube-feeding example, correct feeding decisions follow from correct predictions of stomach or otherwise, whereas missing feeding or feeding into the wrong sites result from erroneous predictions. If feeding into the lung is believed to be far worse than feeding into the intestine, then a higher cut-off should be used to increase the specificity of the test in order to reduce the false positives. Bayesian networks however only deal with uncertainties. To make decisions, we rely on other decision analysis tools, for example *influence diagrams*[19] that include decision nodes (rectangles) and consequence nodes (rectangles with rounded corners), in addition to probability nodes (circles).

7.8
Influence Diagrams

In Decision Sciences, Bayesian networks are a special form of influence diagrams when only chance nodes are present. Let us illustrate with an example. Suppose you have to choose between two weekend activities, a barbecue versus a movie. A sunny weather is compulsive for barbecues to be a success whereas watching movies is better when it drizzles. The only way you can know something about the weather is through the weather forecast report. An influence diagram that captures this decision is shown in Fig. 7.10.

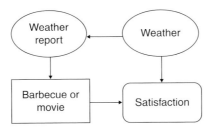

Fig. 7.10 An influence diagram for the weekend activities. *Weather report* and *Weather* are chance nodes, *Barbecue or movie is a* decision node and *Satisfaction* is a consequence node

Fig. 7.11 Decision tree for the weekend activities. Satisfaction ratings usually appear at the end of the branches

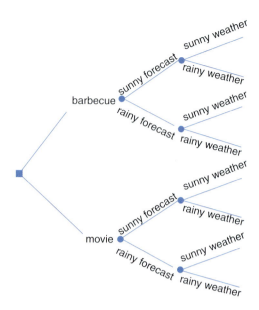

Note that links in influence diagrams take on multiple meanings depending on the context. As in BBNs, the link between uncertain events, for example 'Weather report' and 'Weather', indicates dependence. The link between an uncertain event and a decision, for example from 'Weather report' to 'Barbecue or movie', is however *informational*, indicating that the decision is made with the knowledge of the weather report.

The difference between influence diagrams and decision trees somehow parallels the difference between Bayesian networks and probability trees. For example, compare the subtree in Fig. 7.11 that captures the dependence between sunny forecast and sunny weather versus the sub-network in Fig. 7.10 that denotes the same relationship. Decision trees excel in illustrating the flow of sequential decisions, but become messy quickly as the number of alternatives/decisions increases. By contrast, influence diagrams offer a compact view of the same problem, revealing relations between different decision components that are often obscured in trees. A decision tree representation for the weekend activity decision is shown in Fig. 7.11.

7.9
Limitations

The utility of BBNs relies heavily on accurate structures and parameters. This means their predictions are as good as the data they are built upon. The development of generic algorithms means BBNs can be learned directly from databases. Although the capacity of learning makes using BBNs easier, comes with it the problem of limited applicability. Therefore when using BBNs, it is important to examine their sources and reflect upon the problems at hand. Although expert judgments provide an effective remedy, using expert judgments is often expensive.

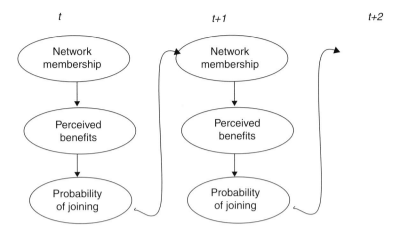

Fig. 7.12 A feedback loop described by a chain of Bayesian networks

Another challenge lies in computational complexity. Although BBNs significantly reduce the number of parameters required to specify a joint probability distribution, the number needed remains one major barrier to their wider penetration. This problem arises for events that have multiple parents, for which, we need information for all possible combinations of parents' states. Valid parametric solutions are only available for certain types of BBN.[20]

Another limitation of BBNs is that they are unable to handle feedback or feedforward loops. Unfortunately, many biological, social and economic systems are cyclic. An example is the situation that outsiders (non-members) decide whether or not to join a social network. It only makes sense to join if the perceived benefits are large enough, which however depend on the number of existing members the network has. That is, the value of the network membership at time $t + 1$ depends on its value at time t. BBNs make static predictions valid for a given time. So to represent problems like this, we need a chain of BBNs, each for a given time (Fig. 7.12). Such representation is cumbersome and computationally inefficient. To solve this, researchers have developed *Dynamic Bayesian Networks* (DBNs) that allow uncertain quantities to have probability distributions dependent upon time.[21] The work on DBNs is ongoing.

7.10
Conclusion

BBNs can combine different types of evidence including expert judgments and 'hard evidence'. They have the capacity to handle incomplete data and capture human reasoning such as 'explaining away'. They are particularly useful when uncertain relationships are complex and non-linear. Computer software (e.g. Netica) relieves, which relieves users from the burden of constructing networks and performing belief updating. A graphical display renders their predictions easy for interpretation and communication.

Acknowledgement The authors wish to thank Norman Fenton and William Marsh for insightful discussions on Bayesian networks.

References

1. Rosenberg W, Donald A. Evidence based medicine: an approach to clinical problem-solving. *BMJ.* 1995;310:1122-1126.
2. Scottish_Intercollegiate_Guidelines_Network. SIGN 50:A guideline developer's handbook. January, 2008.
3. GREAT_Group. Feasibility, safety, and efficacy of domiciliary thrombolysis by general practitioners: Grampian region early anistreplase trial. *BMJ.* 1992;305:548-553.
4. Bayes T. An essay towards solving a problem in the doctrine of chances. *Phil Trans.* 1763;53:370-418.
5. Pocock SJ, Spiegelhalter DJ. Domiciliary thrombolysis by general practitioners. *BMJ.* 1992;305:1015.
6. Edwards W. Dynamic decision theory and probabilistic information processing. *Hum Factors.* 1962;4:59-73.
7. Pearl J. *Probabilistic Reasoning in Intelligent Systems: Networks of Plausible Inference.* San Mateo, Calif: Morgan Kaufmann Publishers; 1988.
8. Lauritzen SL, Spiegelhalter DJ. Local computations with probabilities on graphical structures and their application to expert systems. *J Roy Stat Soc B Met.* 1988;50:157-224.
9. Hanna GB, Phillips LD, Priest OH, Ni Z. Developing guidelines for the safe verification of feeding tube position - a decision analysis approach. A report for the National Health Service (NHS) Patient Safety Research Portfolio 2010.
10. Buntine W. A guide to the literature on learning probabilistic networks from data. *IEEE Trans Knowl Data Eng.* 1996;8:195-210.
11. Dawes RM, Faust D, Meehl PE. Clinical Versus Actuarial Judgment. *Science.* 1989;243:1668-1674.
12. Gilovich T, Griffin D, Kahneman D. *Heuristics and Biases: The Psychology of Intuitive Judgment.* Cambridge: Cambridge University press; 2002.
13. Merkhofer MW, Runchal AK. Probability encoding: Quantifying judgmental uncertainty over hydrologic parameters for basalt. In: Buxton B, ed. *Proceedings of a Conference on Geostatistical Sensitivity and Uncertainty Methods for Groundwater Flow and Radionuclide Transport Modelling.* San Francisco: Battelle Press; 1987.
14. Phillips L. Decision conferencing. In: Edwards W, Miles R, Winterfeldt DV, eds. *Advances in Decision Analysis.* New York: Cambridge University Press; 2007.
15. Phillips LD, Phillips MC. Facilitated Work Groups - Theory and Practice. *J Oper Res Soc.* 1993;44:533-549.
16. Gevaert O, De Smet F, Kirk E, et al. Predicting the outcome of pregnancies of unknown location: Bayesian networks with expert prior information compared to logistic regression. *Hum Reprod.* 2006;21:1824-1831.
17. de Dombal FT, Leaper DJ, Staniland JR, McCann AP, Horrocks JC. Computer-aided diagnosis of acute abdominal pain. *Br Med J.* 1972;2:9-13.
18. Adams ID, Chan M, Clifford PC, et al. Computer aided diagnosis of acute abdominal pain: a multicentre study. *Br Med J (Clin Res Ed).* 1986;293:800-804.
19. Howard RA, Matheson JE. Influence diagrams. In: Howard RA, Matheson JE, eds. *Readings on the Principles and Applications of Decision Analysis II.* Menlo Park: Strategic Decisions Group; 1984.
20. Huang K, Henrion M. Efficient search-based inference for noisy-OR belief networks: TopEpsilon. Uncertainty in Artificial Intelligence 1996:325-331.
21. Ghahramani Z. Learning dynamic Bayesian networks. *Lect Notes Artif Int.* 1998;1387: 168-197.

A Practical Introduction to Meta-analysis

8

Sukhmeet S. Panesar, Srdjan Saso, and Thanos Athanasiou

Abstract In this chapter, we describe how to perform meta-analysis of continuous and dichotomous, stratified and non-stratified data. We also demonstrate how to generate some of the commonly used graphical methods for displaying the results of meta-analysis.

Whilst the Review Manager Software package is an intuitive and easily accessible method for performing meta-analysis, care must be taken to perform a robust review of the literature and adequately explore heterogeneity in order to obtain more reliable results.

8.1
Introduction

In this chapter, we aim to demonstrate, using a practical example from the literature, how to undertake the following aspects of meta-analysis:

- Meta-analysis of dichotomous variables
- Meta-analysis of a continuous variable
- Data stratification
- Use of Funnel plots to assess data heterogeneity

The following example will be completed using the Review Manager Version 5 (Cochrane Collaboration, Oxford, United Kingdom) software package which can be freely downloaded from the Cochrane Collaboration Website (www.cc-ims.net/RevMan/download.htm).[1]

S.S. Panesar (✉)
National Patient Safety Agency, London, UK
e-mail: sukhmeet.panesar@npsa.nhs.uk

T. Athanasiou and A. Darzi (eds.), *Evidence Synthesis in Healthcare*,
DOI: 10.1007/978-0-85729-206-3_8, © Springer-Verlag London Limited 2011

8.2
Background Information and Practical Example

Because of increased life expectancy in Western countries and a higher incidence of coronary artery disease (CAD) in the developing world, surgical revascularization in the elderly is increasing. Advanced age is known to be an independent predictor of stroke, mortality, renal failure, and atrial fibrillation following coronary artery bypass grafting (CABG). More recently, off-pump coronary artery bypass (OPCAB) techniques have been developed due to significant improvements in epicardial and apical suction stabilisation devices allowing surgeons to perform multi-vessel coronary revascularization in a routine fashion by avoiding the invasiveness of cardiopulmonary bypass (CPB). It is thought that the OPCAB technique has better outcomes than CPB. Similarly, the incidence of stroke and atrial fibrillation (AF) following OPCAB surgery is lower than that seen in CPB patients. So what about mortality and the time patients spend in the hospital after the procedure? Does one of the procedures offer better outcomes than the other?

We want to assess whether the OPCAB procedure is associated with a reduced incidence of mortality and length of hospital stay (days) compared to conventional CABG. Is OPCAB surgery the way forward in treating the elderly population?

After a careful literature search and review of the studies, 14 manuscripts satisfy our inclusion criteria.[2] We begin to extract the data onto a pre-piloted table generated in Microsoft Word, as shown in Table 8.1. This table contains all the values we need for the subsequent meta-analysis that we are going to carry out. Of the two variables that we are interested in – mortality and length of hospital stay (days), not all of the 14 studies will include data on both, hence the appearance of blank fields (labelled as 'ND') in the table.

8.3
Getting Started

The data in the table above has to be transferred to the Review Manager programme manually. Double-click the Review Manager icon on your desktop. The following screen should appear as shown in Fig. 8.1.

Select *Create a new review*, then click *OK*. This will reveal the following window (Fig. 8.2).

Select the *Next >* button. The following window will appear (Fig. 8.3). In this window, select the *Intervention review*, then click the *Next >* button. This will reveal Fig. 8.4.

Enter the groups into the above window (Fig. 8.4) as shown, then press the *Next >* button. The following window will appear (Fig. 8.5). Selecting *Finish* will generate the review (Fig. 8.6).

Now begin adding the references for the included studies. In the window below (Fig. 8.7), click on the *References to studies* heading in the navigation tab (A), and then in the main window, click the *Add Study* button under the 'included studies' heading (B). This will reveal Fig. 8.8.

Table 8.1 Included studies

Study	Number of patients		Age		Mortality (number)		Length of hospital stay (mean days±SD)	
	OPCAB	CPB	OPCAB	CPB	OPCAB	CPB	OPCAB	CPB
Boyd (1999)	30	60	>70	>70	0	1	6.30±1.80	7.79±3.90
Ricci (2001)	483	1,389	>70	>70	23	52	ND	ND
Ascione (2002)	219	771	>70	>70	3	16	8.71±8.54	8.76±1.89
Meharwal (2002)	186	389	>70	>70	4	18	5.00±2.00	8.00±3.00
Koutlas (2000)	53	220	>75	>75	0	17	ND	ND
Al-Ruzzeh (2001)	56	87	>75	>75	0	10	ND	ND
Hirose (2001)	104	74	>75	>75	2	0	13.80±8.70	20.00±11.70
Deuse (2003)	53	66	>75	>75	4	6	9.60±5.60	9.70±5.40
Demaria (2002)	62	63	>80	>80	3	10	9.00±8.30	9.60±6.10
Hoff (2002)	59	169	>80	>80	0	8	ND	ND
Beauford (2003)	113	29	>80	>80	1	3	ND	ND
Lin (2003)	17	12	>80	>80	0	1	12.70±2.20	18.10±2.90
Shimokawa (2003)	25	18	>80	>80	0	1	18.60±15.60	37.10±23.40
D'Alfonso (2004)	73	41	>80	>80	5	6	10.00±9.00	9.00±4.00

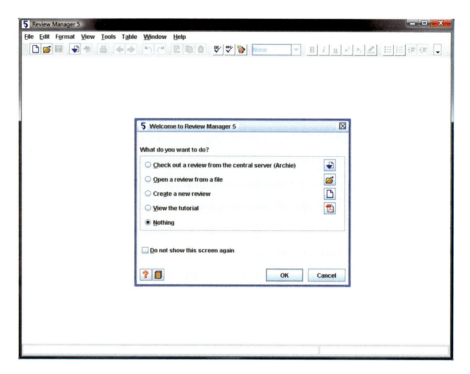

Fig. 8.1 Welcome to review manager 5

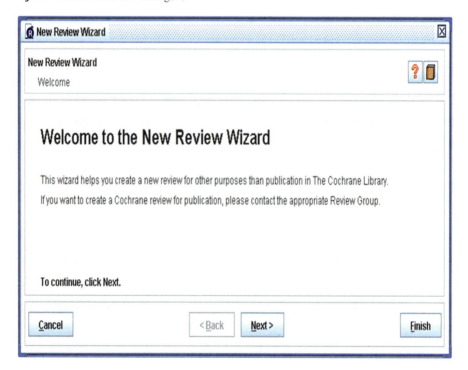

Fig. 8.2 New review wizard

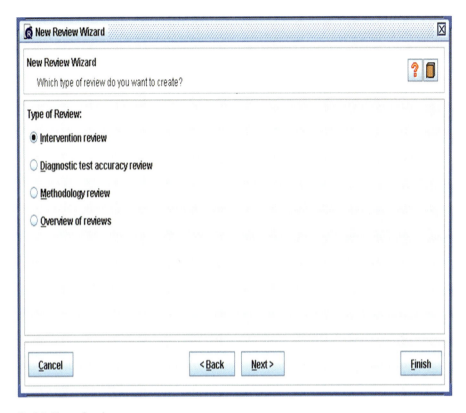

Fig. 8.3 Type of review

Enter the name and date of the study to identify the study as shown in Fig. 8.9.

After you have entered the study identification, click on the *Next >* button in Fig. 8.9 which will reveal the following window (Fig. 8.10). Click on the *Next >* in the following three windows after verifying that the year and data source is correct for the study (Figs. 8.10–8.12).

This will reveal the following window (Fig. 8.13). Select *Add another study in the same selection* and click the *Finish* button. Continue adding studies until all 14 studies are included. After adding all 14 studies, select the *Nothing* option. Review Manager will then return you to the main review window as shown in Fig. 8.14.

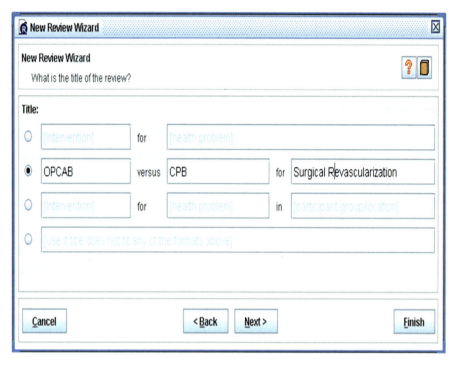

Fig. 8.4 Title of the review

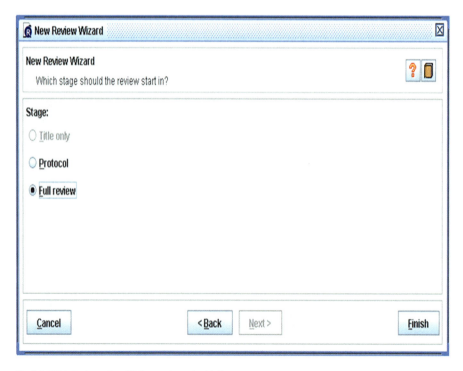

Fig. 8.5 Which stage should the review start in?

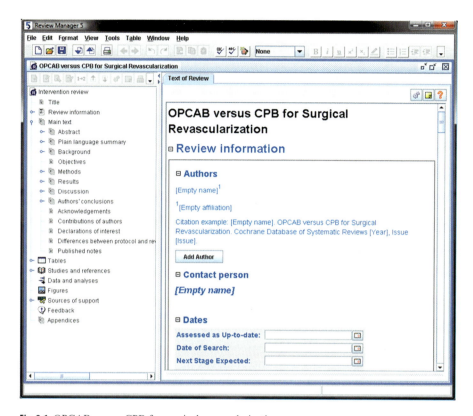

Fig. 8.6 OPCAB versus CPB for surgical revascularization

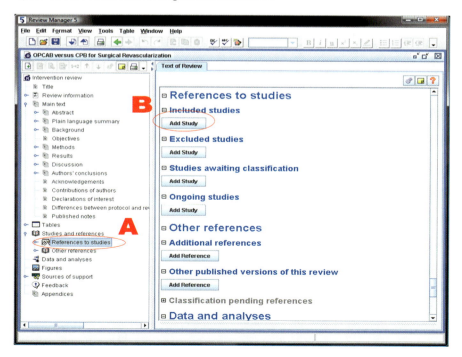

Fig. 8.7 References to included studies

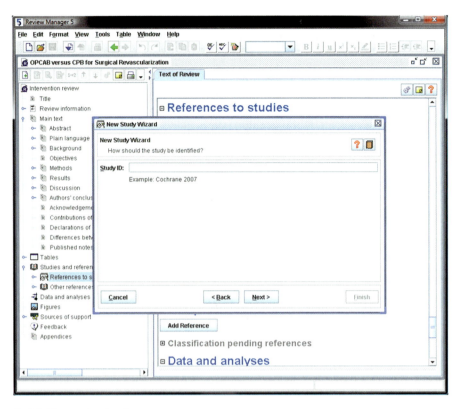

Fig. 8.8 New study wizard

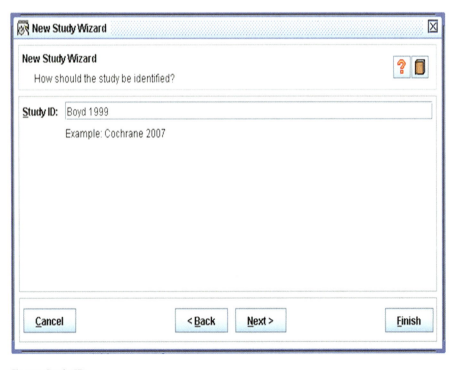

Fig. 8.9 Study ID

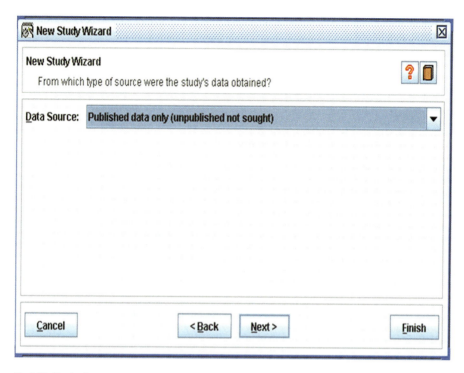

Fig. 8.10 Study data source

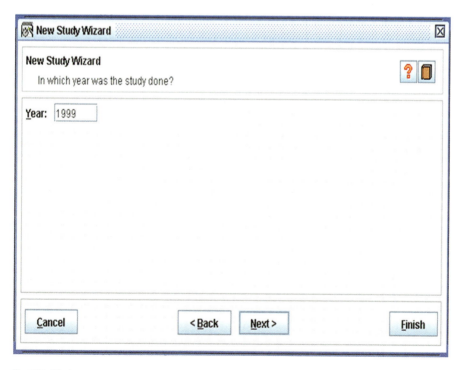

Fig. 8.11 Study year

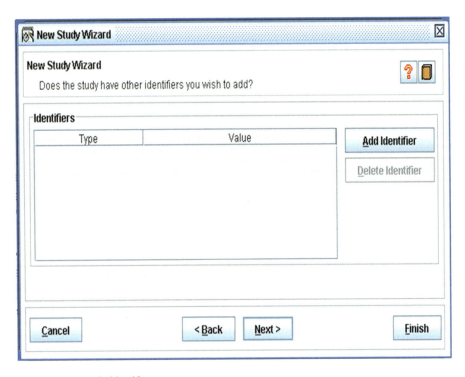

Fig. 8.12 Other study identifiers

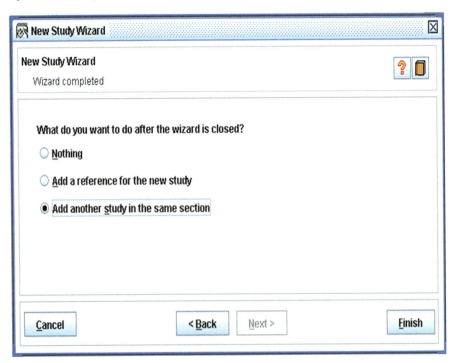

Fig. 8.13 Addition of further studies

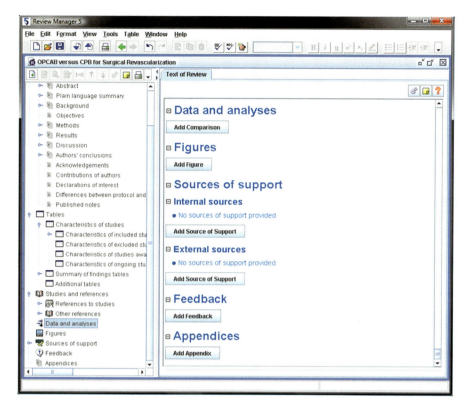

Fig. 8.14 Data and analyses

8.4
Stratification and Meta-analysis of Dichotomous Data

With the right-hand mouse button, select the *Data and Analyses* heading in the navigation tab (Fig. 8.14) (A). In the pop-up menu that is revealed, click on the *Add Comparison* option. The following window will then be shown (Fig. 8.15). Add the title of the comparison into the *Name* box, and then click the *Next >* option. This will reveal the window shown in Fig. 8.16.

In the above window (Fig. 8.16), select *Add an outcome under the new comparison*. This will reveal the following window (Fig. 8.17). Select the type of data, in this case *Dichotomous*, then click *Next>*. This will reveal Fig. 8.18.

Enter the name of the outcomes and groups in the following window as shown, and then, click on the *Next >* button. This will reveal the window shown in Fig. 8.19.

Select the correct statistical method in the *Statistical Method* box, analysis method in the *Analysis Method* box and the summary method in the *Effects Measure* box as shown. Then, click on the *Next >* bow which will reveal Fig. 8.20. As we wish to stratify our data according to age, we need to select the *Add a subgroup for the new outcome* option. This will reveal the window shown in Fig. 8.21.

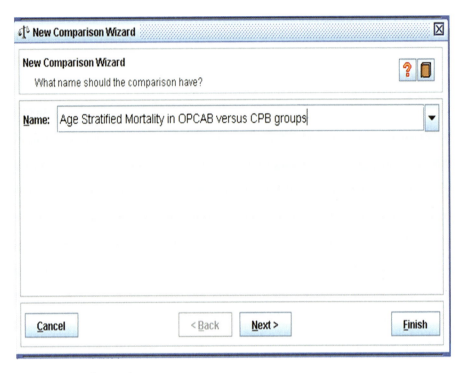

Fig. 8.15 Name of comparison

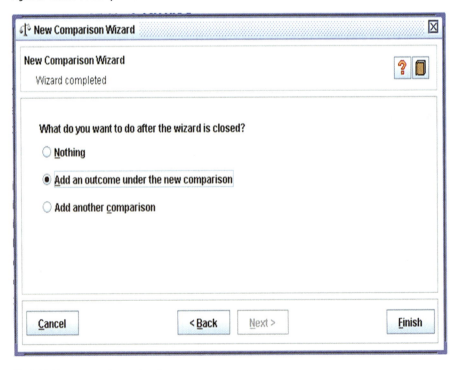

Fig. 8.16 New comparison wizard

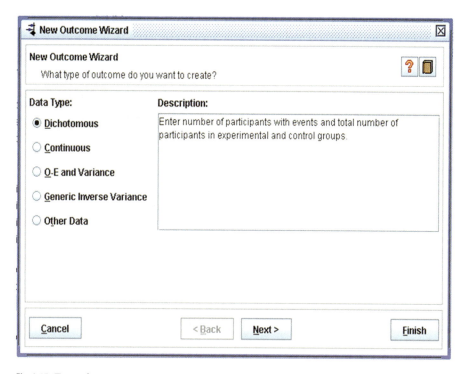

Fig. 8.17 Type of outcome

Fig. 8.18 Name of outcome

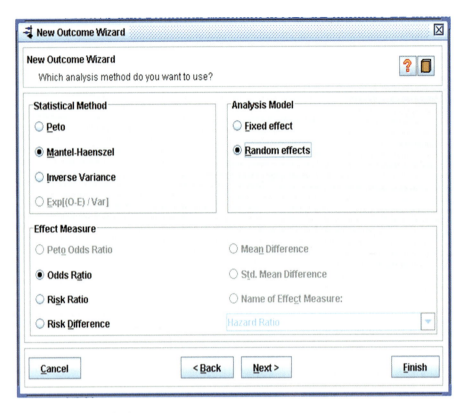

Fig. 8.19 Analysis method

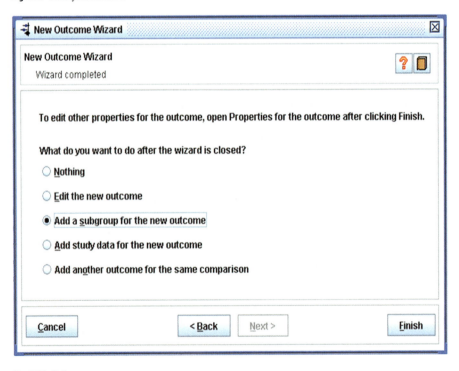

Fig. 8.20 Subgroups

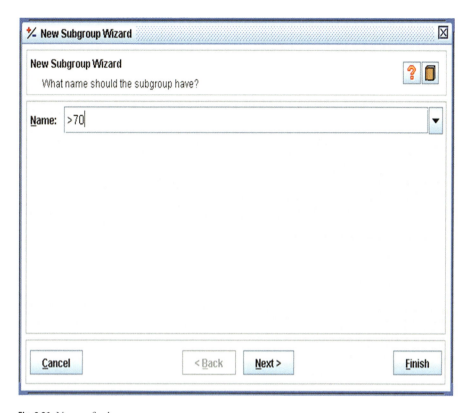

Fig. 8.21 Name of subgroup

Enter the name of the first subgroup (>70) as shown in Fig. 8.21. Afterwards continue to add subgroups (Fig. 8.22) until both the >75 and >80 subgroups have been added.

When all of the subgroups have been included, studies can then be added by selecting the *Add study data for the new subgroup* option (Fig. 8.23) and choosing them from the list revealed in Fig. 8.24.

Alternatively, by clicking on the subgroup in the navigation tab (Fig. 8.25) (A), and then selecting the *Add study data* option, the list shown in Fig. 8.24 will be revealed. Once all the studies have been added to the appropriate subgroups, clicking on any of the subgroups will bring up the table shown in Fig. 8.26. We are now ready to start entering the data.

As the data is entered into the table, Review Manger will generate a Forest plot (Fig. 8.27). The scale of the Forest plot can be changed using the slider at the bottom of the plot (A). The statistical methods used to generate the plot can be changed by clicking on the settings button (B). We will discuss data analysis in more detail in Sect. 8.6.

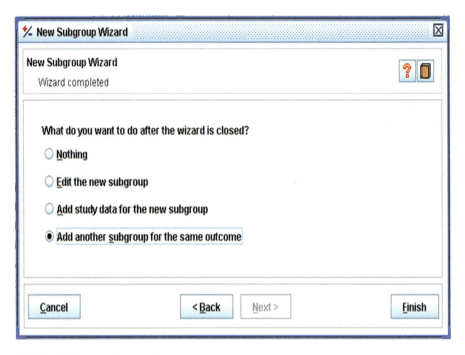

Fig. 8.22 Addition of subgroup to same outcome

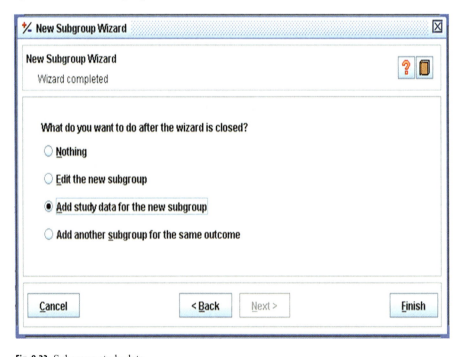

Fig. 8.23 Subgroup study data

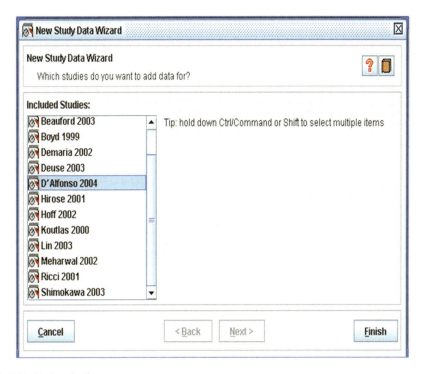

Fig. 8.24 Study selection

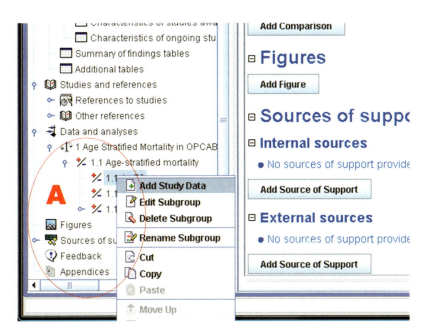

Fig. 8.25 Addition of study data

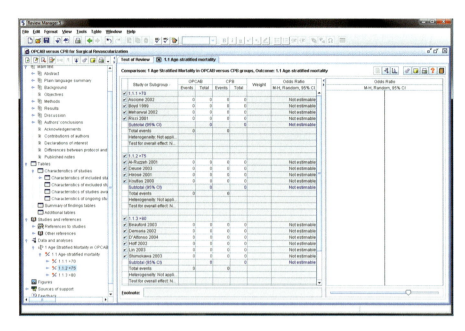

Fig. 8.26 Table of subgroups on review manager

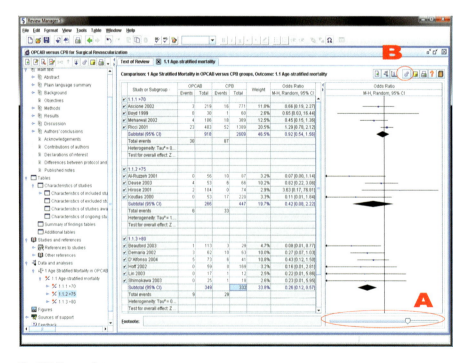

Fig. 8.27 Forest plot

8.5
Analysis of Continuous Variables

The next variable that we will compare is the *Length of hospital stay (days)*, which is a continuous variable. Right click on the *Data and Analyses* heading in the navigation tab, and select *Add Comparison* (Fig. 8.28). This will start the *New Comparison Wizard* (Fig. 8.29).

Follow the steps in the *New Comparison Wizard* as shown previously in Figs. 8.15–8.24. However, as this is a continuous variable, we need to select the *Continuous* option in Fig. 8.30 and select the *Mean Difference* as the summary statistic (Fig. 8.31). Furthermore, as there are not sufficient studies to stratify the data, we do not need to add any subgroup analyses.

The *New Comparison Wizard* will generate the following table (Fig. 8.32). Review Manager will generate a Forest plot for length of hospital stay as we add data (Fig. 8.33), which can be edited as described previously (Fig. 8.27).

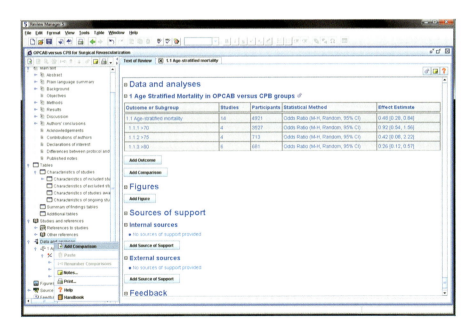

Fig. 8.28 Addition of new comparison

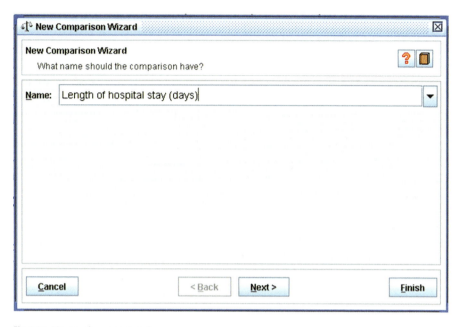

Fig. 8.29 Name of new comparison

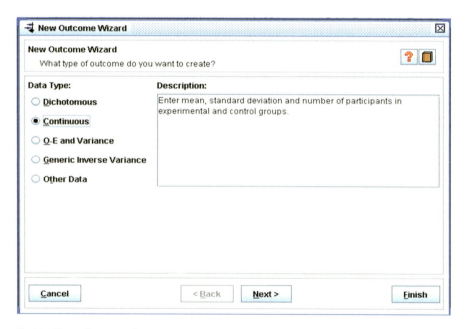

Fig. 8.30 Type of outcome for new comparison

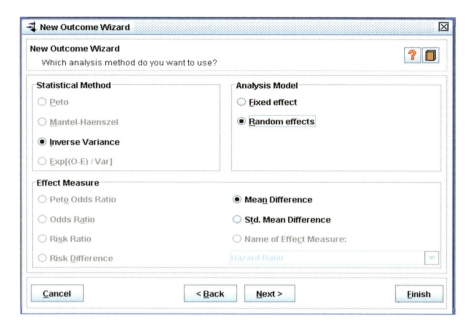

Fig. 8.31 Analysis method for new comparison

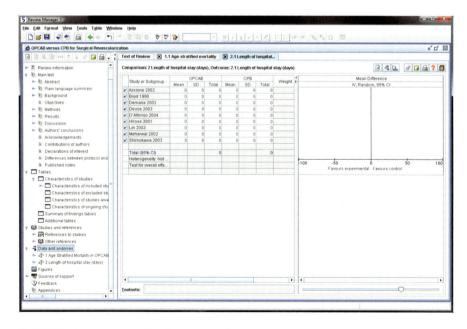

Fig. 8.32 Review manager table of new comparison

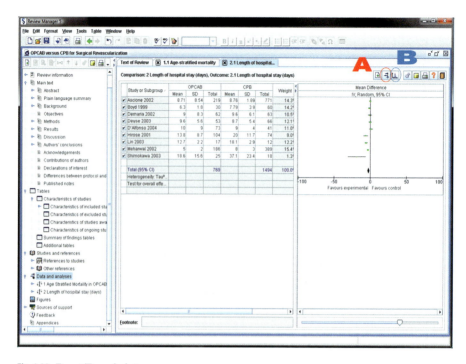

Fig. 8.33 Forest/Funnel plot

8.6
Analysing the Results

Clicking on the Forest Plot (A) in Fig. 8.33 will generate a Forest plot that is suitable for printing/copying to other programmes (Fig. 8.35). Likewise clicking on the Funnel plot button (B) in Fig. 8.33 will generate a Funnel plot (Fig. 8.37). These can be permanently added to the review after editing by clicking the *Add as Figure* button in the bottom right-hand corner of the window (Figs. 8.34–8.37). In a similar way, these figures (Figs. 8.34 and 8.36) can be generated for mortality from the window shown in Fig. 8.27.

Overall mortality was significantly lower in the OPCAB group (OR 0.48 [95% CI 0.28–0.84]) with no significant heterogeneity between the studies. One study in group 03 (Beauford 2003) showed a statistically significant difference in mortality between the OPCAB and CPB groups. Both groups were homogeneous (χ^2-square 20.36, $p=0.09$). Furthermore, we performed a subgroup analysis of the octogenarians in group 03 including 349/1,533 (22.8%) patients in the OPCAB group and 332/3,388 (9.8%) patients in the CPB group. Mortality was significantly lower in the octogenarian OPCAB group (OR 0.26 [95% CI 0.12–0.57], χ^2-square 1.81, $p=0.87$). The results of the analysis are explained in more depth in Fig. 8.34.

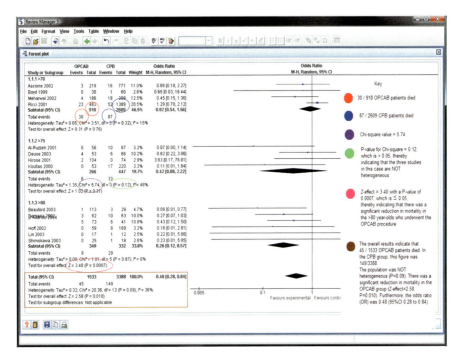

Fig. 8.34 (**a**) Forest plot explained and (**b**) table key

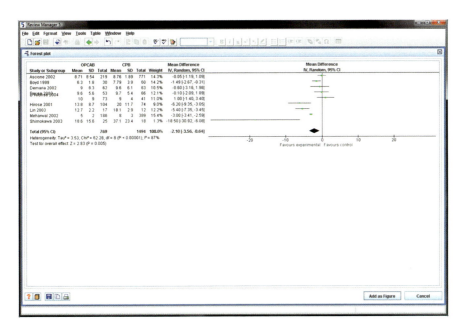

Fig. 8.35 Forest plot explained

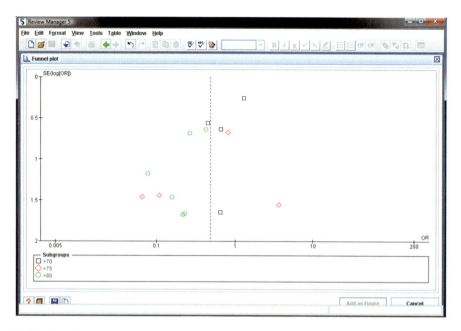

Fig. 8.36 Forest plot

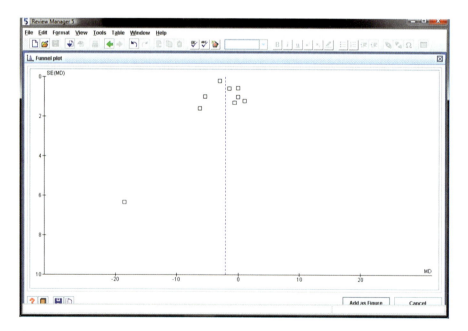

Fig. 8.37 Funnel plot

Figure 8.35 shows a tendency toward shorter hospital stay in the OPCAB group (OR 2.09 [95% CI 3.55 to −0.63], χ^2-square 62.95, $p<0.001$). However, the two groups were heterogeneous.

The funnel plots which represent graphical explorations of heterogeneity and publication bias are shown in Fig. 8.36 (Mortality) and Fig. 8.37 (Length of Stay). The interpretation of these figures is discussed in more depth in Chap. 3.

There is a relatively new concept which can be used to assess risk. As such, a risk of bias for each study can be interrogated and corresponding tables created. Select *Tables* and scroll down to the section on *Risk of Bias* table (Fig. 8.38).

Click the icon next to *Risk of Bias* table, followed by *Add for including other criteria* if you wish to add to the bias in the studies. Once this is done, click *OK* (Fig. 8.39).

Go back to Fig. 8.38 and select Yes, unclear or No for each of the categories that could add to the bias (Fig. 8.40).

Go to Figures, and select *Add Figure* (Fig. 8.41). Select *Add Risk of bias graph* (Fig. 8.42). Click *Next>* and the following screen should appear (Fig. 8.43). Click on *Finish*. Copy the next figure that appears to Figures (Fig. 8.44). Go back to Fig. 8.42, and now select *Risk of bias summary* (Fig. 8.45). Click on *Next>* (Fig. 8.46). Click on *Finish*, and the following figure appears (Fig. 8.47).

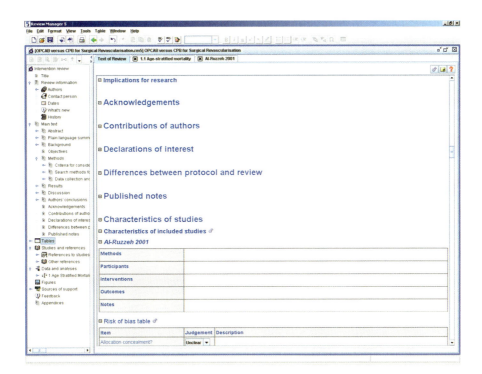

Fig. 8.38 Characteristics of included studies

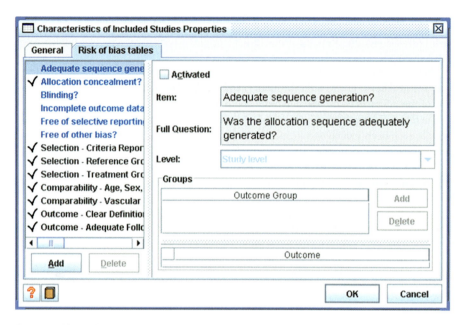

Fig. 8.39 Risk of bias table

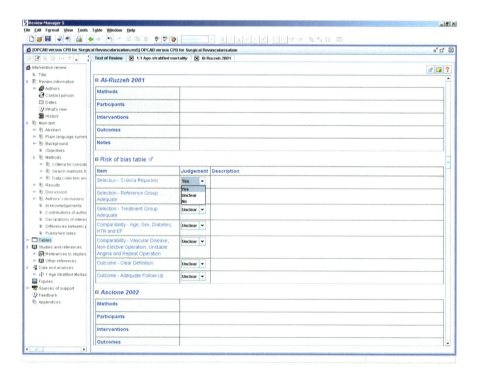

Fig. 8.40 Judgement criteria

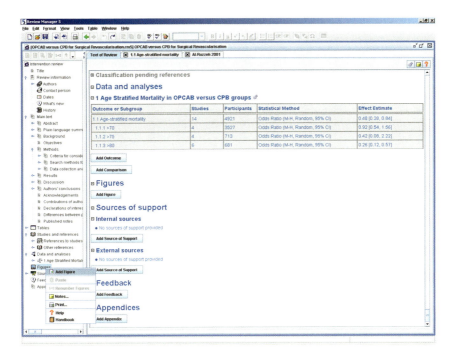

Fig. 8.41 Risk of bias analysis as a figure

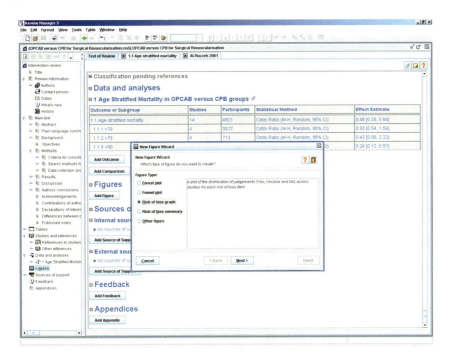

Fig. 8.42 Graph to depict risk of bias

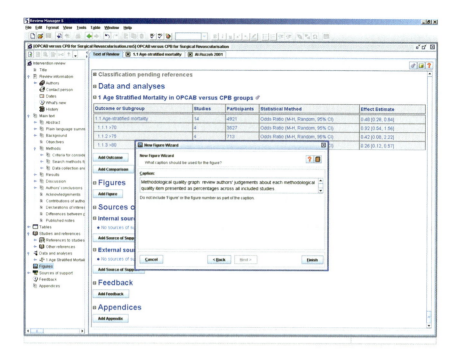

Fig. 8.43 Figure caption

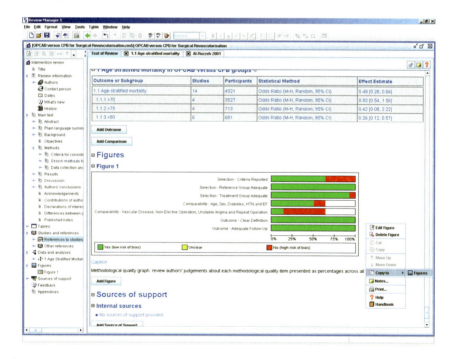

Fig. 8.44 Actual graph

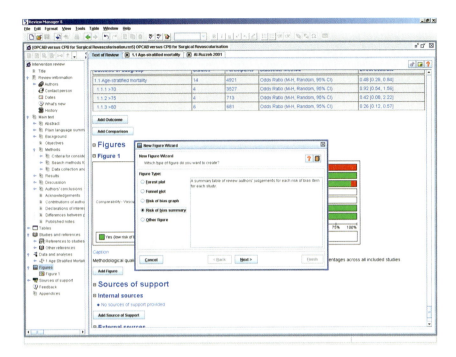

Fig. 8.45 Risk of bias summary

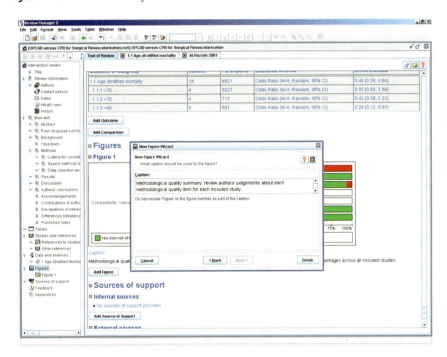

Fig. 8.46 Summary caption

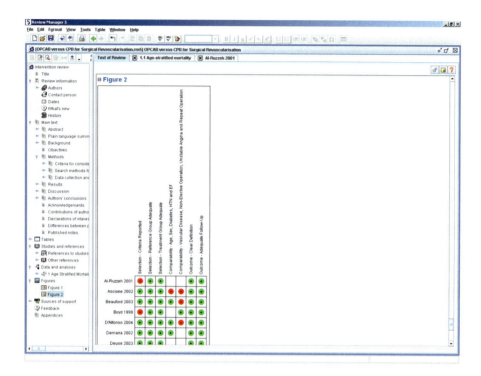

Fig. 8.47 Actual summary

Suggested Reading

Beauford RB, Goldstein DJ, Sardari FF, et al. Multivessel off-pump revascularization in octogenarians: early and midterm outcomes. *Ann Thorac Surg.* 2003;76:12-17; discussion 17.

Lin CY, Hong GJ, Lee KC, et al. Off-pump technique in coronary artery bypass grafting in elderly patients. *ANZ J Surg.* 2003;73:473-476.

D'Alfonso A, Mariani MA, Amerini A., et al. Off-pump coronary surgery improves in-hospital and early outcomes in octogenarians. *Ital Heart J.* 2004;5:197-204.

Shimokawa T, Minato N, Yamada N, et al. Off-pump coronary artery bypass grafting in octogenarians. *Jpn J Thorac Cardiovasc Surg.* 2003;51:86-90.

Deuse T, Detter C, Samuel V, et al. Early and midterm results after coronary artery bypass grafting with and without cardiopulmonary bypass: which patient population benefits the most? *Heart Surg Forum.* 2003;6:77-83.

Ricci M, Karamanoukian HL, Dancona G, et al. On-pump and off-pump coronary artery bypass grafting in the elderly: predictors of adverse outcome. *J Card Surg.* 2001;16: 458-466.

Meharwal ZS, Trehan N. Off-pump coronary artery surgery in the elderly. *Asian Cardiovasc Thorac Ann.* 2002;10:206-210.

Hirose H, Amano A, Takahashi A. Off-pump coronary artery bypass grafting for elderly patients. *Ann Thorac Surg.* 2001;72:2013-2019.

Al-Ruzzeh S, George S, Yacoub M, et al. The clinical outcome of off-pump coronary artery bypass surgery in the elderly patients. *Eur J Cardiothorac Surg.* 2001;20:1152-1156.

Koutlas TC, Elbeery JR, Williams JM, et al. Myocardial revascularization in the elderly using beating heart coronary artery bypass surgery. *Ann Thorac Surg.* 2000;69:1042-1047.

Demaria RG, Carrier M, Fortier S, et al. Reduced mortality and strokes with off-pump coronary artery bypass grafting surgery in octogenarians. *Circulation.* 2002;106(12 Suppl 1): I5-10.

Hoff SJ, Ball SK, Coltharp WH, et al. Coronary artery bypass in patients 80 years and over: is off-pump the operation of choice? *Ann Thorac Surg.* 2002;74:S1340-S1343.

Boyd WD, Desai ND, Del Rizzo DF, et al. Off-pump surgery decreases postoperative complications and resource utilization in the elderly. *Ann Thorac Surg.* 1999;68:1490-1493.

Ascione R, Rees K, Santo K, et al. Coronary artery bypass grafting in patients over 70 years old: the influence of age and surgical technique on early and mid-term clinical outcomes. *Eur J Cardiothorac Surg.* 2002;22:124-128.

References

1. Cochrane Review Manager. Available online at http://www.cc-ims.net/RevMan/download. htm.
2. Panesar SS, Athanasiou T, Nair S, et al. Early outcomes in the elderly: a meta-analysis of 4921 patients undergoing coronary artery bypass grafting-comparison between off-pump and on-pump techniques. *Heart.* 2006;92(12):1808-1816.

A Practical Approach to Diagnostic Meta-analysis

9

Catherine M. Jones, Ara Darzi, and Thanos Athanasiou

Abstract This chapter gives a demonstration of the practical aspects of diagnostic meta-analysis, with emphasis on data entry and manipulation, allocation of variables and code formation, and ensuring the appropriate outcome measures are produced at the end of the analysis. SAS is used to show the manipulation of data in this process. Graphical representation of data and results is shown using Review Manager.

9.1
Objectives

- To be able to assess the quality of diagnostic studies using standard tools and software
- To perform basic hierarchical SROC analysis using SAS
- To understand the process of including covariates into the HSROC model
- To examine the effect of covariates on heterogeneity
- To understand and perform summary receiver operating characteristic analysis (SROC) using Review Manager
- To generate a HSROC curve in Review Manager

9.2
Example

Multidetector computed tomography (MDCT) has evolved over the past decade to the point where coronary artery bypass grafts (CABG) are now being imaged with MDCT as an alternative to invasive coronary angiography (ICA). As angiography is invasive and has

C.M. Jones (✉)
Department of Surgery and Cancer, Imperial College London,
St Mary's Hospital Campus, London, UK
e-mail: Cathjones78@yahoo.com.au

T. Athanasiou and A. Darzi (eds.), *Evidence Synthesis in Healthcare*,
DOI: 10.1007/978-0-85729-206-3_9, © Springer-Verlag London Limited 2011

201

considerable workforce and financial demands, the possibility of performing MDCT in patients after CABG surgery is enticing.

The literature contains many articles comparing MDCT to ICA. We are interested in finding out whether MDCT is as accurate as ICA in diagnosing CABG stenosis and occlusion. We are also interested in whether other factors, such as the symptomatic status of the patient, whether the patients were in the early or late postoperative period, and whether beta blockers were given before the MDCT, influence the results.

For simplicity and clarity in defining our outcomes of interest, we will only include studies that provide data on the accuracy of MDCT with at least eight detectors, with the outcome of interest defined as diagnosing graft occlusion following CABG. Stenosed but not occluded grafts will be considered negative results. The reference standard will be ICA in all the included studies.

9.3
Getting Started

The key steps in a diagnostic meta-analysis will be described below. There are multiple options for how to do the analysis – the most commonly used will be shown in the form of a worked example. Different software can also be used. When it was possible, freely available software has been used.

9.3.1
Data Extraction

After a thorough literature search, 14 studies were appropriate for inclusion in the meta-analysis. (Please note that many more recent articles have since been published – these data are taken from a meta-analysis published in 2007[1]) The relevant data are extracted into a Microsoft Excel Spreadsheet (Table 9.1). Items where the information is not available have been filled in with ND (not defined). Before extracting the data, it is vital to know what information will be used in the analysis. Covariates (characteristics of the study) which may influence the test accuracy should be extracted at this time.

9.4
Quality Analysis Using QUADAS

The first analysis will be quality assessment of the primary studies, performed using the QUADAS tool.[2] Each of the 14 items is allocated as 'yes', 'no' or 'unclear' for each study. To simplify the example, 'yes' will be scored as 1, and 'no' or 'unclear' will be scored as zero. Table 9.2 shows the QUADAS results for the 14 studies in the analysis.

Table 9.1 Excel spreadsheet data file for MDCT example data

Author	Year	n	TP	FN	FP	TN	Sensitivity	Specificity	logDOR	BB	Symptomatic	Late postop
Anders	2006	93	28	0	1	64	0.9828	0.9773	3.3893	1	1	ND
Bartnes	2006	117	11	3	2	101	0.7667	0.9760	2.1252	0	ND	1
Bautista	2005	98	17	0	1	80	0.9722	0.9817	3.2738	0	1	ND
Burgstahler	2006	41	16	0	0	25	0.9706	0.9808	3.2261	1	1	ND
Chiurlia	2005	165	54	0	0	111	0.9909	0.9955	4.3857	1	0	1
Leta	2004	9	4	0	0	5	0.9000	0.9167	1.9956	0	1	ND
Malhotra	2006	209	9	2	0	198	0.7917	0.9975	3.1786	0	ND	1
Martuscelli	2004	251	54	0	0	197	0.9909	0.9975	4.6340	1	1	1
Pache	2006	93	42	0	0	51	0.9884	0.9904	3.9423	1	1	1
Salm	2005	104	25	0	0	79	0.9808	0.9938	3.9090	0	1	1
Schlosser	2004	131	21	0	0	110	0.9773	0.9955	3.9779	1	ND	1
Song M	2005	170	4	1	0	165	0.7500	0.9970	2.9969	1	0	0
Song W	2005	152	34	2	8	108	0.9324	0.9274	2.2459	0	ND	ND
Yamamoto	2006	158	5	0	10	143	0.9167	0.9318	2.1771	1	ND	0

Table 9.2 QUADAS scores for the included studies

Author	Year	n	logDOR	Q1	Q2	Q3	Q4	Q5	Q6	Q7	Q8	Q9	Q10	Q11	Q12	Q13	Q14
Anders	2006	93	3.3893	1	1	1	1	1	1	1	1		1	1	0	1	0
Bartnes	2006	117	2.1252	0	0	1	1	1	1	1	0	1	1	1	1	1	0
Bautista	2005	98	3.2738	1	1	1	0	1	1	1	1	1	1	0	0	1	1
Burgstahler	2006	41	3.2261	1	1	1	0	1	1	1	1	1	1	1	0	1	0
Chiurlia	2005	165	4.3857	1	1	1	1	1	1	1	1	1	1	1	1	0	1
Leta	2004	9	1.9956	1	1	1	1	1	1	1	1	1	1	1	0	0	0
Malhotra	2006	209	3.1786	1	0	1	1	1	1	1	1	0	0	0	0	1	0
Martuscelli	2004	251	4.6340	1	1	1	1	1	1	1	1	1	1	1	1	1	1
Pache	2006	93	3.9423	1	1	1	1	1	1	1	1	1	1	1	1	1	1
Salm	2005	104	3.9090	1	1	1	1	1	1	1	1	1	1	1	1	1	1
Schlosser	2004	131	3.9779	1	1	1	1	1	1	1	1	1	1	1	0	1	1
Song M	2005	170	2.9969	1	1	1	1	1	1	1	1	1	1	1	0	0	1
Song W	2005	152	2.2459	1	1	1	1	1	1	1	1	1	1	1	1	1	1
Yamamoto	2006	158	2.1771	0	0	1	1	1	1	1	1	1	1	1	1	1	0

Univariate analysis of each item against logDOR will be performed to identify any aspect of study design (item scores) which influences the diagnostic accuracy (logDOR). Once items with a significant effect on logDOR are identified (defined in this example by $p<0.10$), multivariate backward elimination analysis against logDOR reduces the model to those items with significance at the 5% level.[3] SPSS 14.0[4] has been used in this example, although any similar software performing univariate regression will suffice.

Export the Excel spreadsheet into SPSS using the 'File' button, then choose 'Open' → 'Data'. Select file type as Excel (.xls), and select your spreadsheet. Make sure that the correct sheet within your Excel file is chosen. If you have used row 1 of the spreadsheet to label the variables, tick the box allowing this to be incorporated into the SPSS data file. The data for our example is shown in Fig. 9.1.

Next, select 'Analyze' → General Linear Model → Univariate. The univariate options are shown in Fig. 9.2. As all the possible options for Q1 are known (i.e., zero or one), choose Fixed Factor for each of the QUADAS items, starting with Q1. Click on the Options

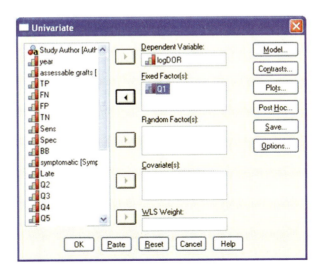

Fig. 9.1 SPSS data file of logDOR and QUADAS results from the 14 primary studies

Fig. 9.2 Univariate analysis box

Fig. 9.3 Options box for univariate analysis

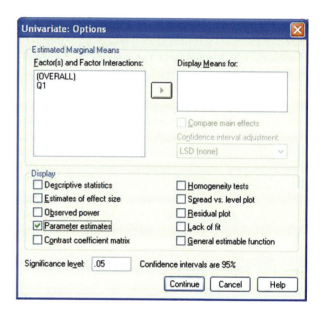

box, and choose to display 'Parameter Estimates' (Fig. 9.3). The parameter estimates, along with the usual output, will be given in the output as in Fig. 9.4. If all the studies score the same value for a particular item, then the univariate analysis cannot be performed (and the item is a redundant variable).

It is the parameter estimate for Q1 (i.e., −1.278) and its standard error (0.581) which are important. The parameter estimate for a given QUADAS item is the estimated value of the log relative diagnostic odds ratio (logRDOR), which is the log of the ratio of DOR values when the item is scored as zero and as one. A new spreadsheet can be created to calculate RDOR values and their confidence intervals (Fig. 9.5). The logRDOR, se(logRDOR) and p value values are transcribed from the SPSS parameter estimates for each item.

The upper and lower limits of the 95% confidence intervals for logRDOR (Lower limit = Estimate − 1.96*SE; Upper limit = Estimate + 1.96*SE) are also easily calculated in the spreadsheet columns. These can then be transformed to RDOR estimates and confidence intervals by using the EXP function (to reverse the logarithmic transformation).

Once the p values are known from the univariate analyses, the items which are significant are entered into a stepwise multivariate regression. A p value less than 0.10 is usually chosen, to incorporate items which may prove significant in the multivariate model. In the example dataset, QUADAS items 1, 2 and 14 are included in the multivariate model. The SPSS output for the multivariate model is shown in Fig. 9.6. In this example, only item 14 influenced the accuracy of the test. This partially explains the heterogeneity of accuracy results across the studies.

Similarly, other covariates can be assessed for influence over accuracy. In our example, beta blocker administration can be analysed for effect. The output shows that the administration of beta blockers has a mildly significant effect on accuracy ($p = 0.085$) and inclusion in a multivariate analysis would be justified (Fig. 9.7).

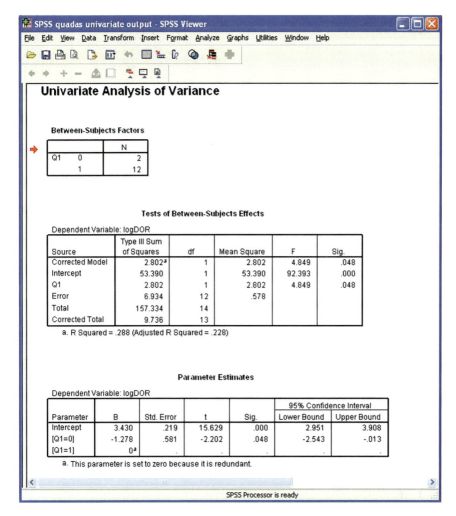

Fig. 9.4 SPSS output document for univariate analysis of QUADAS items against logDOR

Fig. 9.5 Excel spreadsheet for computing RDOR values and confidence intervals

ANOVA^b

Model		Sum of Squares	df	Mean Square	F	Sig.
1	Regression	3.352	1	3.352	6.299	.027^a
	Residual	6.385	12	.532		
	Total	9.736	13			

a. Predictors: (Constant), Q14
b. Dependent Variable: LOGDOR

Coefficients^a

Model		Unstandardized Coefficients		Standardized Coefficients	t	Sig.
		B	Std. Error	Beta		
1	(Constant)	2.682	.298		9.006	.000
	Q14	.989	.394	.587	2.510	.027

a. Dependent Variable: LOGDOR

Excluded Variables^b

Model		Beta In	t	Sig.	Partial Correlation	Collinearity Statistics Tolerance
1	Q1	.334^a	1.296	.222	.364	.778
	Q2	.185^a	.616	.550	.183	.636

a. Predictors in the Model: (Constant), Q14
b. Dependent Variable: LOGDOR

Fig. 9.6 SPSS output for multivariate analysis of QUADAS items against logDOR

9.5
Hierarchical Summary Receiver Operating Characteristic (HSROC) Analysis

Traditional summary receiver operating characteristic (SROC) analysis is simple to perform, particularly in software such as Review Manager 5.0.[5] This will be touched upon briefly later in the chapter. Hierarchical SROC is becoming accepted as the standard method for diagnostic meta-analysis, and so this example will be worked with HSROC.

The NLMIXED procedure in SAS[6] is the most accessible software for most people wanting to perform HSROC analysis. However, it requires acquisition of the SAS software, and a reasonably good understanding of both the SAS syntax and the statistics underlying the HSROC method, as individualised code is required for each analysis. The graphing of the HSROC curve is more straightforward, as it can be performed in Review Manager 5, with the parameter values obtained in SAS entered into the HSROC panel in Review Manager.

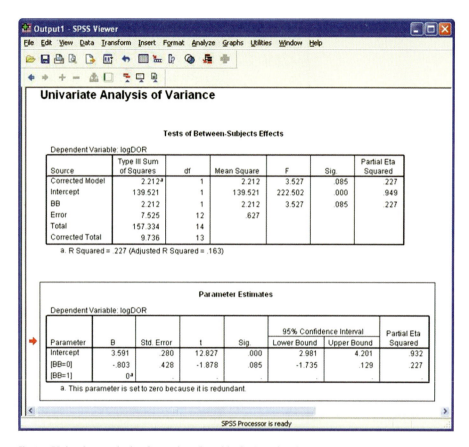

Fig. 9.7 Univariate analysis of covariate (beta blocker) against logDOR

9.5.1
Data Entry and Importing

The data must be assembled differently to how it was in the univariate analysis – the focus is now on the number of positive results, and the true disease status of the patients.

Each dataset in the meta-analysis is allocated a study number and two adjacent rows in the spreadsheet. If a single paper reports different tests or study groups, each dataset is allocated a different study number. In this way, there may be more than one study number per article. In our example this does not occur. Other literature on HSROC contains examples of multiple tests being compared in the same studies.[7]

A separate column (called 'dis' in this chapter) denotes true disease status. The value of dis is 0.5 for patients who are positive for the disease, and –0.5 for those who are negative (according to the gold standard). The number of patients in each 'dis' group in each study is marked in the 'n' column (Fig. 9.8). The number of patients who tested positive on the index test is put in the 'pos' column. In the terminology of a 2×2 table, when dis=0.5, pos=TP and n=(TP+FN). When dis=–0.5, pos=FP and n=(TN+FP).

Fig. 9.8 SAS data entry into Excel spreadsheet

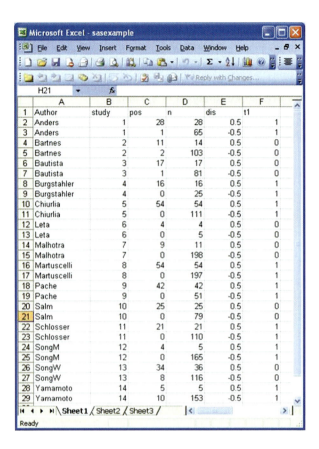

Obviously, when dis is 0.5, the closer 'pos' is to 'n', the fewer the false negative results and the more sensitive the test. Conversely, when 'dis' is –0.5, the smaller the value of 'pos', the fewer false positives are reported. It is also possible to enter covariate data. The 't1' variable in this case represents administration of beta blockers, where a value of 1 indicates that they were given, and zero indicates they were not.

Now that the data is in the right format, it can be imported into SAS. The location of the Excel spreadsheet must match the address given in the DATAFILE line. The file name for the example in this chapter is sasexample.xls (Fig. 9.9).

9.5.2
Basic HSROC Modelling

The difficult part of HSROC analysis in SAS is to understand the multiple levels of analysis. The first level models the number of positives in each study, which is assumed to follow a binomial distribution. However, the model is nonlinear, which limits the available software choices. Both logarithmic and exponential forms are used in the base model, as seen in the SAS code (Fig. 9.10).

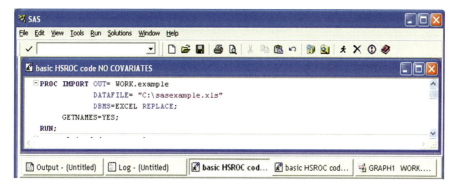

Fig. 9.9 Importing an Excel spreadsheet into SAS

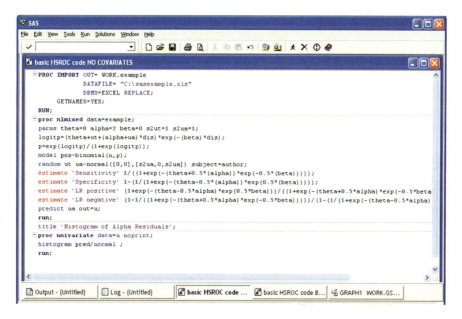

Fig. 9.10 Basic HSROC code for a model with no covariates and a single test

Theta is the random-effects variable for threshold effect (and 'ut' is its random variation variable). Similarly, alpha is the random-effects accuracy variable (and 'ua' is its variation). Beta is the fixed-effects variable which models the shape of the HSROC curve – if there is a significant dependence of accuracy on threshold, the curve will be asymmetric (and beta will be significantly different to zero). A beta variation ('bc') variable can be input into the model to see whether it is asymmetric but, in practice, this can be omitted if there is no evidence of the curve being asymmetric.

The four 'estimate' code lines are the codes used to produce clinically relevant estimates. In this case, estimates of sensitivity, specificity and the positive and negative likelihood ratios have been produced. Other estimates, such as DOR, positive predictive value and negative predictive value, can also be produced. The process is run, and an output produced (Fig. 9.11). The model may fail to converge within the set limit of iterations. In these circumstances, it may be possible to remove covariates from the model (including 'bc' if this has been included). If this is not feasible, changing the optimisation technique may be required (see SAS help notes for more information).

Estimates for theta, alpha and beta are obtained from the SAS output code. Note should also be made of the –2 log likelihood value, as this will be important if further analysis using covariates will be done. The estimates for sensitivity and the other three outcomes are given in the output as well (Fig. 9.12).

The final part of the basic code is production of a histogram of the residual values of alpha across the model. These should follow a normal distribution for the underlying assumptions to be valid. In this case, there is nothing in the histogram to suggest that this

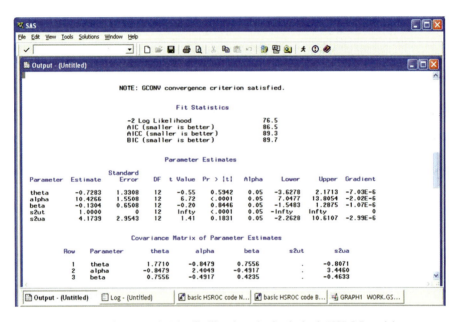

Fig. 9.11 Parameter estimates and –2 loglikelihood results for the basic HSROC model

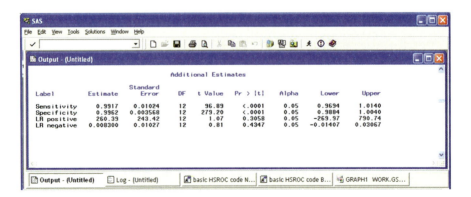

Fig. 9.12 Estimated sensitivity, specificity and likelihood ratios for the basic HSROC model

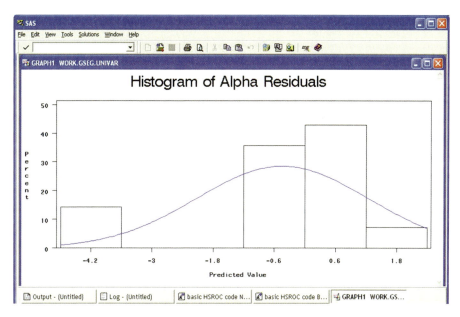

Fig. 9.13 Histogram of alpha residuals to test for underlying normality

assumption is invalid (Fig. 9.13). Once the estimates of theta, alpha and beta are obtained from the output (for example, in this case, theta is estimated to be –0.7283), they can be inputted into Review Manager 5 (see Sect. 9.6).

9.5.3
Covariates in the HSROC Model

The HSROC model is far more flexible than the traditional SROC in assessing the impact of covariates on heterogeneity. In this example, the administration of beta blockers has been included during the data extraction step (Fig. 9.1). Including this covariate into the SAS code is straightforward, as long as the underlying model is understood.

Three new variables are incorporated into the model for the addition of one covariate (Fig. 9.14). 'tc' refers to the variation of threshold parameter due to the effect of beta blockers. 'ac' refers to the variation of the accuracy variable, and 'bc' refers to the effect on the HSROC curve shape. In order for these variables to denote the influence of beta blocker administration, a variable called 't1' has been introduced which is zero if beta blockers are not given, and 'one' when they are. In this way, 'tc', 'ac' and 'bc' only come into effect when beta blockers are administered, making their magnitude solely related to that event. Their start values are assumed to be zero. Sensitivity and the other clinical estimates can be produced for studies using beta blockers, using the altered code accounting for beta blocker administration as a covariate. The output of this model can now be examined (Figs. 9.15 and 9.16).

In the simple model with no covariates, the value for –2LL was 76.5. The model with the covariate has a –2LL value of 67.5. The difference in –2LL values (in this case, 9.0) follows a chi squared distribution with 2 degrees of freedom. The one-tailed probability of

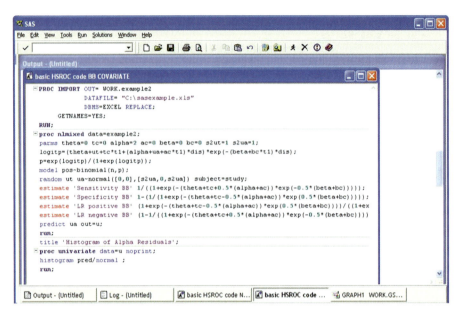

Fig. 9.14 HSROC code for a model with one covariate and a single test

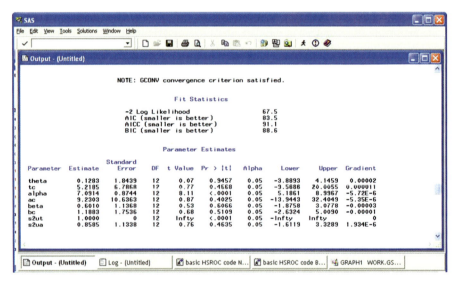

Fig. 9.15 Parameter estimates and −2 loglikelihood results for the HSROC model with one covariate and a single test

randomly having a value of 9.0 or more in a chi squared distribution with 2 degrees of freedom is 0.011. This value (the *p* value) indicates that the administration of beta blockers significantly contributes to the heterogeneity of results of the primary studies.

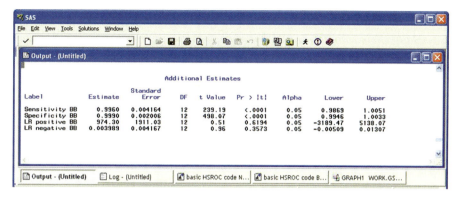

Fig. 9.16 Estimated sensitivity, specificity and likelihood ratios for the HSROC model with one covariate

If the effect of beta blocker administration on curve shape alone is to be investigated, removal of the relevant variable ('bc') from the full model with the beta blocker covariates can be done. The subsequent difference in –2LL values will then generate a *p* value (chi squared distribution with 2 degrees of freedom). Similarly, the effect of beta blockers on test accuracy ('ac') or dependence of test accuracy on threshold ('tc') could also be examined individually.

9.5.4
Convergence

Problems may arise during HSROC analysis with SAS with convergence of the model, especially as the number of variables in the model increases. If convergence does become a problem, the model can be run with and without a shape variable (beta) before covariates are included. If the *p* value is less than 0.10 (calculated by the above method using the –2 Loglikelihood values), then there is evidence that the HSROC is asymmetric, and rather than removing the beta variables from the model, alternative ways to ensure convergence should be sought. These include changing the underlying optimisation technique or increasing the number of allowed iterations.

9.6
Drawing the HSROC Curve

Review Manager 5 (RevMan5) is very useful for creating systematic reviews of diagnostic tests. It allows the SROC curve to be drawn with or without the hierarchical parameters from the SAS analysis entered into the curve equation; thus, a traditional SROC curve requires nothing but data entry into RevMan 5 and subsequent analysis. If the bivariate SROC approach is being performed, those parameters may alternatively be entered into the model for the curve.

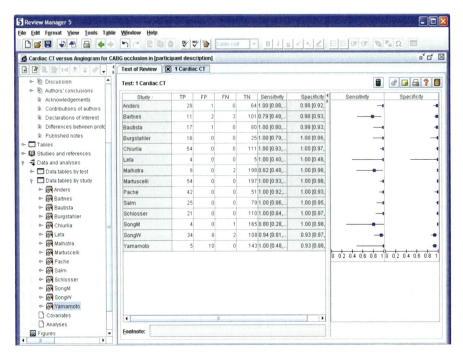

Fig. 9.17 Data entry into RevMan 5 with Forest plot

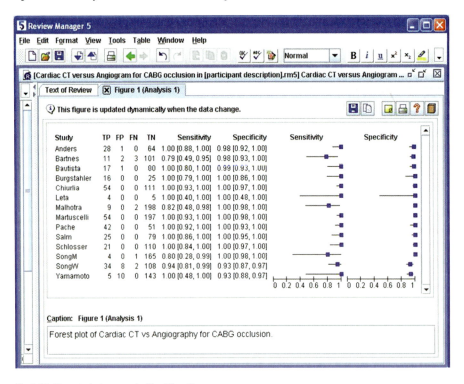

Fig. 9.18 Forest plot screen in RevMan 5

Basic knowledge of RevMan is assumed here. If you have not used RevMan before, do not worry – it comes with user manuals, and is itself user-friendly. Once the review has been created in RevMan, register the studies (14 in our example) and for each study, allocate values for TP, FN, FP and TN (note that the SAS data entry approach will not be valid here). Make sure that the values correspond to those in the original data extraction – FN and FP may be reversed from the spreadsheet (as in this example) (Fig. 9.17). From this, create an Analysis (the name does not matter, it is your choice) and perform a Forest plot to gain an overall view of the data (Fig. 9.18). The plot can then be saved as pdf, eps or other file types. Alternatively, it can be copied and pasted into a Paint programme, and then saved as a jpeg, bitmap or other image type.

The next step in RevMan is to create the HSROC curve, using the parameters for theta, beta and alpha (referred to as lambda) obtained from the SAS output (Figs. 9.19 and 9.20). In this example, the accuracy is very close to perfect and the curve is nearly the perfect square. The diagonal is drawn onto the curve by default, and represents the accuracy of a random test. If beta blocker administration is a covariate, its contribution to heterogeneity of study results can be graphically demonstrated in RevMan 5 through covariate curves (Fig. 9.21).

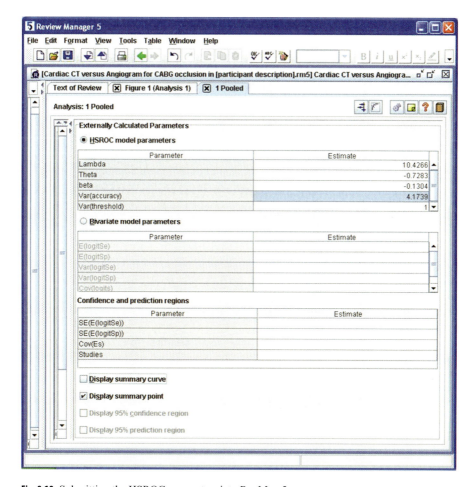

Fig. 9.19 Submitting the HSROC parameters into RevMan 5

Fig. 9.20 The HSROC curve for the example (no covariates)

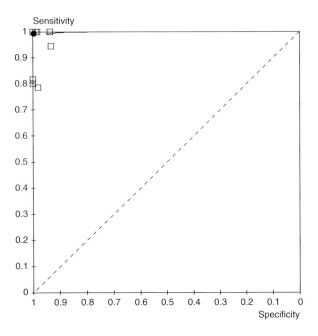

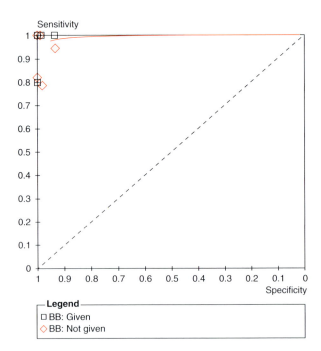

Fig. 9.21 The HSROC curve for the example, using beta blocker administration as a covariate

9.7
Conclusion

Diagnostic test meta-analysis is complex, with multiple steps required to fully analyse the data. Mastering the SAS code, RevMan 5 application and QUADAS tool is required for an accurate meta-analysis using these methods. However, if the clinical question is relevant, and the literature search, data extraction, quality assessment, HSROC and curve generation are sound, the results of the analysis produce meaningful and useful information.

References

1. Jones CM, Athanasiou T, Dunne N, et al. Multi-detector computed tomography in coronary artery bypass graft assessment: a meta-analysis. *Ann Thorac Surg.* 2007;83:341-348.
2. Whiting P, Rutjes AW, Dinnes J, Reitsma J, Bossuyt PM, Kleijnen J. Development and validation of methods for assessing the quality of diagnostic accuracy studies. *Health Technol Assess.* 2004;8:iii, 1-234.
3. Westwood ME, Whiting PF, Kleijnen J. How does study quality affect the results of a diagnostic meta-analysis? *BMC Med Res Methodol.* 2005;5:20.
4. SPSS for Windows, Rel. 14.0.0. 2005. Chicago: SPSS Inc. 2005.
5. Review Manager (RevMan) [Computer program]. Version 5.0. Copenhagen: the Nordic cochrane centre, the cochrane collaboration. 2008.
6. SAS/STAT 9.1. Cary, NC: SAS Institute. 2004.
7. Macaskill P. Empirical Bayes estimates generated in a hierarchical summary ROC analysis agreed closely with those of a full Bayesian analysis. *J Clin Epidemiol.* 2004;57:925-932.

Practical Examples of the Application of Decision Analysis in Healthcare

10

Christopher Rao, Ara Darzi, and Thanos Athanasiou

Abstract In this chapter, we use examples adapted from the published literature to illustrate the practical application of decision analytical methods. For both examples, we use the TreeAge Pro Suite software package (TreeAge Software inc., Williamstown, Massachusetts, USA). By using these methods, we hope that the reader will be able to construct more complex decision analytical models to address clinical problems in their own practice.

10.1
Introduction

In this chapter, we use examples adapted from the published literature to illustrate practical application of the decision analytical methods discussed in Chap. 5. In the first example, we adapt a complex decision analytical model from the literature[1] to compare percutaneous coronary artery stenting with surgical revascularisation. In this example, we demonstrate the basic principles of model construction and analysis. In the second example, we use an adapted example from the literature[2] comparing different methods of mitral valve replacement to demonstrate more advanced decision analytical methods. An overview of the aims of this chapter is shown in Box 10.1.

For both examples, we use the TreeAge Pro Suite software package (TreeAge Software inc., Williamstown, Massachusetts, USA) for two reasons; firstly, it is more accessible to the 'novice' analyst with its intuitive visual interfaces requiring little prior specialist computing or statistical knowledge. Secondly, the practical application of decision analytical methods using other programmes such as Excel (Microsoft Corporation, Redmond, Washington, USA) has already been discussed in other texts[3]. A free trial version of the TreeAge Pro Suite software package that will allow the reader to work through these examples and gain a basic understanding of practical decision analysis is available for download from the TreeAge website (www.TreeAge.com).

C. Rao (✉)
Department of Surgery and Cancer, Imperial College London,
St Mary's Hospital Campus, London, UK
e-mail: christopher.rao@imperial.ac.uk

T. Athanasiou and A. Darzi (eds.), *Evidence Synthesis in Healthcare*,
DOI: 10.1007/978-0-85729-206-3_10, © Springer-Verlag London Limited 2011

10.2
Example 1: Coronary Revascularisation

10.2.1
Background Information

Ischaemic heart disease is a major cause of morbidity and mortality worldwide. As the symptoms of ischaemic heart disease are caused by blockage or narrowing of the heart's blood vessels, the symptoms can be treated by improving the blood flow to the muscle of the heart. In this simplified adaption of a published economic analysis,[1] we compare the quality-adjusted life year (QALY) payoff in the first year following two different interventions. The first is *coronary artery bypass grafting* (*CABG*) where an operation is performed to bypass the diseased segments of the heart arteries with veins or arteries from the patient's legs, arms or chest wall. The second is *percutaneous transluminal coronary angioplasty with stenting* (*PTCA*) where the arteries of the heart are first unblocked using a specially adapted wire, and then held open with a metal tube or *stent*. Whilst fewer patients have recurrence of symptoms following CABG, procedural mortality is lower following PTCA. What is the best course of action? In this example, we use a simplified version of a published economic analysis[1] to illustrate the principles of constructing and analysing a decision analytical model. To fully assess which strategy is the most effective, a complicated model is required that considers a number of outcomes over a period of several years. Consequently, this example is designed to illustrate the principles of decision analysis and not to inform practice, for which we refer readers to the published analysis on which our example is based[1]. The model parameters used in this model are given in Table 10.1. An overview of the structure of the model 1 is shown in Fig. 10.1. Box 10.2 explains how to correct mistakes made during the examples.

Box 10.2   Correcting Mistakes in TreeAge

During the course of these examples, any mistakes can be corrected by clicking on the *Edit* menu and *Undo*; alternatively, hold down the *Ctrl* + *Z* keys.

To delete parts of the tree, they must be selected by clicking on the *Options* menu and then *Select Subtree*; alternatively, hold down the *Ctrl + B* keys. They can then be deleted by cutting the selected portions of the tree. This can be done by clicking on the *Edit* menu and then *Cut*; alternatively, hold down the *Ctrl + X* keys.

Table 10.1 Model parameters used in Example 1

Parameter	Value	Range	Distribution
Utility parameters			
Asymptomatic utility	0.860	0.774–0.946	Triangular
Symptomatic utility	0.858	0.772–0.944	Triangular
Path probabilities			
PTCA symptom recurrence rate	0.0677	0.0284–0.1535	Triangular
CABG symptom recurrence rate	0.0247	0.0098–0.0573	Triangular
PTCA procedural mortality	0.0075	0.0026–0.0281	Triangular
CABG procedural mortality	0.0224	0.0059–0.0610	Triangular

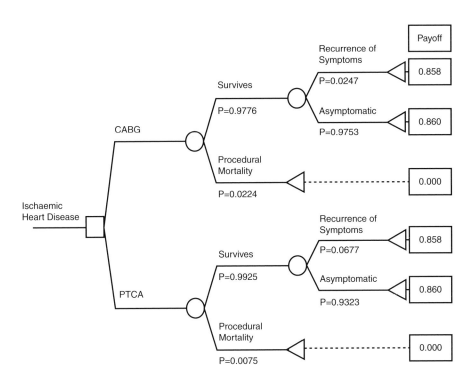

Fig. 10.1 The structure of the model used in Example 1

10.2.2
Constructing a Decision Tree

Start by opening TreeAge.

In the Main tree window, a single unnamed decision node will be visible

To name the decision node, left click on the area above the node; the name can be changed in the future by left clicking on area above the node again (Fig. 10.2).

Choices can be added to the decision node by left clicking on the node. Left clicking on the node once adds two choices. Every subsequent left click on the node adds one further choice (Fig. 10.3).

In the same way that we named the decision node, we can name the chance nodes (Fig. 10.4).

Possible outcomes can be added to the chance nodes in the same way that we added all the possible choices to the decision node. Left clicking on the node once adds two chance outcomes. Every subsequent left click on the node adds one further chance outcome (Fig. 10.5).

When the tree is complete (Fig. 10.5), most of the final nodes will be converted into terminal nodes, with payoffs attached to them. This can be done by right clicking on the node. This reveals a menu of options. Select the *Change Node Type…* option; alternatively, select the chance node by left clicking on it and select the change node type button (⊠), click on the *Options* menu and then *Change Node Type…* from the pull-down menu or hold down *Ctrl + T* keys. This will bring up the following menu (Fig. 10.6).

Select *Terminal*, and then click on *OK*. The following box will appear (Fig. 10.7).

Whilst it is possible to enter numerical payoffs, by naming the payoffs, we will be able to use the same payoffs for different outcomes. We will also be able to change the numerical value of payoffs more easily and perform sensitivity analysis. In our example, we have

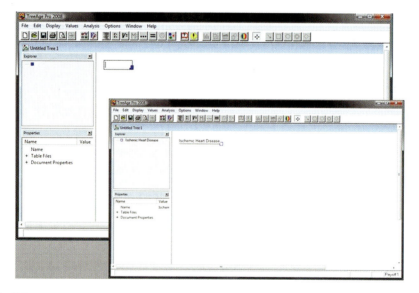

Fig. 10.2

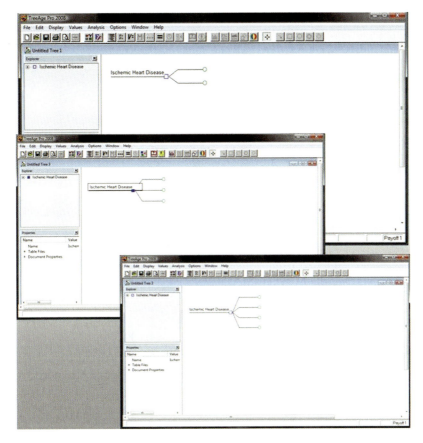

Fig. 10.3

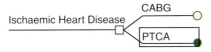

Fig. 10.4

called the utility associated with the symptom free health state *u_asymp* and the utility associated with the symptomatic health state *u_symp*. Enter *u_symp* into the box *Payoff 1:*.

Entering a variable name that has not been previously defined will automatically reveal the following window (Fig. 10.8).

Select the *Define numerically* (*at root*) tick box. Enter the default value in the *Value* box and high and low values for sensitivity analysis in the *Low value* and *High value* box. Then click *OK*.

When this process is completed for all the terminal nodes (Fig. 10.9), we can begin to enter the path probabilities.

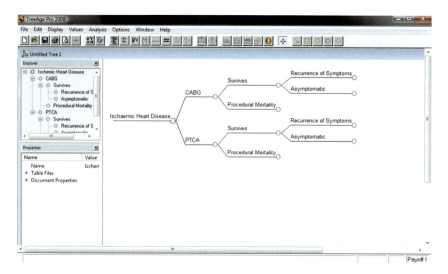

Fig. 10.5

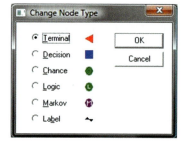

Fig. 10.6

Fig. 10.7

Fig. 10.8

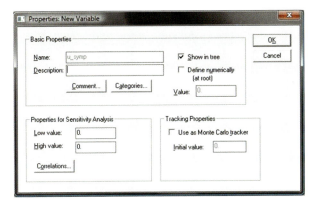

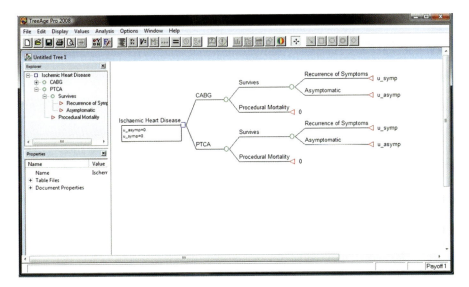

Fig. 10.9

Whilst it is possible to give the path probabilities numerical values, it is easier to name the path probabilities for the same reasons that it is easier to name the payoffs associated with terminal nodes. The path probabilities at each chance node must add up to 1. The easiest way to ensure that they add up to exactly 1 is to assign 1 of the outcomes of each chance node the path probability '#'. The path probability '#' represents 1 minus the sum of all the other path probabilities at that chance node.

Path probabilities are added by simply left clicking underneath each branch that follows a chance node (Fig. 10.10), and then typing the name of the variable. For example, in our model, we have named the preoperative death rate following CABG, *p_periop_cabg*.

In the same way, entering an unknown variable into the payoff window (Fig. 10.7) automatically brings up the new variable window (Fig. 10.8). Entering an unknown variable as a probability will bring up the new variable window (Fig. 10.8). It can then be defined in the same way that the payoffs can be defined.

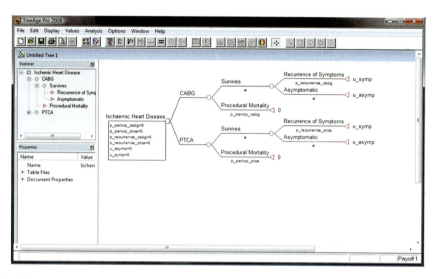

Fig. 10.10

We can edit the values of the variables after we have defined them by clicking on the *Values* menu and then clicking on *Variables and Tables*. Alternatively, press *Ctrl + D*. This will reveal the following menu (Fig. 10.11).

Click on the *Variables List* in the top left hand corner to reveal the list of variables defined in the tree. Double clicking on any of the variables will reveal the variable window shown in Fig. 10.12. This window can also be reached by clicking on the *Edit Properties...* button.

If the TreeAge Excel Expansion module and Microsoft Excel is available, then the variables can be more easily edited by selecting all the variables in the variables and tables window (Fig. 10.11). This can be done by either by pressing and holding the *shift* button and left clicking the top and then bottom variable, or by pressing and holding the *ctrl* button and selecting each variable individually. Once all of the variables have been selected, press the *Edit in Excel* button. This will automatically start Microsoft Excel, and the variables can be entered into a spreadsheet in the following way (Fig. 10.13).

The variables can then readily be edited. New variables can easily be added by entering the name and the values associated with the new variable underneath the existing variables in the same format.

When all new variables have been added and editing has been completed, highlight all of the variables as shown (Fig. 10.13). Click on the *Add-Ins* menu tab, and then click on the *TreeAge* drop down menu, then on the *Add or Update Variables* option. If this action has been successful, the following window will appear (Fig. 10.14).

Finally, before we are ready to analyse our decision analytical model, we must change the numerical format of the results. This can be done by right clicking anywhere in the main tree window and selecting *Preferences...* from the menu that is revealed. Alternatively, click on the preference button (🔳) in the tool bar, press the *F11* key or click on the *Edit* menu and then *Preferences...* All of these paths will bring up the preference menu (Fig. 10.15).

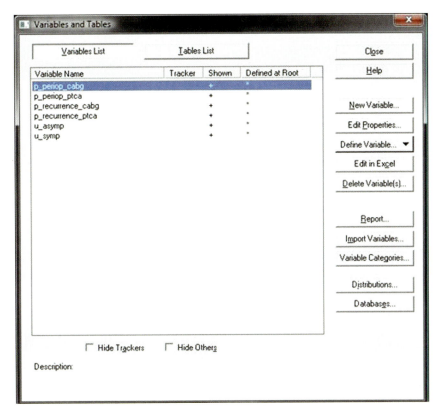

Fig. 10.11

Fig. 10.12

Click on the *Calculation Method* option. Choose the *Simple (single payoff)* option from the *Method* pull-down menu. Ensure that *1* is selected in the *Use payoff* pull-down menu. Then select the *Numeric Format*. This will open the window shown below (Fig. 10.16).

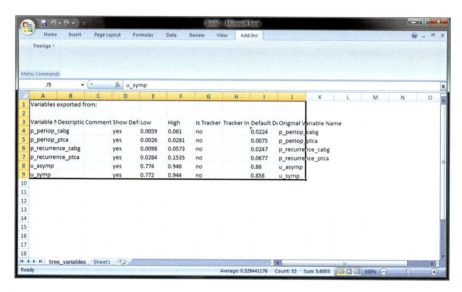

Fig. 10.13

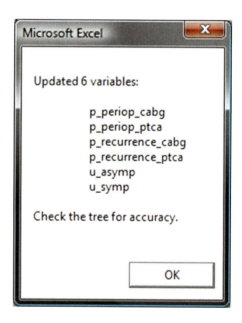

Fig. 10.14

Select the number of decimal places required for the results. From the *Units* pull-down model, select *None*. The results of analysis are utility values and consequently have no units. When this is completed, press *OK*. This will return us to the preferences menu. Press *OK* to return us to the tree.

We are now ready to start analysing our decision analytical model.

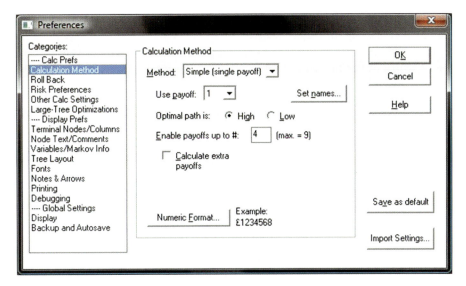

Fig. 10.15

Fig. 10.16

10.2.3
Analysing a Decision Tree

The expected value at any node in the decision tree can be calculated by selecting the node by left clicking on it, selecting the *Analysis* menu and then *Expected Value*. Alternatively, hold down the *Ctrl + E* keys.

If we calculate the expected value at the *Asymptomatic* node of the *CABG* subtree, the following results (Fig. 10.17) are obtained

In a similar way, we can calculate the path probability at any node by clicking on it and then selecting on the *Analysis* menu and then *Path Probability*. If we do this at the same node, the *Symptom Free* node of the *CABG* subtree, the following results (Fig. 10.18) are obtained.

We can roll back the whole tree by clicking on the roll back button (◧) in the tool bar; alternatively, click on the *Analysis* menu and then *Roll Back,* or hold down the *Ctrl* + *R*.

The following results (Fig. 10.19) are obtained.

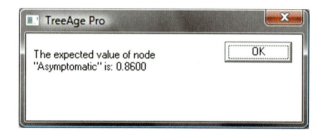

Fig. 10.17

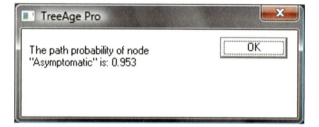

Fig. 10.18

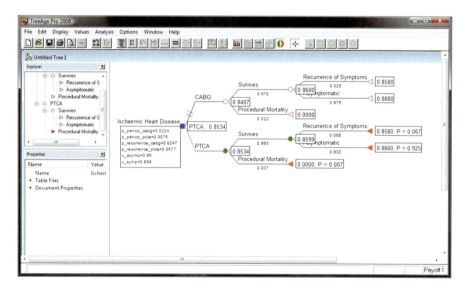

Fig. 10.19

Fig. 10.20

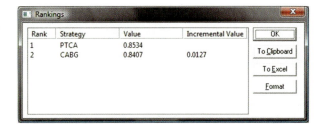

Finally, for information on the difference between the expected value of each strategy (Fig. 10.20), they can be ranked by clicking on the *Analysis* Menu and *Rankings*. This information can be exported to either the clipboard or Microsoft Excel by clicking on the appropriate button.

10.2.4
Univariate and Multivariate Sensitivity Analysis

We are able to perform univariate and two-way sensitivity analysis to investigate the uncertainty associated with our model parameters.

In order to perform univariate sensitivity analysis, click on the univariate sensitivity analysis button (▦). Alternatively, click on the *Analysis*, then *Sensitivity Analysis*, then *One Way…* or simply press *F5*. This will bring up the sensitivity analysis window (Fig. 10.21). Choose the variable on which you wish to perform univariate sensitivity analysis. The *High value* and *Low value* will automatically be set to the high and low values that we defined earlier. Choose the *Number of Intervals* and press then *OK*.

The results will be displayed as shown bellow (Fig. 10.22).

Fig. 10.21

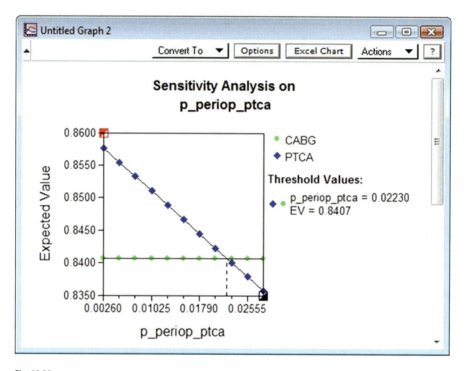

Fig. 10.22

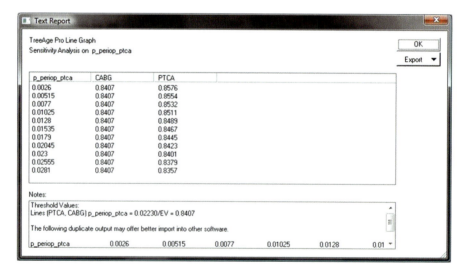

Fig. 10.23

By pressing the *Actions* button and then the *Text Report* option, the information displayed graphically in Fig. 10.22 can be displayed in written form (Fig. 10.23). This can be exported to the clipboard or Excel by pressing the *Export* button.

It is possible to export the graph to Excel in order to edit it further (Fig. 10.24), by pressing the *Excel Chart* button in Fig. 10.22.

Two-way sensitivity analysis can be performed by pressing the two-way sensitivity button (▣). Alternatively, click on the *Analysis* menu, then on *Sensitivity Analysis*, then on *Two Way...* Alternatively, press *Shift + F5*. This will reveal the two-way sensitivity menu (Fig. 10.25).

Choose the required variables from the *Variable* pull-down menus, and change the *Number of Intervals* to 10. The *Low value* and *High value* will automatically be set to the values specified earlier. By pressing *OK,* the following diagram will be produced (Fig. 10.26). A test report for this graph can be produced in a similar way to the other graphical reports by pressing the *Text Report* buttons.

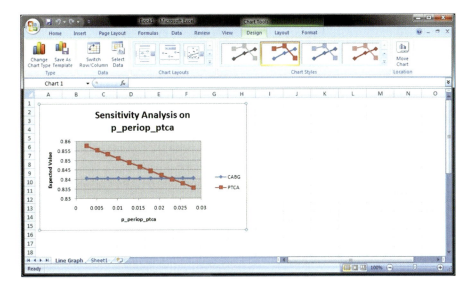

Fig. 10.24

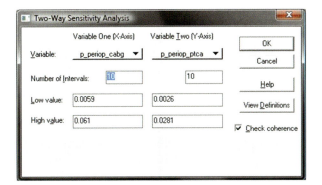

Fig. 10.25

Fig. 10.26

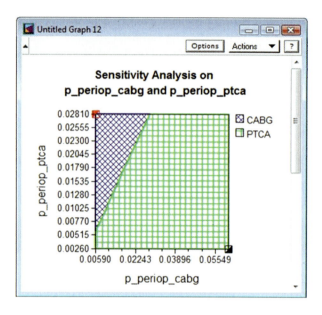

10.2.5
Probabilistic Sensitivity Analysis

When the tree has been constructed, we need to define distributions for each of the variables. To define a variable in TreeAge, click on *Values*, then on *Distributions...*, alternatively, press *Ctrl + Shift + D*. This will reveal the following window (Fig. 10.27).

Click on the *New...* button. The following window will be revealed (Fig. 10.28).

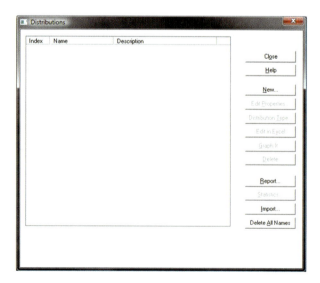

Fig. 10.27

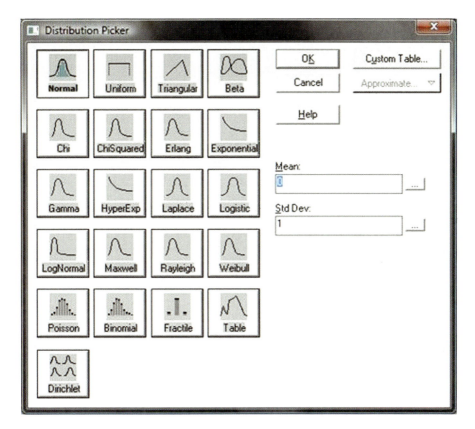

Fig. 10.28

A distribution type can be selected by clicking on it. Most distributions frequently used in decision analysis are available in TreeAge. In this model, we will use triangular distributions. Click on the triangular distribution button (△). The following window will be revealed (Fig. 10.29).

We will start by defining the preoperative mortality rate following CABG. Enter '0.0059' into the *Min:* box, '0.0224' into the *Likeliest:* box, and '0.0610' into the *Max:* box. When this has been completed, press the *OK* box. The following window will appear (Fig. 10.30). Enter a name and description for the distribution, and then press *OK*.

The distribution will then appear in the list of distributions (Fig. 10.31.). Distributions can be assigned to the other variables in the same way; however, in a similar way to how we defined the variables, it is easier to define the distributions in Excel.

This can be done selecting the distributions in Fig. 10.31 that have already been defined and then clicking on the *Edit in Excel* button. The following window will appear, and the distributions should be entered manually as shown (Fig. 10.32).

When all new variables have been added and editing has been completed, highlight all of the variables as we did previously for the variables (Fig. 10.13). Click on the *Add-Ins* menu tab, then click on the *TreeAge* drop down menu on the *Add or Update Distributions* option. If this action has been successful, the following window will appear (Fig. 10.33).

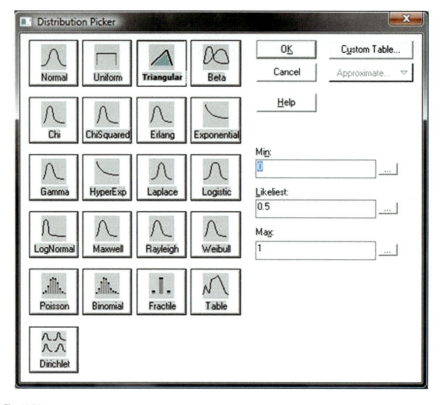

Fig. 10.29

Fig. 10.30

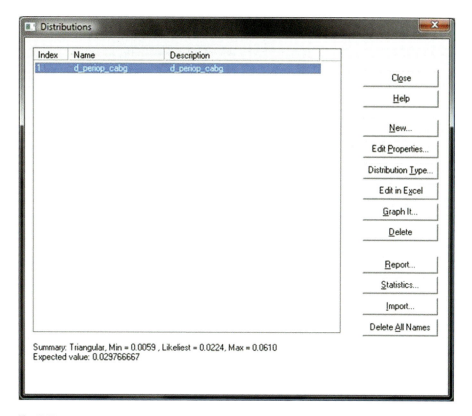

Fig. 10.31

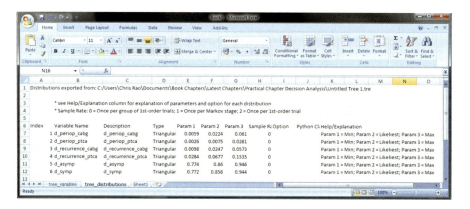

Fig. 10.32

Fig. 10.33

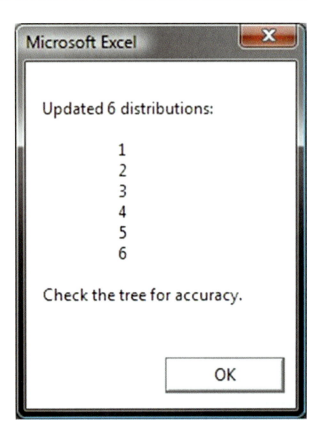

When all of the distributions have been defined (Fig. 10.34), we can start to connect them to the variables. It is easiest way to do this in Excel as described before.

When the variables have been entered into Excel as shown in Fig. 10.35, update the variables in TreeAge. We can now perform a probabilistic sensitivity analysis.

In this example, we are able to perform a second-order Monte Carlo simulation as we have defined distributions from which the variables will be sampled. Click on the decision node and press the Markov simulation button from the tool bar (⊞); alternatively, press *F7* or select the *Analysis* menu and then select *Monte Carlo Simulation,* then *Two-Dimensional (Sampling + Trials)....* The following window will be revealed (Fig. 10.36).

TreeAge can perform Monte Carlo simulation either for a theoretical cohort of patients using expected values of the distributions or for individual patients using microsimulation. In most cases, it is appropriate to perform Monte Carlo simulation for a theoretical cohort of patients as it is computationally more efficient. Enter 1,000 into the *Number of samples (and model recalculations)* box. When this has been completed, select *Begin.* The following results are generated (Fig. 10.37).

Clicking the *Sats Report...* button reveals the following window (Fig. 10.38). Note that according to the results of this model, the largest payoff is gained by the PTCA option.

Graphs of the payoffs and incremental outcomes (Fig. 10.39) can be produced by pressing the *Graph* button in Fig. 10.37. These results can also be exported to Excel (Fig. 10.40).

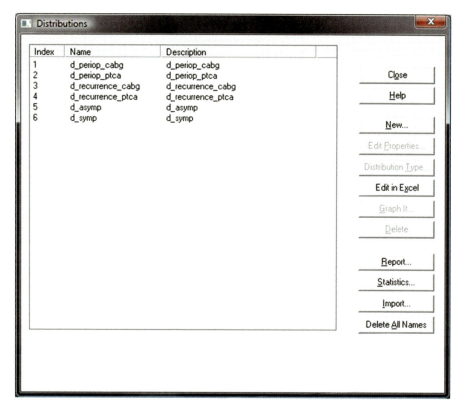

Fig. 10.34

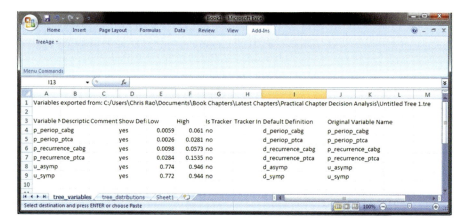

Fig. 10.35

Fig. 10.36

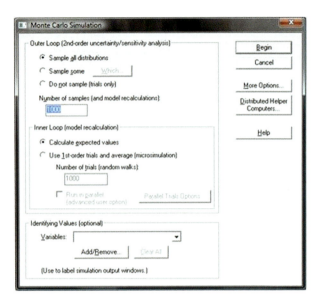

Fig. 10.37

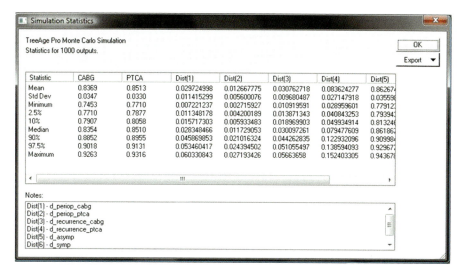

Fig. 10.38

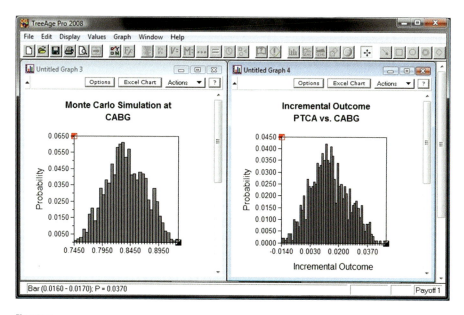

Fig. 10.39

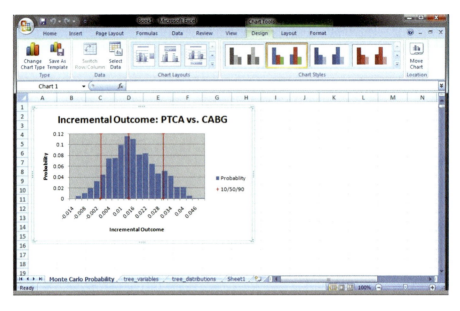

Fig. 10.40

10.3
Example 2: Mitral Valve Replacement

10.3.1
Background Information

The commonest cause of death after mitral valve replacement is heart failure. It has been hypothesised that this is because the mitral valve apparatus is commonly excised during operations to replace the mitral valve, and that these structures play a vital role in maintaining the structure and function of the heart. It has been suggested that preservation of the mitral valve apparatus would reduce the incidence of heart failure and consequently improve the survival of patients after mitral valve replacement[2].

In the following example based on an example from the literature[2] we evaluate what effect mitral valve apparatus preservation has on the quality and length of life in the first 10 years after mitral valve replacement. In order to answer this question, we will construct the following simple simulation (Fig. 10.41). Patients start in the 'ALIVE' state. Each

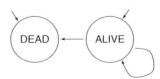

Fig. 10.41 A basic Markov model

Table 10.2 Model parameters used in Example 2

Parameter	Value	Range/SD	Distribution
Transition probabilities			
Cardiac-related mortality without preservation			
Year 1	0.1090		
Year 2	0.0233		
Year 3	0.0263		
Year 4	0.0144		
Year 5	0.0205		
Year 6	0.0205		
Year 7	0.0205		
Year 8	0.0205		
Year 9	0.0205		
Year 10	0.0205		
Cardiac-related mortality preservation			
Year 1	0.0575	0.0214–0.1500	Triangular
Year 2	0.0117	0.0046–0.0288	Triangular
Year 3	0.0127	0.0054–0.0291	Triangular
Year 4	0.0067	0.0031–0.0143	Triangular
Year 5	0.0093	0.0047–0.0187	Triangular
Year 6	0.0093	0.0047–0.0187	Triangular
Year 7	0.0093	0.0047–0.0187	Triangular
Year 8	0.0093	0.0047–0.0187	Triangular
Year 9	0.0093	0.0047–0.0187	Triangular
Year 10	0.0093	0.0047–0.0187	Triangular
Baseline population mortality			
Year 1	0.0130		
Year 2	0.0147		
Year 3	0.0162		
Year 4	0.0180		
Year 5	0.0202		
Year 6	0.0226		
Year 7	0.0252		
Year 8	0.0289		
Year 9	0.0334		
Year 10	0.0384		

cycle they can then remain in the 'ALIVE' state or move to the 'DEAD' state either by dying of a causes related to their cardiac pathology, or by dying of causes of death unrelated to their cardiac pathology. The following tables show the parameters that will be used in this example (Tables 10.2 and 10.3)

Table 10.3 Model parameters used in Example 2

Parameter	Value	Range/SD	Distribution
Utility parameters			
Postoperative utility without preservation			
Year 1	0.7111	0.1503	Normal
Year 2	0.6794	0.1436	Normal
Year 3	0.6794	0.1436	Normal
Year 4	0.6794	0.1436	Normal
Year 5	0.6794	0.1436	Normal
Year 6	0.6794	0.1436	Normal
Year 7	0.6794	0.1436	Normal
Year 8	0.6794	0.1436	Normal
Year 9	0.6794	0.1436	Normal
Year 10	0.6794	0.1436	Normal
Postoperative utility with preservation			
Year 1	0.7833	0.0703	Normal
Year 2	0.7483	0.0672	Normal
Year 3	0.7483	0.0672	Normal
Year 4	0.7483	0.0672	Normal
Year 5	0.7483	0.0672	Normal
Year 6	0.7483	0.0672	Normal
Year 7	0.7483	0.0672	Normal
Year 8	0.7483	0.0672	Normal
Year 9	0.7483	0.0672	Normal
Year 10	0.7483	0.0672	Normal

10.3.2
Constructing a Markov Model

In the main tree window, construct the following tree (Fig. 10.42).

Now change the chance nodes at the end of the tree into Markov nodes. This can be done by right clicking on the node and selecting *Change Node Type...* from the menu that is revealed; alternatively, select the chance node by left clicking on it and select the change node type button (⊠), click on the *Options* menu and then *Change Node Type...* from the pull-down menu or hold down *Ctrl + T* keys. This will bring up the following menu (Fig. 10.43).

Select *Markov*, and then click on *OK*. Complete this process for both of the chance nodes (Fig. 10.44).

We now have to add Markov states to each of the Markov simulations. This is done by left clicking on the Markov node once to add two Markov states and clicking on it again to add further states in a similar way to how options are added to a decision node or chance occurrences are added to a chance node (Fig. 10.45).

Fig. 10.42

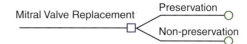

Fig. 10.43

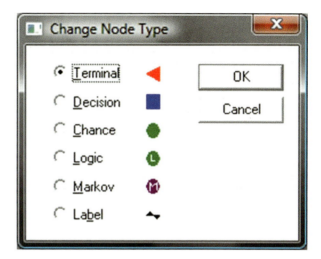

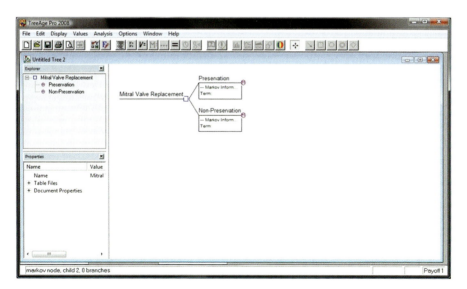

Fig. 10.44

After this is done, we need to designate Markov states that are absorbing states, in this case death. This can be done by changing the node associated with that state from a chance node to a terminal node in the same way as described in the first example (Fig. 10.46).

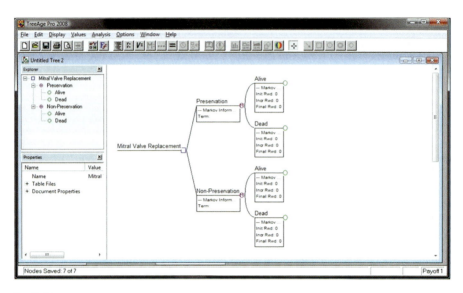

Fig. 10.45

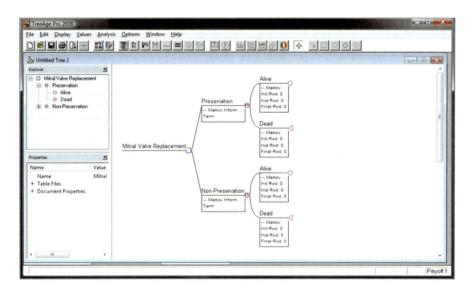

Fig. 10.46

We now need to model the state transition that can take place from the 'alive' state. Our Markov simulation is very simple, and there are only two possible outcomes that can take place. A patient can either die, or they can continue to live. Practically, we model this by adding chance outcomes to the chance node associated with the alive node. This is done simply by left clicking on the chance node in same way that we have done previously (Fig. 10.47).

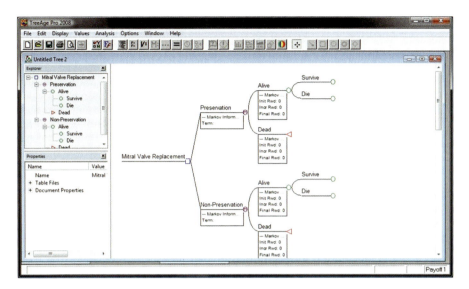

Fig. 10.47

Once we have completed this process for all the Markov transitions, we need to define where the patient in the simulation will start the next Markov cycle. This can be done by changing the chance node associated with the Markov transition into a terminal node in the same way described previously.

When this has been done, the 'Jump To' menu automatically appears (Fig. 10.48). Select the Markov transition state that we wish the patient to start the next cycle in from the menu and then press *OK*. In the case of the *Survive* transition from the *Alive* state, we want our patient to start the next cycle in the *Alive* state. In the case of the *Die* transition from the *Alive* state, we want our patient to start the next cycle in the *Death* state.

After this has been successfully completed, the Markov state that the patient will jump to from the *Alive* state after making the transition *Live* will be displayed after the terminal node (Fig. 10.49).

When this process has been completed for all of the Markov transitions (Fig. 10.50), the structure of the decision analytical model is complete and we are ready to start defining our model parameters.

We will start by defining the termination conditions. In this simulation, we want the time horizon to be 10 years; consequently, we want our simulation to finish when ten cycles have been performed. The tenth cycle is called 'Stage 9' using the nomenclature used in TreeAge as the programme calls the first cycle 'Stage 0'. To do this, double left click on the *Markov Termination* box hanging underneath the Markov node; alternatively, click on *Values* and then click on *Markov Termination…* after selecting the Markov simulation by left clicking on it. The following window will appear (Fig. 10.51).

Delete the default termination condition, and enter _stage = 10. This will terminate the Markov simulation after ten cycles (0–9) have occurred. When this has been done, click on *OK*. Complete this for both Markov Simulations.

Fig. 10.48

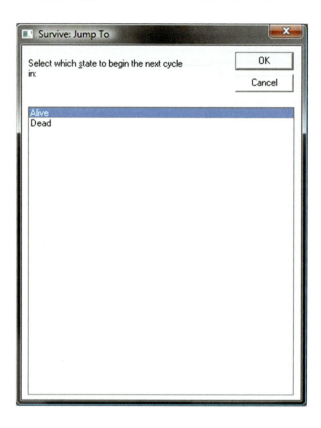

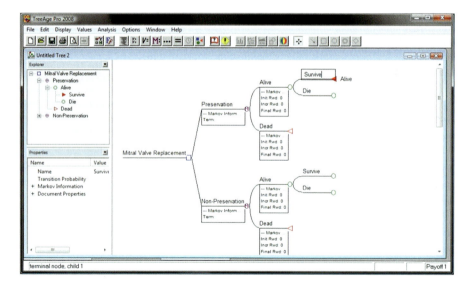

Fig. 10.49

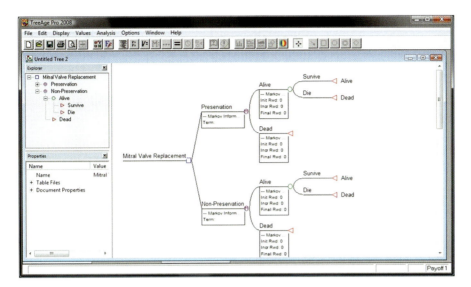

Fig. 10.50

Fig. 10.51

We must now define the rewards associated with each of the Markov states. This can be done by double left clicking on the *Markov State info* box hanging under each of the Markov states; alternatively, click on *Values* and then click on *Markov State Information...* after selecting the Markov state by left clicking on it. The following window will appear (Fig. 10.51).

The *Initial (stage 0):* box is the reward that will be applied to all the patients who start the simulation in that state. The *Incremental:* box is the reward that will be applied to patients who enter or return to the state each cycle. The *Final (after term):* box is the reward that will be applied to each patient who finishes the simulation in that state. Enter 0 into all three boxes for the *Dead* state in all the simulations. Enter *u_p* into the first two boxes for the *Alive* state in the *Preservation* simulation and *u_np* into the first two boxes for the *Alive* state in the *Non-Preservation* simulation. When this has been completed, click on *OK* (Fig. 10.52).

Fig. 10.52

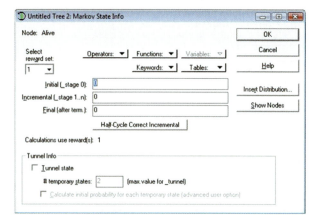

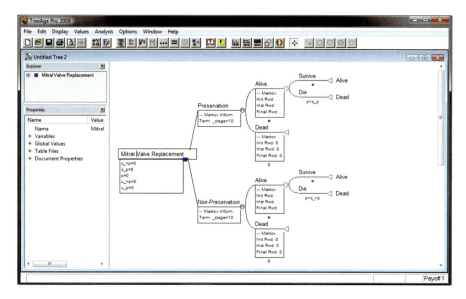

Fig. 10.53

As we have entered an undefined variable into our decision analytical model, the *New Variable* window will appear (Fig. 10.8). Click on the *Define numerically (at root)* check box, then click on *OK*. We can now define the variable at a later stage as described in the previous example using Excel. As there is no payoff associated with the Dead state, we do not need to enter payoffs; however, we do need to enter transition probabilities. Enter the transition probability *p* representing baseline population mortality, and the transition probabilities *c_p* and *c_np* representing cardiac mortality in the *Preservation* and *Non-Preservation* cohorts, respectively, as shown in Fig. 10.53. When the *New Variable* window appears (Fig. 10.8), click on the *Define numerically (at root)* check box and then click on *OK*.

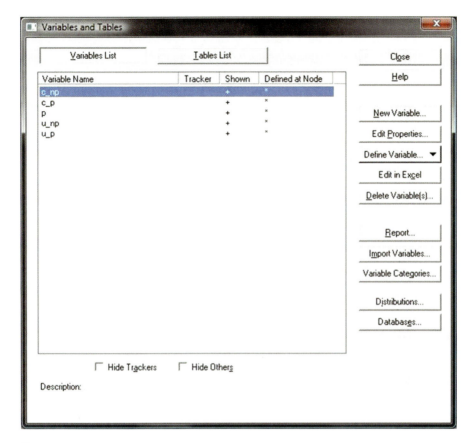

Fig. 10.54

10.3.2.1
Cycle-Dependant Model Parameters

The cardiac mortality is highest in the first year after the operation and declines with time; however, the baseline mortality increases as the cohort of patients gets older. Likewise, the health-related quality of life declines as the patient gets older and patient co-morbidities increase. Whilst it would be possible to define the variable that we have already entered into our model with static numerical variables or distributions, this would not reflect what actually happens to patients who undergo mitral valve replacement. Consequently, in this section, we will explain how to define model parameters, or the distributions that define model parameters using tables. This will allow the model parameters or distributions to change with time.

First of all we must create distributions to reflect the uncertainty associated with the cardiac mortality in the *preservation* group and utility in both groups. For the purpose of this example, we will assume that there is no uncertainty associated with either the population baseline mortality or the cardiac mortality in the *non-preservation group.* Create two normal distributions called *d_u_np* and *d_u_p* with the TreeAge default values for the mean (0) and standard deviation (1) to define the utility of the *non-preservation* and *preservation* state, respectively. Create a triangular distribution called *d_c_p* with the TreeAge default definitions for the minimum (0), likeliest (0.5) and maximum (1) to represent the cardiac mortality in the *preservation* group. The TreeAge default definitions can be changed at a later stage.

We must now create tables to define the baseline population mortality (*t_p*), the cardiac mortality in the non-preservation group (*t_c_np*), the standard deviation and mean of the utility in the *preservation* (*t_sd_u_p, t_x_u_p*) and *non-preservation* group (*t_sd_u_np, t_x_u_np*), and the minimum, likeliest and maximum cardiac mortality in the *preservation* group (*t_min_c_p, t_lik_c_p, t_max_c_p*).

To create a table in TreeAge, click on the *Values* menu and then *Variables and Tables...*, alternatively press *Ctrl* + *D*. This will open the following window (Fig. 10.54).

Click on the *Tables List* button at the top of the window; the following window will appear (Fig. 10.55).

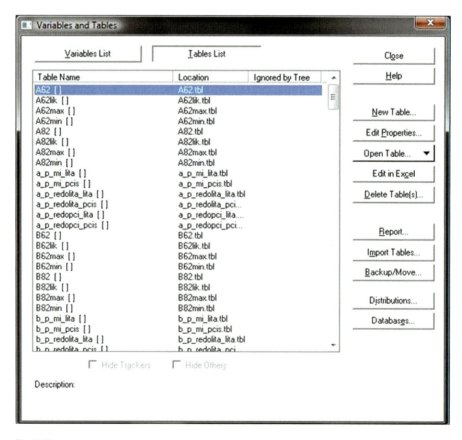

Fig. 10.55

If you have not used the programme before, the main list will be empty. Table files are saved separately from the individual decision analytical model and can be reused in all models.

Click on the *New Table* button. The following window (Fig. 10.56) will appear. Enter the name of the new table (*t_p*) into the *Name:* and the *File:* box and the press *OK*.

The new table will now appear in the list of tables (Fig. 10.57).

To enter values into the table, click on the *Open Table* button, then select *Edit Table* from the pull-down menu. The following window will appear (Fig. 10.58).

Enter the first value from Table 10.2, and then click on *OK*. The first value will appear in the table window (Fig. 10.59).

A quicker way to edit the table is to select the table in the main *Variables and Tables* window (Fig. 10.57) and then click the *Edit in Excel* button. The following spreadsheet is generated (Fig. 10.60).

Enter the data from Tables 10.2 and 10.3 and then highlight it as shown (Fig. 10.61) before clicking on the *TreeAge* menu, then *Add or Update Table.*

When this operation has been successfully completed, the following window will appear (Fig. 10.62).

Click on *OK*. If we have already defined some of the variables in the table, the following window will appear (Fig. 10.63). Click on *Yes.*

To use our table to define a variable, open the *Variables and Tables* window (Fig. 10.64) as described above and select the variable *p*. Then click on the *Define Variable…* button and select *Default for Tree* from the pull-down menu. The following window will be revealed. Enter *t_p[_stage]* into the box *p*. Then press *OK*. This means that during every cycle, TreeAge will look up the index value of the value of the table *t_p* that corresponds to the

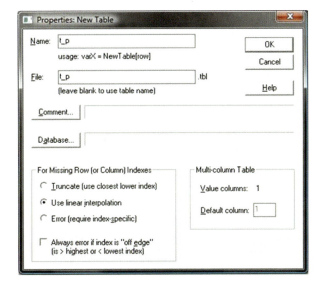

Fig. 10.56

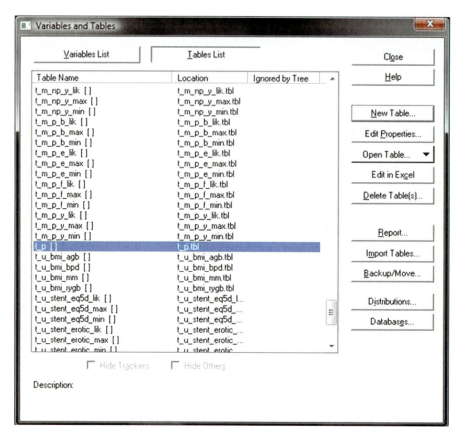

Fig. 10.57

Fig. 10.58

Fig. 10.59

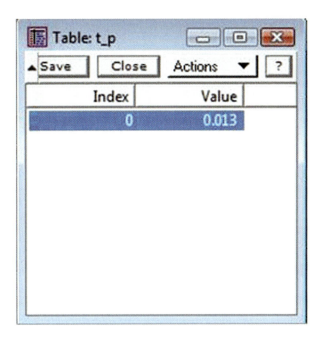

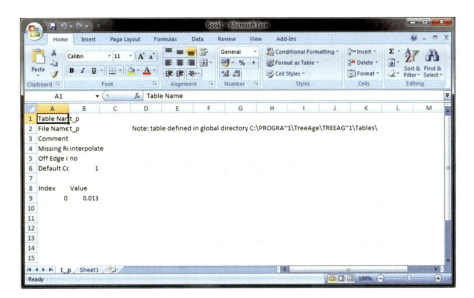

Fig. 10.60

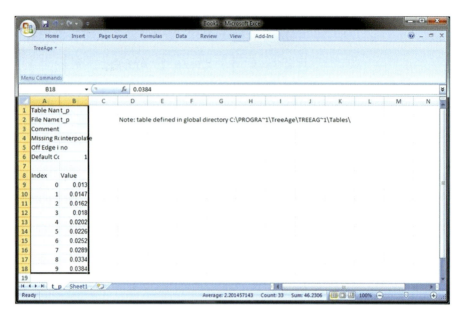

Fig. 10.61

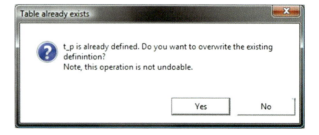

Fig. 10.62

Fig. 10.63

Fig. 10.64

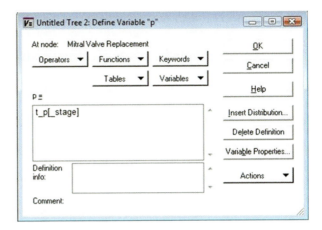

cycle number and use the associated value from the table as the value for *p*. We must now define all of the other tables, summarised below using the same method (Table 10.4).

Now, using Excel defines the distributions and parameters used in this model as demonstrated (Figs. 10.65 and 10.66).

Finally, before we are ready to analyse our decision analytical model, we must change the numerical format of the results. This can be done by right clicking anywhere in the main tree window and selecting *Preferences*... from the menu that is revealed. Alternatively, click on the preference button ( ) in the tool bar, press the *F11* key or click on the *Edit* menu and then *Preferences*... All of these paths will bring up the preference menu (Fig. 10.67).

Click on the *Calculation Method* option. Choose the *Simple (single payoff)* option from the *Method* pull-down menu. Ensure that *1* is selected in the *Use payoff* pull-down menu. Then select the *Numeric Format*. This will open the window shown below (Fig. 10.68).

Select the number of decimal places required for the results. From the *Units* pull-down model, select *Custom suffix*. Enter *QALYs* into the *Suffix:* box. When this is completed, press the *OK*. This will return us to the preferences menu. Press *OK* so as to return us to the tree. We are now ready to start analysing our decision analytical model.

10.3.2.2
Discounting

In this decision analytical model, we will discount the results of the Markov simulation. To do this, instead of simply entering *u_p* as the payoff in the *Markov State info* box of the *preservation* state, enter *discount(u_p; d_rate; _stage)*. The variable *d_rate* represents the discount rate. Define the discount rate using the triangular distribution *d_d_rate*, with minimum value 0, likeliest value 3.5, and maximum value 6.

Table 10.4 Model parameters used in Example 2

	t_p	t_c_np	t_x_u_p	t_sd_u_p	t_x_u_np	t_sd_u_np	t_min_c_p	t_lik_c_p	t_max_c_p
0	0.013	0.109	0.7833	0.0703	0.7111	0.1503	0.0214	0.0575	0.15
1	0.0147	0.0233	0.7483	0.0672	0.6794	0.1436	0.0046	0.0117	0.0288
2	0.0162	0.0263	0.7483	0.0672	0.6794	0.1436	0.0054	0.0127	0.0291
3	0.018	0.0144	0.7483	0.0672	0.6794	0.1436	0.0031	0.0067	0.0143
4	0.0202	0.0205	0.7483	0.0672	0.6794	0.1436	0.0047	0.0093	0.0187
5	0.0226	0.0205	0.7483	0.0672	0.6794	0.1436	0.0047	0.0093	0.0187
6	0.0252	0.0205	0.7483	0.0672	0.6794	0.1436	0.0047	0.0093	0.0187
7	0.0289	0.0205	0.7483	0.0672	0.6794	0.1436	0.0047	0.0093	0.0187
8	0.0334	0.0205	0.7483	0.0672	0.6794	0.1436	0.0047	0.0093	0.0187
9	0.0384	0.0205	0.7483	0.0672	0.6794	0.1436	0.0047	0.0093	0.0187

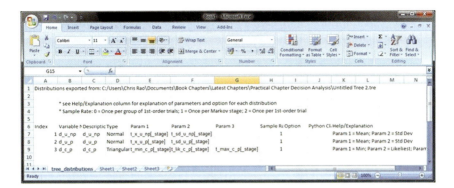

Fig. 10.65

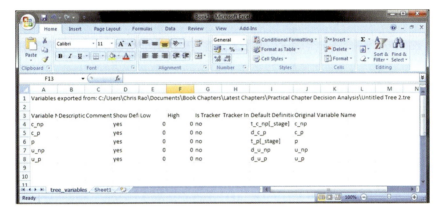

Fig. 10.66

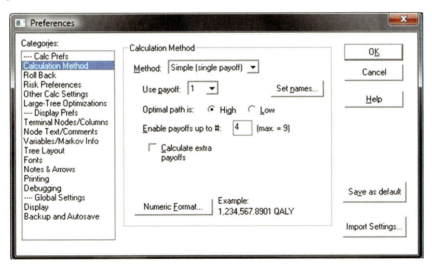

Fig. 10.67

Fig. 10.68

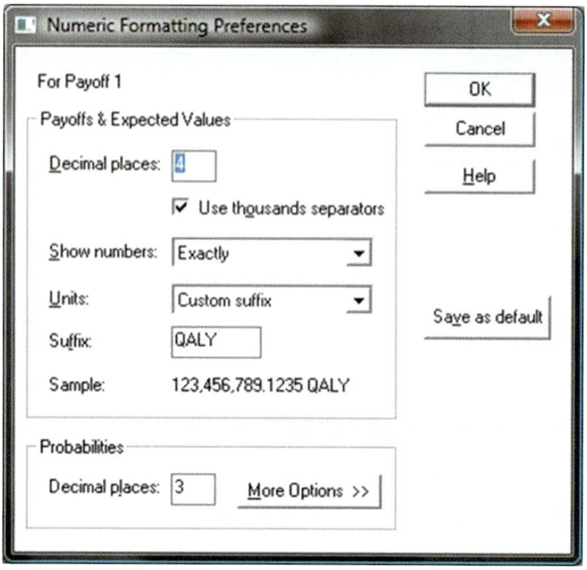

10.3.3
Analysing a Markov Model

We are now ready to start analysing the tree. The tree can be rolled back (Fig. 10.69), and the outcomes can be ranked in the same way as in Example 1.

It is also possible to perform univariate in the same way as in Example 1; however, as we used a Markov simulation, we are able to extract information from the decision analytical model in Example 2 that we were unable to extract in Example 1. Click on the decision node and press the Markov simulation button from the tool bar (⬚); alternatively, press *F7* or select the *Analysis* menu and then select *Monte Carlo Simulation,* then *Two-Dimensional (Sampling + Trials)....* The following window will be revealed (Fig. 10.70).

Choose *Calculate expected values* in the *Inner Loop (model recalculation)* box. Then, press the *Begin* button to start the Markov simulation.

The results of the Markov simulation will then be displayed (Fig. 10.71). This can take some time depending on the speed of the computer, the complexity of the model, the number of trials and whether the inner loop consists of calculation of the expected values or microsimulation. As it can take some time to perform a Markov simulation, it is prudent to save simulations so that analysis can be performed again or further graphs and figures extracted at a later date.

By pressing the *Stats shown for:* button the results can be seen for both the *Preservation* and *Non-Preservation* cohort.

Clicking the *Stats Report...* button displays a summary of the results of the Markov simulation (Fig. 10.72). This information can be exported to Excel or a text file by clicking the *Export* button.

Graphs showing the distribution of the payoffs and incremental payoffs can be constructed in both TreeAge and Excel in the same way that they were produced in Example 1.

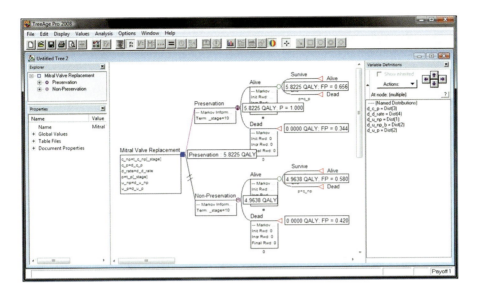

Fig. 10.69

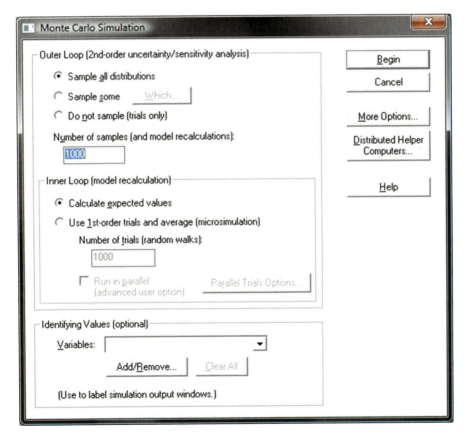

Fig. 10.70

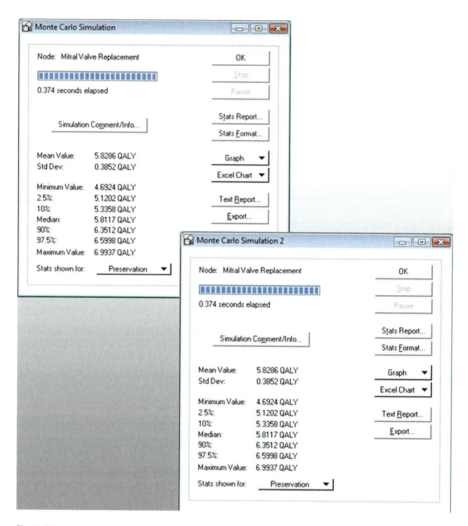

Fig. 10.71

Further information can be gained by selecting one of the Markov nodes, for example, the *Preservation* node. A Markov cohort analysis can then be performed.

This can be done by clicking on the *Analysis* menu and then on *Markov Cohort (Full Detail)*; alternatively press *Shift + F6*. This will reveal the following window (Fig. 10.73).

By selecting the *Graph* button, graphs can be generated showing for the selected cohort the probability a patient is in each of the states for each cycle, the rewards earned by patients in each of the states for each cycle, the average reward per patient earned by the whole cohort for each cycle, the average cumulative reward per patient for each cycle, and the survival curve for the selected cohort (Fig. 10.74).

A text report can be generated by selecting the *Text Report* button in the graph. In the same way as all previous figures, Excel charts can also be generated for all of these graphs.

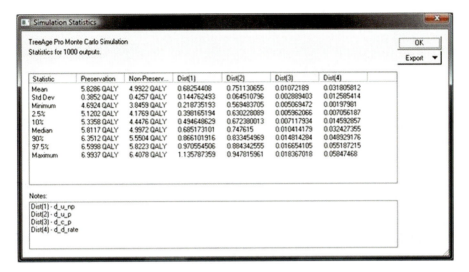

Fig. 10.72

Fig. 10.73

Finally, exporting graphs to Excel is a powerful aid to analysis as the user can manipulate these graphs in order to display on the same graph information about all of the Markov cohorts simultaneously (Fig. 10.75).

10.4
Summary

In this chapter, we have demonstrated how to construct a basic decision analytical model, how to conduct sensitivity analysis and how to perform Markov simulation using practical examples. By using these methods, we hope that the reader will be able to construct more complex decision analytical models to address clinical problems in their own practice.

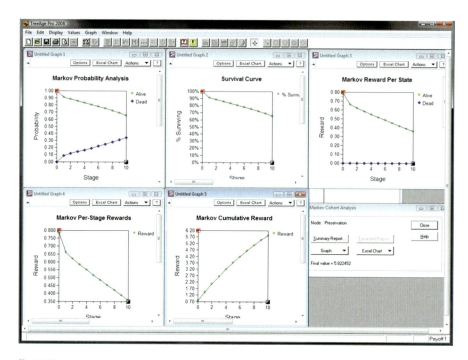

Fig. 10.74

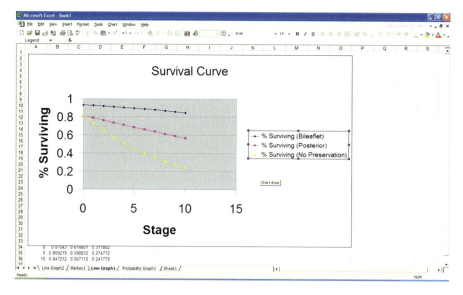

Fig. 10.75

References

1. Rao C, Aziz O, Panesar S, et al. Cost effectiveness analysis of minimally invasive internal thoracic artery bypass versus percutaneous revascularisation for isolated lesions of the left anterior descending artery. *BMJ*. 2007;334:621.
2. Rao C, Hart J, Chow A, et al. Does preservation of the sub-valvular apparatus during mitral valve replacement affect long-term survival and quality of life? A microsimulation study. *J Cardiothorac Surg*. 2008;3:17.
3. Briggs A, Sculpher M, Claxton K. *Decision Modelling for Health Economic Evaluation*. Oxford: Oxford University Press; 2006.

A Practical Example of Cost-Effectiveness Analysis

11

Christopher Rao, Sejal Jiwan, and Thanos Athanasiou

Abstract In this chapter, we describe the practical application of cost-effectiveness analysis using an example adapted from the published literature. Analysis was performed using the decision analytical software package *TreeAge Pro Suite* (TreeAge Software inc., Williamstown, Massachusetts, USA). By using these methods, and the methods described in Chap. 10, we hope that the reader will be able to construct more complex models to assess the cost-effectiveness of medical technology and practice.

11.1
Introduction

Cost-effectiveness analysis has been widely applied in healthcare research to evaluate whether the effectiveness of an intervention justifies additional expenditure. In this chapter, we describe the practical application of important aspects of cost-effectiveness analysis using an example adapted from the published literature.[1] We will demonstrate how to construct and analyse cost-effectiveness models. We will also describe how to produce the common graphical methods used in the literature to present the results of cost-effectiveness analysis.

Analysis was performed using the decision analytical software package *TreeAge Pro Suite* (TreeAge Software inc., Williamstown, Massachusetts, USA). It is suggested that Examples 1 and 2 in Chap. 10 should be completed first before the reader attempts the example in this chapter as we rely on the familiarity with TreeAge acquired completing the examples in chapter 10 during the following example.

C. Rao (✉)
Department of Surgery and Cancer, Imperial College London,
St Mary's Hospital Campus, London, UK
e-mail: christopher.rao@imperial.ac.uk

T. Athanasiou and A. Darzi (eds.), *Evidence Synthesis in Healthcare*,
DOI: 10.1007/978-0-85729-206-3_11, © Springer-Verlag London Limited 2011

11.2
Background Information

The large veins of the leg are commonly used to bypass the diseased segments of arteries in the heart during coronary artery bypass operations. Removing these veins for use in coronary artery bypass procedures often requires a long incision to be made from the ankle to the groin. Over the past decade, minimally invasive alternatives have been developed where the vein is harvested through either one or two small transverse incisions above and or below the knee, depending on the length of conduit required.

The reduced surgical trauma resulting from the smaller incisions made during minimally invasive harvesting has been shown to significantly reduce many of the common complications of great saphenous vein harvesting. Patient satisfaction following minimally invasive harvesting is also significantly greater than following conventional harvesting. In this example, based on a published study, we investigate whether the greater clinical effectiveness justifies the increased cost of minimally invasive vein harvesting.[1] The model used in this example is summarised in Fig. 11.1, and the parameters used in this model are shown in Table 11.1.

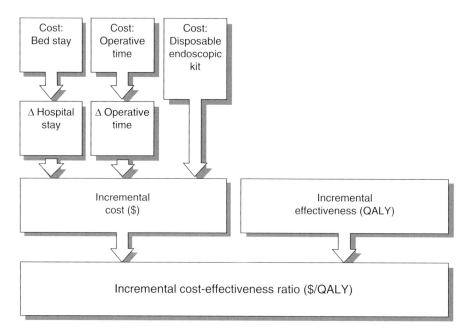

Fig. 11.1

Table 11.1 Model parameters

Parameter	Value	Range/SD	Distribution	Variable name	Distribution name
Cost parameters ($)					
Cost of bypass surgery in first year postoperatively	6,231.0	5,607.89–6,852.78	Triangular	c_cabg	d_c_cabg
Cost of disposable endoscopic equipment	742.50	659.99–825.01	Triangular	c_minv	d_c_minv
Cost of a cardiothoracic bed day	613.80	257.40–902.88	Triangular	c_bed	d_c_bed
Cost of a minute of cardiothoracic theatre time	21.78	10.89–32.67	Triangular	c_op	d_c_op
Model parameters					
Incremental operative time for minimally invasive vein harvesting (min)	15.26	0.01–30.51	Triangular	t_op	d_t_op
Incremental hospital stay of conventional vein harvesting (d)	1.04	0.16–1.92	Triangular	t_bed	d_t_bed
QALY payoff					
Utility after bypass surgery	0.860	0.774–0.946	Triangular	u_cabg	d_u_cabg
Increment utility after minimally invasive vein harvesting	0.0232	0.0035–0.0427	Triangular	u_minv	d_u_minv

11.3
Constructing a Cost-Effectiveness Analysis

Constructing a decision analytical model in order to perform a cost-effectiveness analysis is very similar to constructing any other decision analytical model. The primary difference between a decision analytical for cost-effectiveness analysis and any other decision analytical model is that every outcome has two payoffs associated with it, one for cost and one for effect. In order to perform a cost-effectiveness analysis, we must first change the tree preferences in the same way that we have done in previous examples.

In the *Preferences* window (Fig. 11.2), select *Calculation Method* from the menu on the left. Change the calculation method to a Cost-effectiveness analysis by selecting *Cost-Effectiveness* from the *Method*: menu (Fig. 11.3). We now need to define a willingness to pay or cost-effectiveness threshold. Click on the *CE Decision Rules/Parameters...* button. The following window will be revealed (Fig. 11.4). Type the willingness to pay/cost-effectiveness threshold into the *Willingness to pay*: box and then press *OK*.

We now need to change the numerical format of our output parameters. Click on the *Numeric Format...* button in the preferences button.

Select the *Cost* button in the *Numeric Formatting* window (Fig. 11.5). The following window is revealed. Change the preferences as shown (Fig. 11.6). Then press *OK*.

In a similar way, change the Effectiveness and Cost-effectiveness parameters to the ones shown in Figs. 11.7 and 11.8 by pressing the *Effectiveness* and *Cost/Eff...* buttons in the *Numeric Formatting* window (Fig. 11.5).

When this has been completed, select the *Close* button in the *Numeric Formatting* window (Fig. 11.5). We are now ready to start building our decision analytical model.

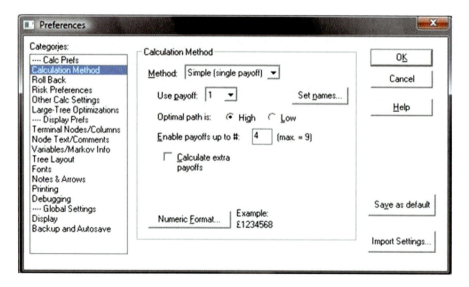

Fig. 11.2 Model Structure

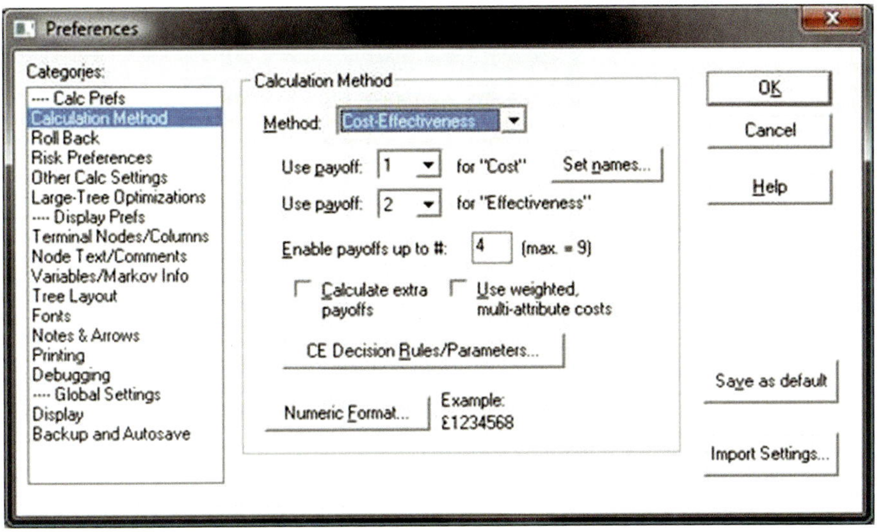

Fig. 11.3

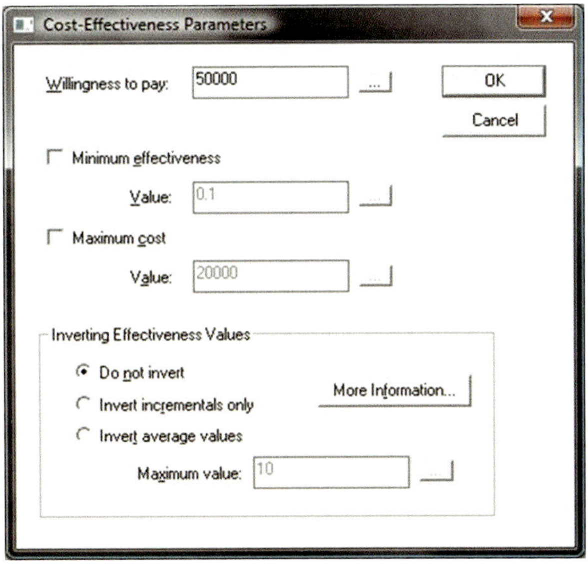

Fig. 11.4

Using the techniques demonstrated in Chap. 10, construct the following decision model (Fig. 11.10). Variables (Fig. 11.11) and Distributions (Fig. 11.1) should also be entered as shown. A summary of variable and distribution names is shown in Table 11.1. When entering the payoffs associated with each terminal node, enter the cost parameters into the first (*Cost:*) box and the effects parameters into the second (*Effects:*) box as shown below (Fig. 11.9).

Fig. 11.5

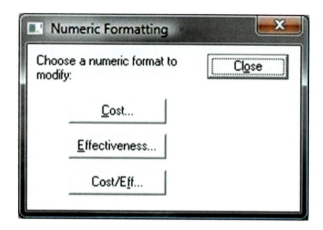

Fig. 11.6

11.4
Analysing a Cost-Effectiveness Analysis

Now that we have finished constructing our decision analytical model, we are ready to start the analysis.

Select the decision node and start a Monte Carlo simulation as described in the previous chapter. The following window will appear (Fig. 11.13).

Select *Calculate expected values*, in the *Inner Loop (model recalculation)* box, and then press the *Begin* button. The following Monte Carlo simulation is generated (Fig. 11.14).

Fig. 11.7

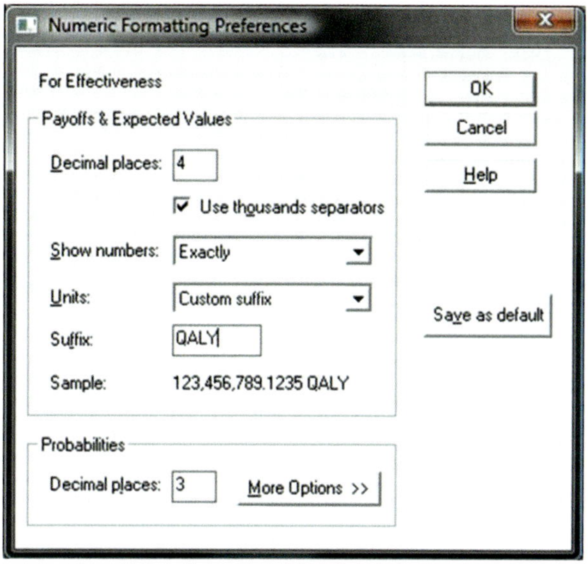

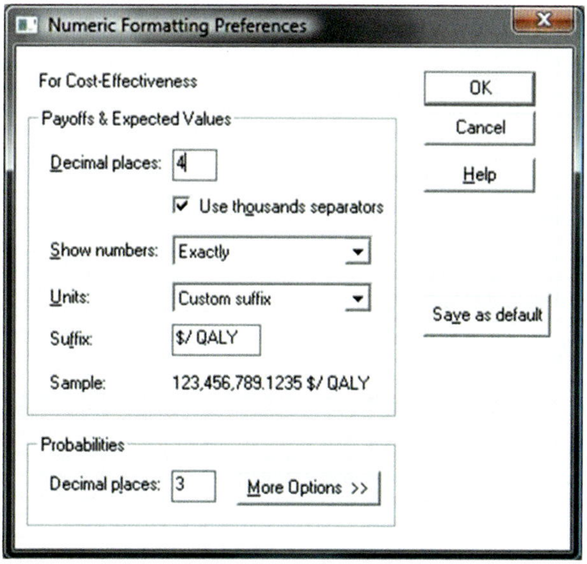

Fig. 11.8

Information on the *Conventional Open Method* can be obtained by selecting this option from the menu button at the bottom of the window. A fuller text report, which can be exported to other applications as described in previous examples can be obtained by selecting the *Stats Report...* button. The following window will appear (Fig. 11.15).

Selecting *Net monetary benefits* and then pressing *OK* reveal the results shown in Fig. 11.16. Selecting *Cost-effectiveness* reveals the results shown in Fig. 11.17.

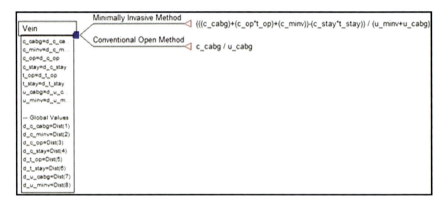

Fig. 11.9

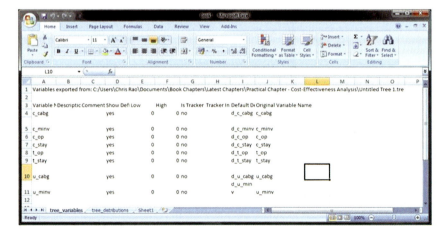

Fig. 11.10

Fig. 11.11

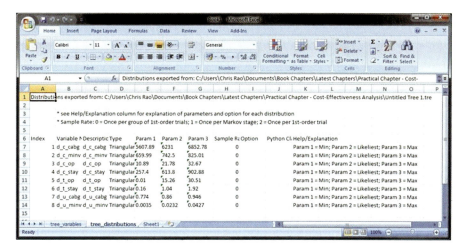

Fig. 11.12

Fig. 11.13

11.5
Graphical Exploration of the Results of a Cost-Effectiveness Analysis

Clicking on the *Graph* button in the *Monte Carlo Simulation* window (Fig. 11.14) reveals a menu of options for displaying the results of the cost-effectiveness analysis graphically. The majority of these graphs can be exported to Excel as described in previous examples.

Graphs of the distribution of costs, effects (Fig. 11.18) and cost-effectiveness ratios (Fig. 11.19) can be generated by clicking on the *Distribution of Costs, Distribution of*

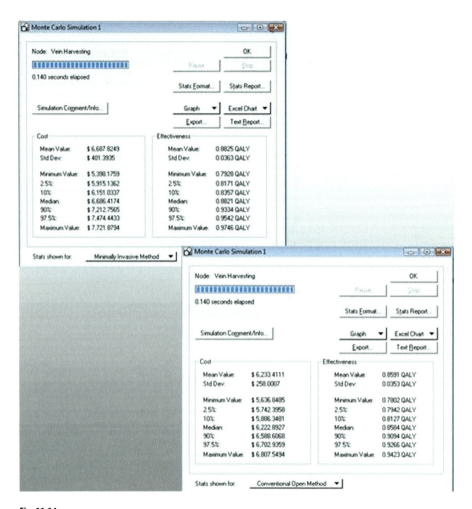

Fig. 11.14

Fig. 11.15

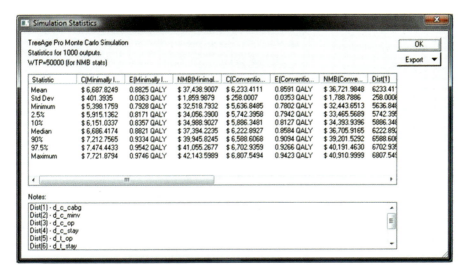

Fig. 11.16

Fig. 11.17

Effectiveness Values or *Distribution of C/E Ratios*, from the graph menu revealed by pressing the *Graph* button in the *Monte Carlo Simulation* window (Fig. 11.14) and then selecting the outcome for which we want to generate the distribution.

Graphs of the distribution of incremental costs, effects and cost-effectiveness ratios (Fig. 11.21) can be generated by clicking on the *Distribution of Incremental*, then *Incremental Costs…*, *Incremental Effectiveness…*, or *Incremental CE Ratios…*, from the

Fig. 11.18

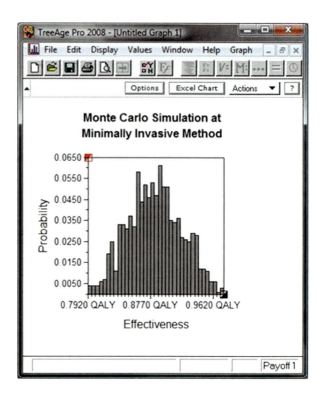

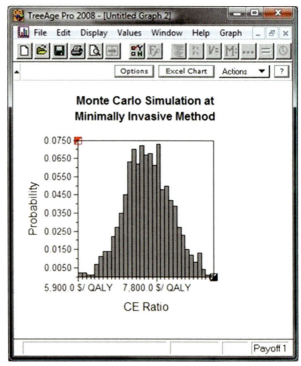

Fig. 11.19

Fig. 11.20

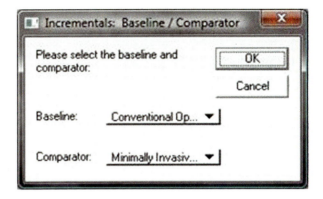

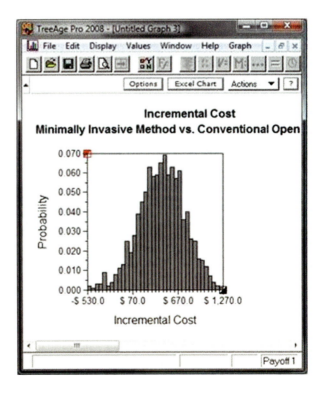

Fig. 11.21

graph menu revealed by pressing the *Graph* button in the *Monte Carlo Simulation window* (Fig. 11.14). On selecting the required incremental distribution, the following window (Fig. 11.20) will appear. Choose which strategy is the control from the *Baseline:* menu and the intervention from the *Comparator:* menu and then press *OK*.

A Scatter plot for the cost and effects of the interventions (Fig. 11.22) can be generated by clicking on the *CE Scatterplot* from the graph menu revealed by pressing the *Graph* button in the *Monte Carlo Simulation* window (Fig. 11.14).

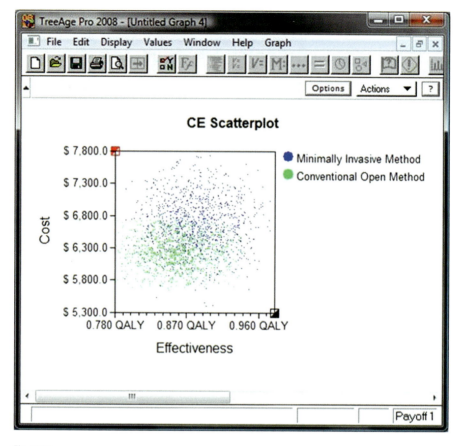

Fig. 11.22

A Scatter plot for the incremental cost and effects of the interventions (Fig. 11.24) can be generated by clicking on the *ICE Scatterplot + Isos…* from the graph menu revealed by pressing the *Graph* button in the *Monte Carlo Simulation* window (Fig. 11.14).

On selecting this option, the following window (Fig. 11.23) will appear.

Choose which strategy is the Control from the *Baseline:* menu and the intervention from the *Comparator:* menu, enter the willingness to pay/cost-effectiveness threshold in the *Willingness to pay:* box and then press *OK*. This will generate the graph (Fig. 11.24)

Acceptability curves (Fig. 11.27) can be generated by clicking on *Acceptability Curve…*, from the graph menu revealed by pressing the *Graph* button in the *Monte Carlo Simulation* window (Fig. 11.14). This will reveal the following window (Fig. 11.25). Click *Yes*.

This will reveal the following window (Fig. 11.26).

Set the range of values for the cost-effectiveness/willingness to pay threshold into the *Low:* and *High:* boxes. Enter the number of intervals into the *Interval:* box. Select both comparators. Clicking *OK* will generate the distribution (Fig. 11.27).

Fig. 11.23

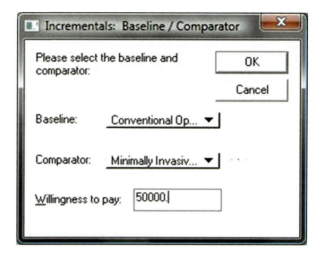

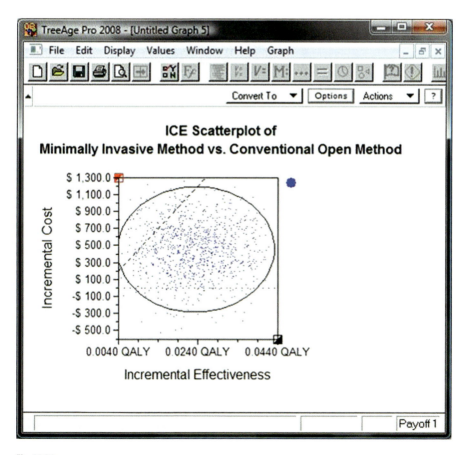

Fig. 11.24

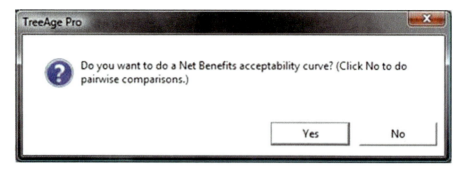

Fig. 11.25

Fig. 11.26

Graphs of the net monetary benefit and willingness to pay (Fig. 11.29) can be generated by clicking on the *Net Benefits* then *vs. WTP*..., from the graph menu revealed by pressing the *Graph* button in the *Monte Carlo Simulation* window (Fig. 11.14). This will reveal the following window.

Enter the settings shown into the *Net Benefit Curve Parameters* window (Fig. 11.28). Pressing *OK* will generate the following curve.

Graphs of the incremental net monetary benefit and willingness to pay (Fig. 11.30) can be generated by clicking on the *Net Benefits* then *vs. WTP*..., from the graph menu revealed by pressing the *Graph* button in the *Monte Carlo Simulation* window (Fig. 11.14). In the *Net Benefit Curve Parameters* window (Fig. 11.28), select *Graph comparative (incremental) NB:*. Choose the control strategy from the Baseline: menu and then the intervention from the list above. Pressing *OK* will generate the following graph.

Comparative graphs of the net monetary benefit (Fig. 11.32) can be generated by clicking on the *Net Benefits*, then *Distribution of Average NBs* the *Comparative*..., from the

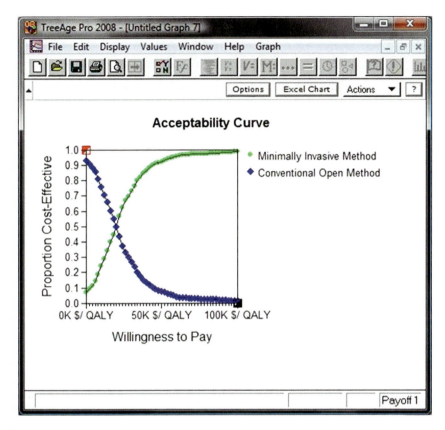

Fig. 11.27

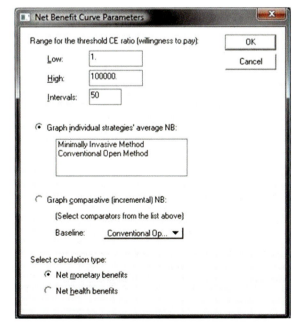

Fig. 11.28

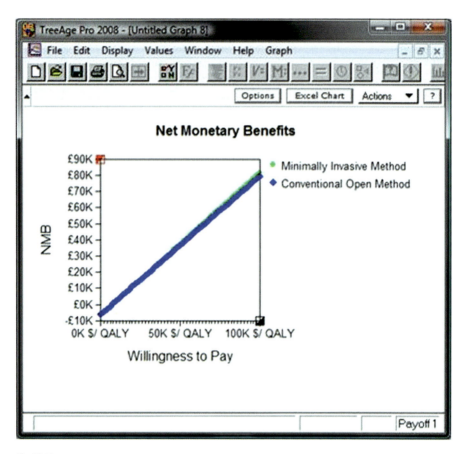

Fig. 11.29

graph menu revealed by pressing the *Graph* button in the *Monte Carlo Simulation* window (Fig. 11.14). This will reveal the following window.

Enter the settings shown above in the *Comparative Net Health Benefits* window (Fig. 11.31). On pressing *OK*, the following graph will be generated (Fig. 11.32).

The Distribution of the incremental net monetary benefit (Fig. 11.34) can be generated by clicking on the *Net Benefits* then *Distribution of Incremental NBs...*, from the graph menu revealed by pressing the *Graph* button in the *Monte Carlo Simulation* window (Fig. 11.14). This will reveal the following window (Fig. 11.33).

Enter the settings shown above into the *Incremental Net Health Benefits* window (Fig. 11.33). On pressing *OK*, the following graph will be generated (Fig. 11.34).

Analysis using a minimum significant difference threshold (Fig. 11.35) can be generated by clicking on the *Minimum Significant Difference...*, from the graph menu revealed by pressing the *Graph* button in the *Monte Carlo Simulation* window (Fig. 11.14). The following window will be revealed (Fig. 11.36).

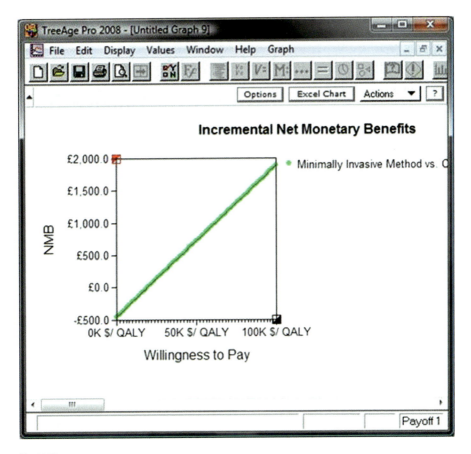

Fig. 11.30

Fig. 11.31

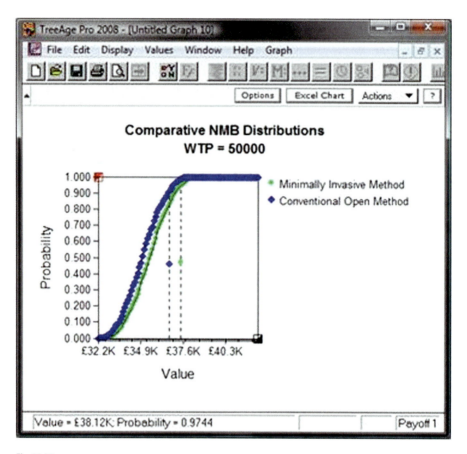

Fig. 11.32

Fig. 11.33

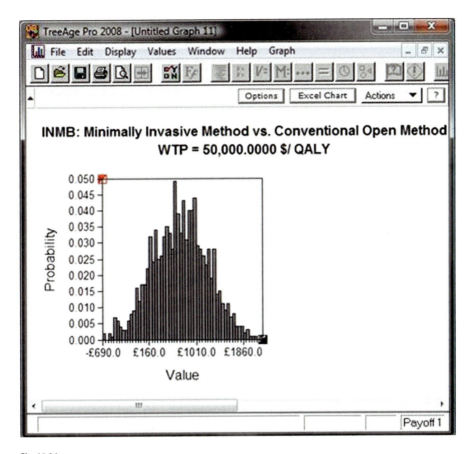

Fig. 11.34

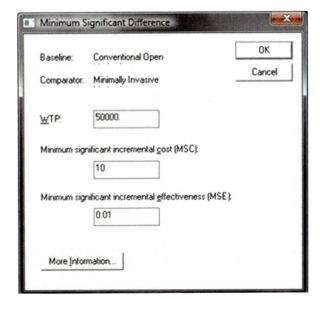

Fig. 11.35

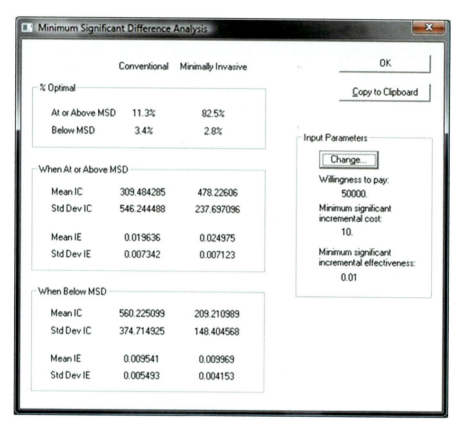

Fig. 11.36

Entering the willingness to pay threshold/cost-effectiveness threshold into the *WTP*: box, the minimum significant incremental cost into the *Minimum significant incremental cost (MSC)*: box, the minimum significant incremental effectiveness into the *Minimum significant incremental effectiveness (MSE)*: box and the clicking *OK* will generate the analysis (Fig. 11.36). The input parameters can be changed by clicking the *Change* button.

11.6
Summary

In this chapter, we have demonstrated how to perform cost-effectiveness analysis and how to produce the common graphical methods used to present the results of cost-effectiveness analysis. By using these methods, and the methods described in Chap. 10, we hope that the reader will be able to construct more complex models to assess the cost-effectiveness of medical technology and practice.

Reference

1. Rao C, Aziz O, Deeba S, et al. Is minimally invasive harvesting of the great saphenous vein for coronary artery bypass surgery a cost-effective technique? *J Thorac Cardiov Surg.* 2008;135: 809-815.

Exploring Bayesian Belief Networks Using Netica®

12

Zhifang Ni, Lawrence D. Phillips, and George B. Hanna

Abstract Bayesian belief networks (BBNs) are graphical tools for reasoning with uncertainties (see Chap. 7). They can be used to combine expert knowledge with hard data and making sense of uncertain evidence. The computation of Bayesian inference is complex. In this chapter, we provide a step-to-step guide of how to construct and use Bayesian networks by using Netica software.

12.1
Objectives

This chapter aims to demonstrate:

- How to construct Bayesian Belief networks (BBNs)
- How to discretize continuous data
- How to learn parameters from Microsoft Excel files
- How to perform belief updating
- How to perform sensitivity analyses

We used Netica 4.08 for MS Windows (95/98/NT4/2000/XP/Vista, copyright 1992–2008 by Norsys Software Corp). A free trial version can be found at: http://www.norsys.com/download.html.

Z. Ni (✉)
Department of Surgery and Cancer, Imperial College London,
St Mary's Hospital Campus, London, UK
e-mail: z.ni@imperial.ac.uk

T. Athanasiou and A. Darzi (eds.), *Evidence Synthesis in Healthcare*,
DOI: 10.1007/978-0-85729-206-3_12, © Springer-Verlag London Limited 2011

12.2
Background

Nasogastric feeding is in widespread use in the National Health Service (NHS) of United Kingdom. The correct location of a feeding tube is in the stomach. In fact, blindly inserted tubes can end up in oesophagus, lung or intestine, among other places. The current gold standard for checking tube location is chest x-ray but a pH test of tube aspirates is most commonly used. Nevertheless, pH test lacks precision and accuracy – using the test can lead to feeding errors, including non-stomach feeding and missing feeding when the tube is correctly placed in the stomach. Aspirate pH also depends on whether or not a patient receives feeding or acid inhibitor medication that could increase gastric pH.

Given these intertwined uncertainties, what can we do to improve the accuracy of aspirate pH? In what follows, we show how Bayesian belief networks (BBN) can be employed to provide insights into safe feeding using nasogastric tubes [1].

12.3
Getting Started

Construction of BBNs requires (1) a list of uncertain variables, (2) the possible values (states) of discrete variables and/or the possible ranges of value of continuous variables, (3) the dependent relationship between these variables and (4) conditional probabilities that quantify the dependences. For the current problem, we have four uncertain variables i.e. the location of the tube (or node 'tube site' in the BBN model, see below), the value of the pH test ('pH'), the feeding and medication status ('feeding' and 'medication') of the patient. Among these, 'pH' is a continuous variable that takes any value between 0 and 14 (The range could be different (smaller) depending on the type of pH paper/strip being used). We are however most interested in two threshold values, i.e., whether or not pH exceeds 4 and/or 6. This leads to three ranges: below 4 (between 0 and 4), between 4 and 6, and above 6 (between 6 and 14). Table 12.1 summarises this information.

We also assume that the acidity of tube aspirates depends on the actual tube site (i.e., whether the tube is in the stomach or intestine), as well as on the medication and feeding status of a patient. With this understanding, we model 'pH' as a child (or descendant) of 'tube site', 'medication' and 'feeding'. We also assume, for simplicity, that the three parent

Table 12.1 Summary of Bayesian belief network 'pH'

Uncertain variable	Type	State (Range)
pH	Continuous	below 4/between 4 and 6/above 6
tube site	Discrete	Stomach/intestine
feeding	Discrete	Fed/unfed
medication	Discrete	Present/absent

nodes are independent of each other. This discussion implies a 2-level BBN that looks like Fig. 12.1, with the three parent nodes on top and the child node at the bottom.

Although BBNs as in Fig. 12.1 convey explicitly the structure of the problem, it would be more useful if we can quantify the relationships (the strength of the dependences) between the variables. That is, what is the level(s) of pH when the three parent nodes have different states or values. Once this information becomes available, we can perform backward reasoning and infer from the pH the probability distribution of tube sites.

Assume we can get such information from a well-maintained database in Excel named 'pHdata.xls'. Each row corresponds to a record of pH from pH meter (pH meter is gold standard for testing pH values), tube location from a chest x-ray, as well as feeding and medication statues (Fig. 12.2).

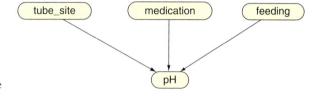

Fig. 12.1 Screenshot of BBN 'pH' with complete structure

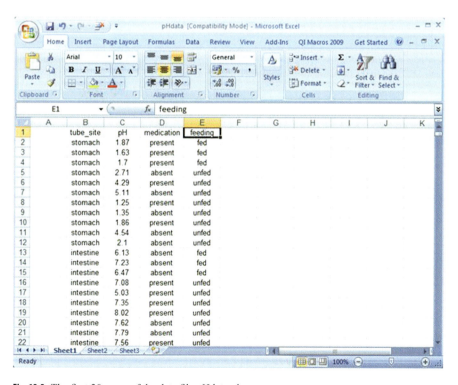

Fig. 12.2 The first 20 cases of the data file pHdata.xls

For simplicity, we consider only two possible tube sites, i.e., stomach and intestine. This database allows us to compute the frequencies (When a pH happens to be a threshold value, i.e., 4 or 6, we assume it falls into the lower inclusive range, i.e., pH=4 counted as an occurrence within 0–4 and pH=6 as one within 4–6) of pH under different combinations of values of medication, feeding and tube site. A snapshot is shown in Table 12.2:

This information also allows us to examine the assumed conditional independence between tube site, medication and feeding. The correlation statistics are shown in Table 12.3. Based on the conventional standard, the correlations are non-significant.

In what follows, we show how to build Bayesian networks using Netica software, based on data contained in 'pHdata.xls' (Table 12.2).

12.4
Building a BBN Using Netica

A trial version of Netica for Windows can be downloaded from http://www.norsys.com/download.html.

Install by following instructions. After successful installation, launch Netica[2] by double-clicking the desktop short-cut icon '⬛'. A dialog window pops up asking for activation code. Click (Unless otherwise specified, a 'click' refers to a left-click) on *Limited mode* button on the right. A blank screen is presented to the user (Fig. 12.3):

Table 12.2 The frequency table of pH computed from 'pHdata.xls'

Tube site	Medication	Feeding	pH between 0 and 4	pH between 4 and 6	pH between 6 and 14
Stomach	Present	Fed	44%	42%	14%
Stomach	Present	Unfed	49%	25%	26%
Stomach	Absent	Fed	53%	40%	7%
Stomach	Absent	Unfed	73%	14%	13%
Intestine	Present	Fed	8%	12%	80%
Intestine	Present	Unfed	2%	5%	94%
Intestine	Absent	Fed	12%	7%	81%
Intestine	Absent	Unfed	3%	9%	88%

Table 12.3 Checking dependence between tube site, medication and feeding

Correlation between	Medication and feeding	Feeding and tube sites	Medication and tube sites
Spearman's rho	0.011	0.120	0.050
p value	0.671	0.095	0.064

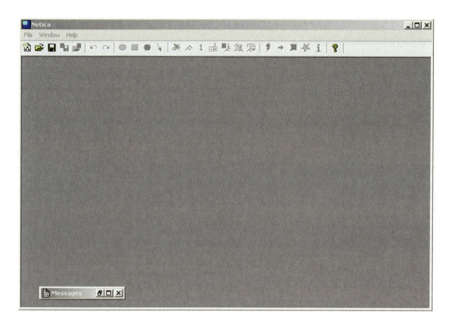

Fig. 12.3 Launching Netica

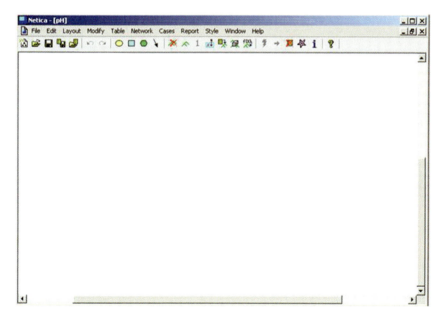

Fig. 12.4 A BBN named 'pH' is ready to be specified

Establish a new model by either clicking once on the tool button 📇 or selecting *File\ New Network* from the menu bar. A new network appears on the screen, which is automatically named 'Untitled-1'. Select *File\Save* to rename it as 'pH.neta' (Fig. 12.4)

Click on '◻' to expand the main window (i.e., the working space) to its full-size.

12.4.1
Specifying Uncertain Variables

Click once on '$\bigcirc$' in the tool bar and then click once anywhere on the main window to create an uncertain node. Repeat the same operation for four times. Alternatively, double-click '$\bigcirc$' to multi-select the function and click for four times at four different places on the main window; then click once '$\bigcirc$' to unselect the function. Four nodes appear in the main window, each representing one uncertain event. Netica automatically names them, 'A', 'B', 'C' and 'D' (Fig. 12.5).

Double-click 'A' to define the node (including its name and states). Alternatively, click once on the node, then right-click and select *Properties...* from the drop-down menu. This activates the so-called 'node dialog box' (Fig. 12.6).

12.4.2
Specifying Discrete Variables

Rename 'A' as 'tube_site' by using the *Name* field. Netica uses this field to identify the nodes. The names are case-sensitive. Based on the way it is created, 'A' is a *Nature* node (i.e., an uncertain event) and has *Discrete* states. To specify what these states are, input 'stomach' in the *State* field; click on *New* to save and continue; input the next state 'intestine'. All states can be viewed any time by clicking '$\blacktriangledown$' next to *State*. Select and *Delete* unwanted states (Fig. 12.7).

Click *Okay* to exit.

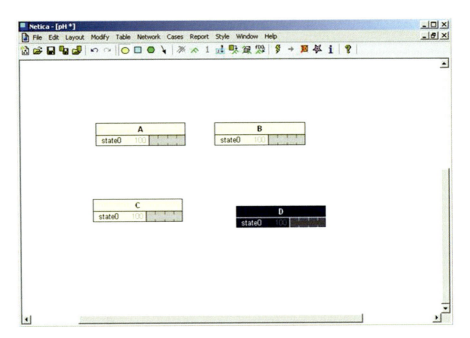

Fig. 12.5 Four uncertain variables (or nodes) are added to BBN pH

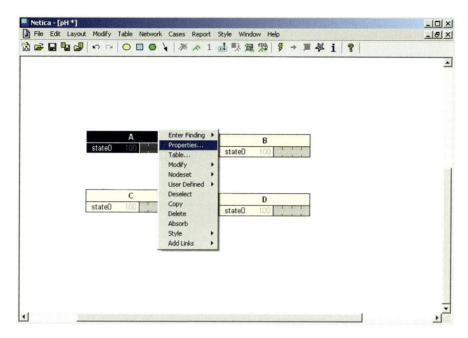

Fig. 12.6 Specifying node properties

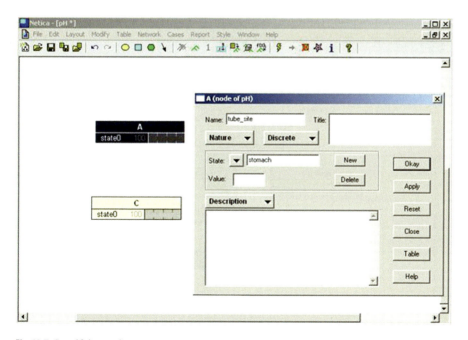

Fig. 12.7 Specifying node states

The node 'tube_site' appears on the main window with 'stomach' and 'intestine' as its possible states (Fig. 12.8).

Repeat the same process for 'B' and change it to 'medication' which is either 'present' or 'absent'. Repeat the same process again for 'C' and change it to 'feeding' which is either 'fed' or 'unfed' (Fig. 12.9):

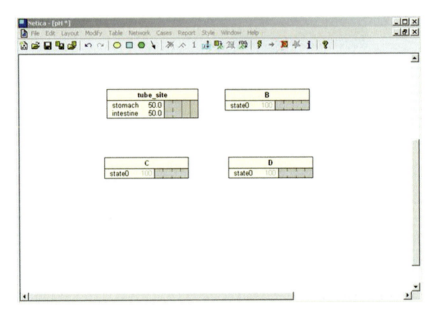

Fig. 12.8 Node pH is specified

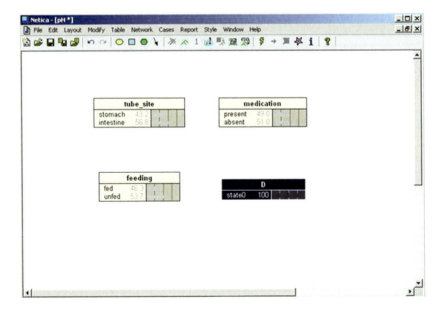

Fig. 12.9 BBN pH with all discrete variables specified

12.4.3
Specifying Continuous Variables

Different from the rest, pH is continuous rather than discrete in the sense that it can take any value within a given range. To specify such variables, first discretize it by defining thresholds and value ranges. As discussed, the three ranges of interests are between 0 and 4, between 4 and 6 or between 6 and 14. Discretization can be done manually or *learned* directly from data. We discuss manual input in this section and model learning (including states and parameters) in Sect. 12.5

Double-click 'D' to activate the node dialog box. Rename it as 'pH'. Click on *Discrete* to change it to *Continuous* (Fig. 12.10).

Use *Delete* to delete the default state (State 0) (Fig. 12.11).

Input '0'–'4' in the *Range* field. Click *New* to store this range, and define the other two ranges (Fig. 12.12).

After all ranges have been defined, click *Okay* to return to the window (Fig. 12.13).

12.4.4
Specifying Dependences

Double-click '↘'. With the cursor changed to take the same shape, click once on node 'tube_site' and then once on node 'pH'. This links the two nodes together with the first node ('tube_site') as the parent and the second ('pH') as the child. Repeat the same process for 'medication' and 'pH' and then for 'feeding' and 'pH'.

Click once on '↘' button to unselect the function and arrange the nodes so that they display a two-level structure (Fig. 12.14).

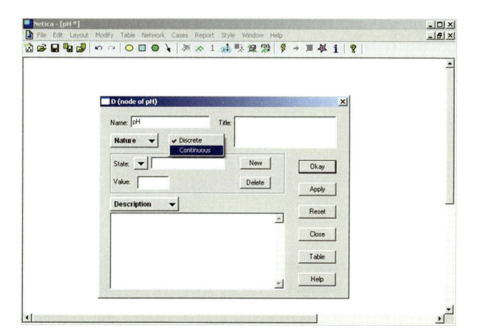

Fig. 12.10 Specifying the continuous variable pH

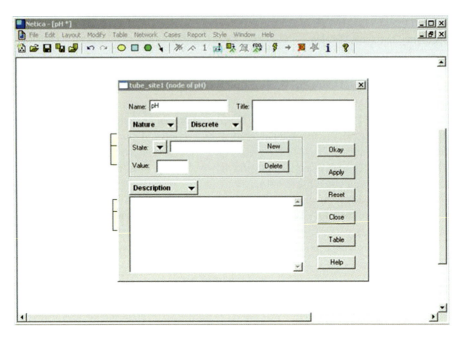

Fig. 12.11 Updating the states (ranges) of 'pH'

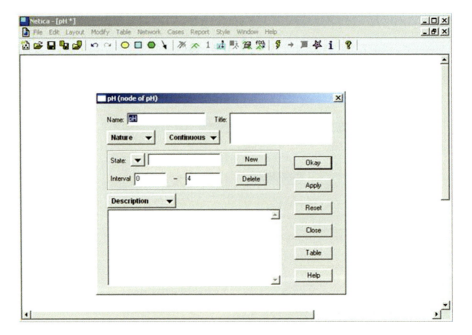

Fig. 12.12 Discretizing a continuous variable

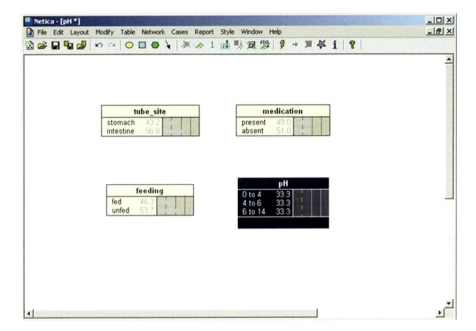

Fig. 12.13 BBN pH with all variables specified

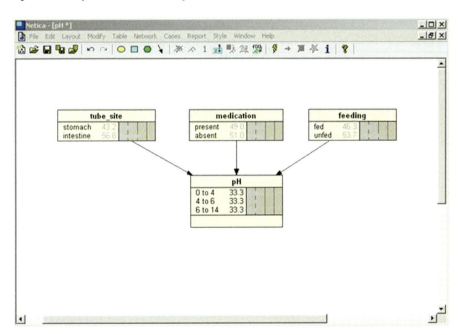

Fig. 12.14 BBN 'pH' with all variables specified and linked

12.4.5
Specifying Parameters

Double-click 'pH' to activate the node dialog box. Click *Table*. A new window appears for inputting conditional probabilities (Fig. 12.15).

The default mode of probabilities is *%Probability*. This means every number is taken as a percentage and the sum of each row must be *exactly* 100. Specify the probabilities according to the frequency Table 12.2 (Fig. 12.16).

Click *Apply* to store the input. Netica automatically checks whether the probability percentages in each role add up to 100. If not, an error dialog box appears demanding the problem to be solved.

Click *Okay* to return to the main window.

Click on ' ⚡ ' in the tool bar to compile the model. Alternatively, choose *Network\ Compile* from the menu. Once compiled, the colour of the belief bars changes from grey to black (Fig. 12.17).

Netica can represent uncertain events in different ways. The one shown so far is the default 'Belief Bars' representation. To try out other styles, select from the *Style* menu. For instance, Fig. 12.18 shows a BBN using both 'Belief Bars' and a 'Labelled Box' (pH).

The model is now ready for making inferences, which we discuss in more detail in Sect. 12.6

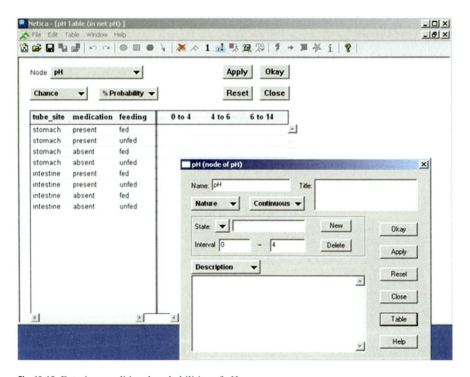

Fig. 12.15 Entering conditional probabilities of pH

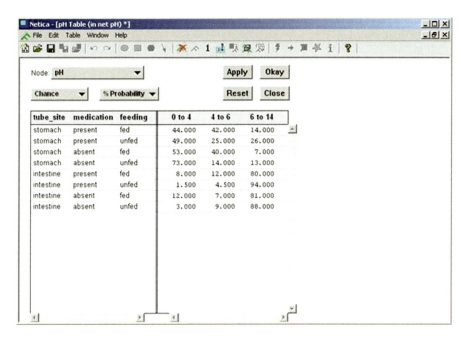

Fig. 12.16 The conditional probability table (CPT) captures the dependence of pH on tube_site, medication and feeding

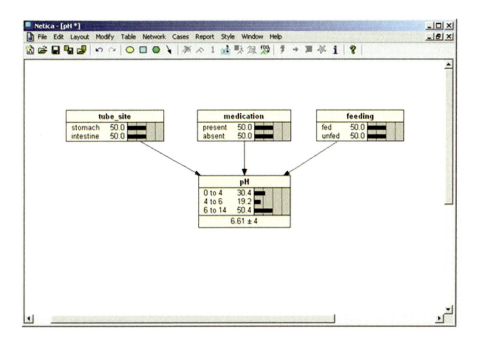

Fig. 12.17 BBN pH is compiled and ready for making predictions

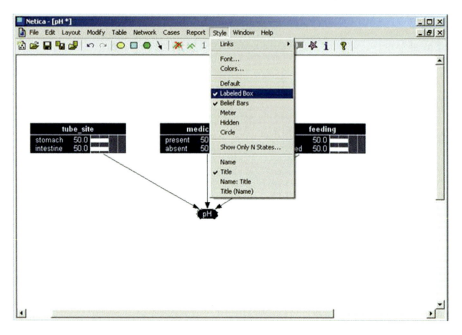

Fig. 12.18 Changing node appearances

12.5
Model Learning

Netica allows users to derive, or *learn*, a model directly from data. In what follows, we demonstrate learning of continuous variables and conditional probabilities from Excel. To perform the following task, create an Excel file named 'pHdata.xls' that is similar to Fig. 12.2. Make sure the names and/or the states of the uncertain variables as stored in the *Name* and *States* field in Netica are exactly the same to the ones stored in the database.

12.5.1
Learning States

Return to network shown in Fig. 12.19.

Double-click 'pH' to activate the node dialog window. Make sure the only state remaining for pH is its range, i.e., between 0 and 14. Delete any other states (Fig. 12.20).

Click *Okay* to exit the window.

Click once on 'pH' to select the node. Select *Modify\Discretize Nodes* from the menu bar (Fig. 12.21).

Browse the computer to locate the data file 'pHdata.xls' (Fig. 12.22).

Click *Open*.

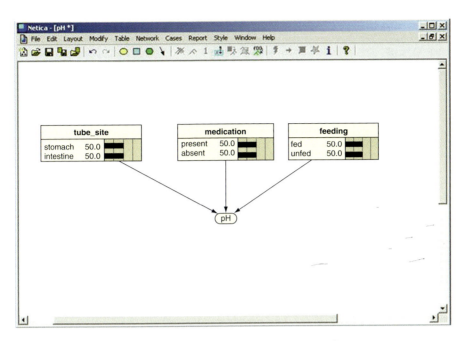

Fig. 12.19 Node pH shown as a 'labelled box' whereas the rest as 'belief bars'

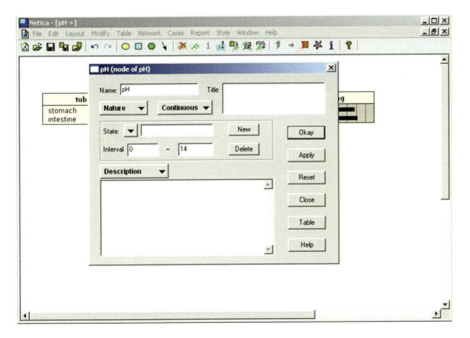

Fig. 12.20 Updating the states of pH

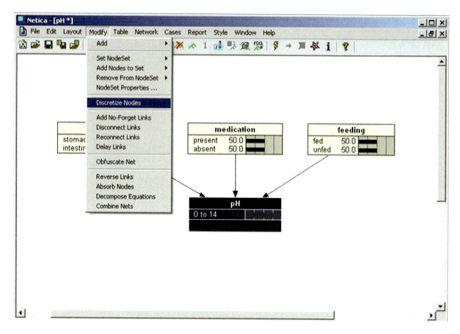

Fig. 12.21 Discretizing a variable by using data files

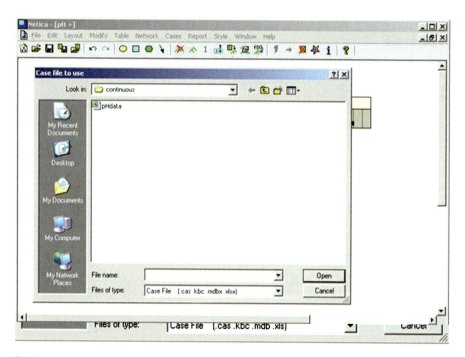

Fig. 12.22 Opening a database for learning the states (ranges)

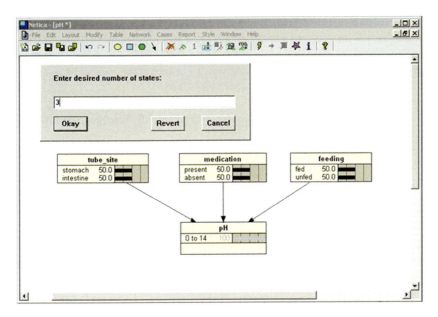

Fig. 12.23 Specifying the number of ranges (states)

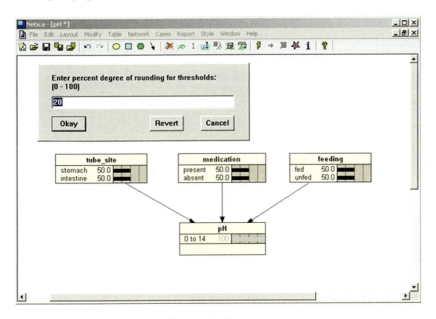

Fig. 12.24 Entering the degree of rounding thresholds

A dialog box appears. Determine the degree of discretization by changing the number of states (ranges) from '*5*' to '*3*'. Click *Okay* (Fig. 12.23).

A second dialog box appears. Use 20% as the "percentage degree of rounding the thresholds".

Click *Okay* (Fig. 12.24).

With successful learning, Netica automatically selects two thresholds for defining the three ranges. For our data, the two thresholds are 4 and 7.2 such that pH has roughly the same chances (33.3%±20%) of being observed as falling into 0–4, 4–7.2 and 7.2–14. Note that the upper-bound of pH has been changed to 9.3 instead of the original 14, to reflect the true upper limit of pH stored in 'pHdata.xls' (Fig. 12.25).

To change the thresholds, double-click 'pH' to activate the node dialog box. Click on '▼' button next to *States*. Select the range we want to modify from the drop-down menu. Change the upper-bound back to 14.

Click *Okay* to return to the main window (Fig. 12.26).

12.5.2
Learning Parameters

Go to *Cases\Incorp Case File* (Fig. 12.27).

Open 'pHdata.xls' (as in Fig. 12.22). A dialog window appears asking for degree of learning. The default value is 1, meaning that all information in this database will be learned once (Fig. 12.28).

Click *Okay*.

Netica search through the file to find information corresponding to the existing nodes and states and update the conditional probability tables accordingly.

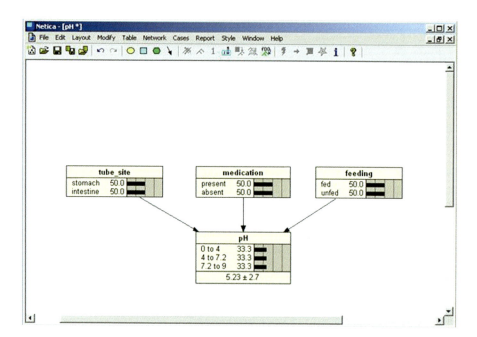

Fig. 12.25 BBN pH with node pH learned from data

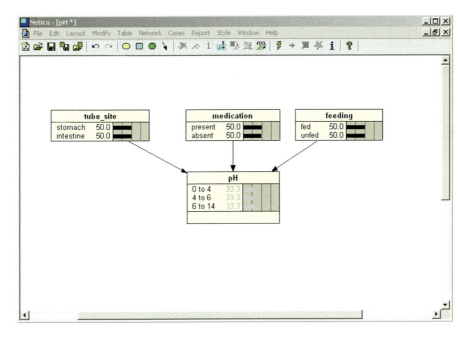

Fig. 12.26 Changing the cutoffs of pH back to 4 and 6

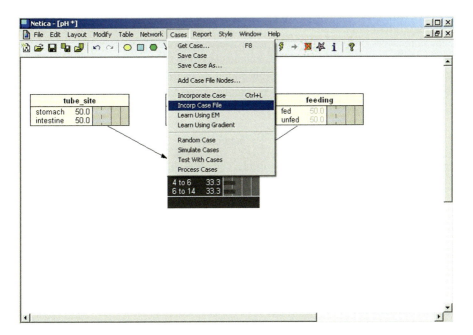

Fig. 12.27 Learning conditional probabilities in Netica

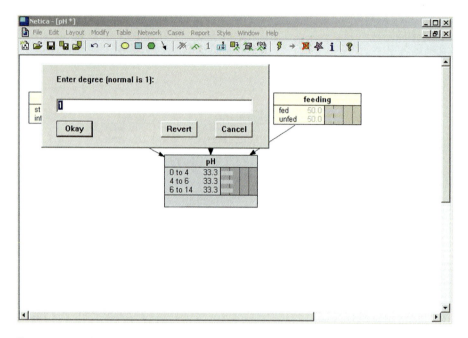

Fig. 12.28 Enter degree of learning conditional probabilities

Successful learning can lead to updating of all parameters, including prior and conditional probabilities. Prior probabilities refer to the distribution of root nodes (i.e., nodes without predecessors, including 'tube_site', 'feeding' and 'medication' in this example).

Click ' ⚡ ' button to compile the learned network (Fig. 12.29):

Note that the learned conditional probabilities differ from the frequencies. This is due to the learning algorithm employed by Netica. Users can reduce the discrepancy by

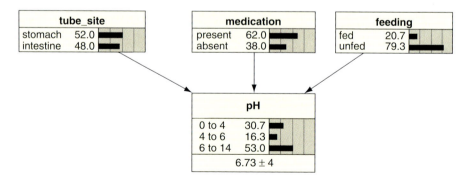

Fig. 12.29 Screenshot of BBN 'pH' learned from 'pHdata.xls'

increasing the degree of learning, say to 500 (every row/case is learned 500 times as 500 identical cases).

12.6
Using Bayesian Belief Networks

One advantage of Bayesian networks is that model parameters can be adjusted to capture characteristics of individual cases, in the form of prior distributions and findings.

To illustrate, imagine for Patient A, we observe a pH reading of 5.5 but have no insights of her feeding and medication history. Which of the two hypothesized tube sites is more likely, stomach or intestine?

In this case, a flat (even) distribution is used to capture lack of knowledge. Double-click 'tube_site' and click *Table*. Input 50 and 50 in the table, indicating the belief that the tube is equally likely to be in the two tube sites (Fig. 12.30).

Click *Okay*. Repeat this for 'medication' and 'feeding'.

Alternatively, click 'tube_site'. Right-click and select *Enter Finding\Likelihood* from the drop-down menu (Fig. 12.31).

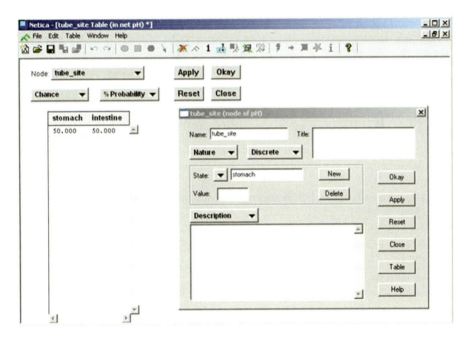

Fig. 12.30 Updating prior probabilities by direct data entry

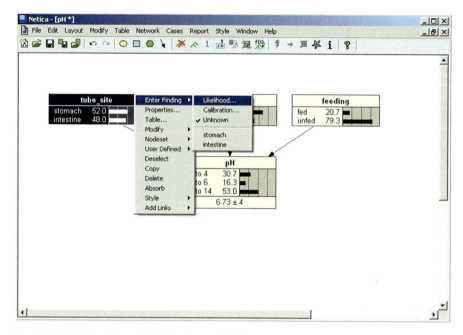

Fig. 12.31 Updating prior probabilities by entering findings

A dialog window appears asking users to specify the probability of the first state (Fig. 12.32).

Type in '0.5' as the probability of 'tube_site=stomach'. Click *Okay*.

Type in '0.5' as the probability of 'tube_site=intestine'. Click *Okay*.

Repeat this for 'medication' and 'feeding'.

To inform Netica that the pH reading for Patient A is 5.5, which lies within the range of '4 to 6', we simply click once on this state of 'pH' (Fig. 12.33).

Alternatively, right-click on node 'pH' and select *Enter Finding\4 to 6* in the drop-down menu. We observe that as a result, the probability of stomach intubation increases from the original 50–78.8%.

To remove a finding, we click on the corresponding state to unselect it, or enter a different finding. To remove all the *entered findings*, right-click and select *Remove Findings* from the drop-down menu. Note that in the case of prior probabilities, only entered findings can be removed this way but not findings directly typed into the probability table (Fig. 12.34).

What if all we know is that pH *cannot* take certain values? Netica calls such findings *negative findings*. To enter a negative finding, first remove all existing findings of pH, then hold down the *Shift* key ⇧ while clicking one by one on all the state(s) we want to exclude (e.g., '4 – 6') (Fig. 12.35).

We can see that knowing a pH to be either low (less than 4) or high (more than 6) is not very informative as the probability of stomach intubation only changes slightly to 43.2% from the initial 50%.

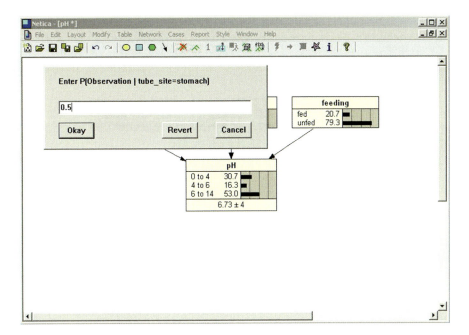

Fig. 12.32 Entering finding for each state

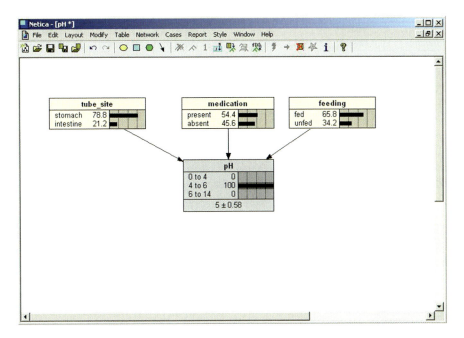

Fig. 12.33 BBN 'pH' when a pH between 4 and 6 has been observed

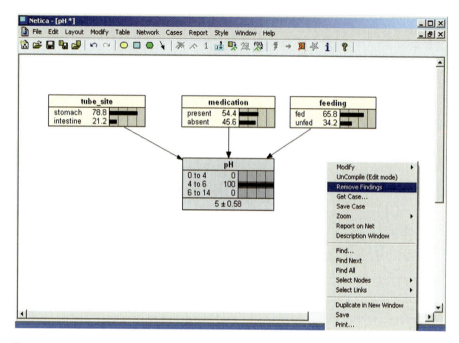

Fig. 12.34 Removing all entered findings

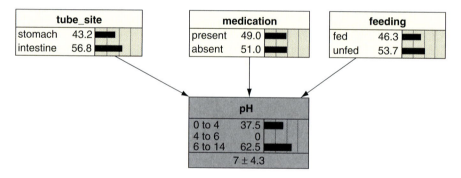

Fig. 12.35 Predicting tube_site with a negative finding

12.7
Sensitivity Analyses

Sensitivity analyses are crucial to examine the impact of uncertainties. Suppose we want to examine how sensitive 'tube_site' is to pH, feeding and medication states.

Click once to select node 'tube_site', which becomes the target node for sensitivity analyses. Select *Network\Sensitivity to Findings* from the menu bar (Fig. 12.36).

A report is generated and displayed in the *Message* window (Fig. 12.37).

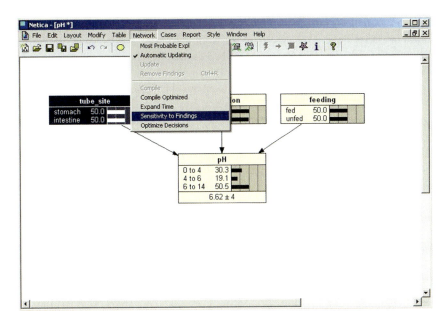

Fig. 12.36 Testing the sensitivity of tube site to pH

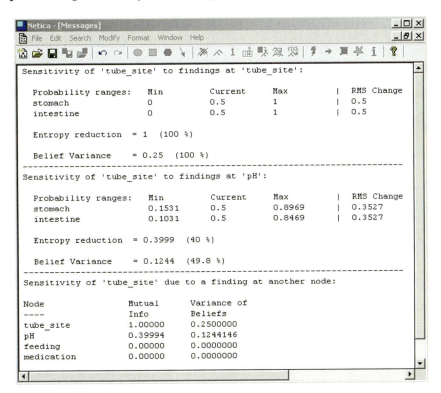

Fig. 12.37 Output of the sensitivity analysis

For each node in the model (including the target node), Netica reports the range of probabilities the target node takes (specified by 'Min' and 'Max' values) given *all* possible values taken by this node. For instance, Fig. 12.37 shows that the chance that the tube is in the stomach ranges from 15.31% (Min=0.1531) to 89.69% (Max=0.8969), compared to the current 50% (Current=0.5), in response to all possible values of pH.

A single number that summarises sensitivity to findings is stored under *Mutual Information* at the end of the analysis report. The larger the number, the more sensitive the target variable ('tube_site') is to a given variable. Not surprisingly, mutual information is one for 'tube_site' which is the target node. Among the rest, tube sites are most sensitive to pH (mutual information=0.39994) but not to medication or feeding (mutual information=0).

References

1. Hanna GB, Phillips LD, Priest OH, Ni Z. Developing guidelines for the safe verification of feeding tube position - a decision analysis approach. A report for the National Health Service (NHS) Patient Safety Research Portfolio; 2010.
2. Norsys_Software_Corp. Norsys Tutorial. Norsys Software Corporation 1995-2010:2010.

Index